# LIVER CANCER: NEW RESEARCH

# LIVER CANCER: NEW RESEARCH

FELIX LEE
EDITOR

**Nova Biomedical Books**
*New York*

For permission to use material from this book please contact us:
Telephone 631-231-7269; Fax 631-231-8175
Web Site: http://www.novapublishers.com



**Library of Congress Cataloging-in-Publication Data**
*Available upon request.*

ISBN 1-59454-182-5

*Published by Nova Science Publishers, Inc. ✣New York*

# Contents

# Preface

Primary liver cancer occurs when cancerous, or malignant, cells begin to grow in the tissues of liver. Although many cancers are on the decline, the incidence of primary liver cancer in the United States increased more than 70 percent between 1975 and 1995. The increase is linked to rising rates of hepatitis B and C infection - the leading causes of liver cancer. Far more common than primary liver cancer, however, is cancer that occurs when tumors from other parts of the body spread, or metastasize, to the liver. The liver is especially vulnerable to invasion by tumor cells and with the exception of the lymph nodes, is the most common site of metastasis. There are two main kinds of liver cancer. Heptoma and cholangiocarcinoma. Heptoma is cancer of the hepatocytes, the main functioning liver cell. Hepatoma is primary liver cancer which usually grows in the liver as a ball-like tumor, invading the normal tissue surrounding it. Cancer of the bile duct cells is called cholangiocarcinoma. Cholangiocarcinoma originates in the bile ducts and is often caused by infestation with the liver fluke Clonorchis, a parasite. The cancer grows along the bile ducts in sheets or lines, and is difficult to find on X-ray studies. This book presents the latest new research developments from around the world in the field of liver cancer.

In Chapter 1, an overview is presented which summarizes novel findings in the rapidly evolving field of liver cancer. Malignant epithelial tumors of the liver involving the hepatocyte lineage comprise hepatocellular carcinoma (HCC) and its variants, fibrolamellar (hepatocellular) carcinoma (FL-HCC), several types of mixed tumors, hepatoblastoma (HBL), and a novel entity, transitional liver cell tumor (TLCT). Carcinogenic pathways, patterns of growth, invasion, and metastatic spread of these lesions display considerable differences. HCC is one of the most common malignancies worldwide, whereas HBL is a very rare pediatric tumor. HCC is frequently a terminal complication of chronic, mainly viral-induced inflammatory and fibrotic liver disease. In contrast, HBL, FL-HCC and TLCT typically develop in nonfibrotic livers, but HBL is more frequently associated with a broad array of malformations in other organs. Cancerogenesis in HCC involves several groups of altered genes (mainly the p53, RB1, TGF-beta, and APC/WNT pathways), whereas in HBL the WNT/beta-catenin signaling protein network seems to be predominantly involved. Growth, differentiation and expansion of these tumors, depends on an altered expression of several growth factors/oncogenes modulated by distinct protease systems, and on angiogenesis/antiangiogenesis factors. Invasion and spread of HCC involves changes of cell adhesion molecules, cellular junction proteins, factors of cellular remodeling, proteins affecting cell polarity, proangiogenic proteins, and metalloproteinases acting on the extracellular matrix. Several factors have been identified that regulate the metastatic behavior of HCC, while less is still known about gene products affecting the metastatic spread of HBL and related tumors.

The focus of Chapter 2 is on the molecular and biological mechanisms that transpire during the development of colorectal liver metastases. In addition, this chapter evaluates novel therapeutic strategies targeting liver metastases, angiogenesis and apoptosis. Metastatic development is the primary cause of cancer treatment failure and is responsible for nearly all deaths from colorectal cancer. For the majority of patients, by the time primary colorectal cancers are diagnosed, sub-clinical or clinically relevant liver metastases have already occurred. The formation of liver metastases represents a highly selective sequence in which a subpopulation of cells within a tumor express genes that allow them to progress through distinct steps and spread to distant organs. Modification of gene expression in these cells leads to transformation, growth, angiogenesis, and invasion, and dissemination, survival in systemic circulation and attachment in the organ of metastases. Existing therapies directed at metastatic disease of the liver have had minimal impact on outcome. Contemporary treatment regimens are not likely to appreciably alter the natural history of liver metastases. Consequently, understanding the molecular and biologic mechanisms of liver metastases may allow for the development of therapeutic strategies designed to prevent and treat liver metastases.

The treatment of metastatic colorectal cancer to the liver has evolved over the past decade. Chapter 3 explores the methods used and although surgical resection remains the gold standard, only 15% to 20% of newly diagnosed patients are candidates for curative resection. To extend indications for curative treatment of 'unresectable' colorectal liver metastases, other therapeutic modalities are being developed such as loco regional chemotherapy with tumor 'down staging', two stage liver resections after portal vein embolization and the use of loco-regional ablative therapy. Within the latter category, radio frequency thermal ablation (RFA) has recently gained popularity with reported early survival results equivalent to liver resection in selected cases using either percutaneous image-guided, laparoscopic or open radio frequency thermo ablation techniques. Published reports have shown an overall survival in the range of 67% at 2 years and 33% at 3 years respectively. These results however, are hampered by the short follow up period in the majority of cases and are generally reported in conjunction with RFA of other tumor types.

More importantly, this chapter's main goal is to underline the role of liver resection as the first line therapy in the management of hepatic metastatic colorectal cancer within the context of an increasing utilization of new treatment modalities such as the thermal ablative therapy, which has not yet been completely evaluated in the long term. A review of the published literature as well as a discussion on the effect of RFA on liver function, per operative lactate production and the impact on residual liver functional reserve are presented.

Chapter 4 establishes the strategies for inferior phrenic arteriography and transcatheter arterial chemoembolization (TACE) in patients with hepatocellular carcinoma (HCC) including when to perform, how to perform, and hemodynamic changes of the inferior phrenic artery (IPA).

The contents of Chapter 5 pertain to the oncogene, mdm-2, which is over-expressed in a fraction of hepatocellular carcinomas (HCC), suggesting that it is important in tumor pathogenesis. HBV encoded x antigen (HBxAg) is also closely associated with the development of HCC. To determine whether mdm-2 over-expression in HCC correlates with HBxAg, expression, HCC tissues from HBV carriers were stained for HBxAg and mdm-2 by immunohistochemistry. Mdm-2 was over-expressed in the nuclei of tumor cells in 25 of 37 HCC tissues examined (67%), and its over-expression correlated with that of HBxAg in the cytoplasm of the same cells. Using different HBxAg mutants, it was shown that HBxAg trans-activation function correlated with elevated endogenous mdm-2 mRNA levels. HBxAg also trans-activated the mdm-2 promoter in an exogenously added reporter gene construct in p53 null Hep3B cells. These results suggest that mdm-2 is frequently over-expressed in HBV associated HCC, and that it appears to be a transcriptional target for HBxAg. Hence, HBxAg mediated trans-activation may contribute importantly to the up-regulated expression of mdm-2 in HCC.

The focus of Chapter 6 is that of new drugs on the market, namely, Tamoxifen, which has been used successfully as adjuvant therapy in the treatment of breast cancer since the 1970's. Epidemiological investigations showed this drug might increase the incidence of new primary malignancies, such as liver, endometrial or colorectal cancers. Life-time dosing of rats with tamoxifen showed there was a dose dependent increase in the incidence of hepatocellular carcinomas in the treated animals. Since human liver tumors often take decades to develop, it was hoped that by understanding the mechanisms of carcinogenicity in rodents, it might be possible to assess the risks to women taking this class of drug. In rats, tamoxifen dosing leads to hepatic DNA damage, detected by techniques such as $^{32}$P-postlabeling. Little or no such damage could be detected in non-target organs such as kidney, lung or spleen. Tamoxifen is converted by CYP's, to the putative active metabolite, α-hydroxytamoxifen that, following conjugation with sulfate, gives an electrophile that is highly reactive towards DNA. Using insect baculovirus expressed human CYPs, in combination with liquid chromatography-mass spectrometry, it was shown that only CYP3A4 was able to carry out α-hydroxylation. With [$^{14}$C] tamoxifen as substrate and employing the highly sensitive technique of accelerator mass spectrometry, only CYP3A4 was able to catalyze the covalent binding of this drug to DNA. However, Phase 2 glucuronidation conjugates α-hydroxytamoxifen to a stable non-toxic glucuronide. This glucuronidation reaction in human liver is over 50 fold higher than in rats and protects against the toxicity. The evidence presented suggests that in women, tamoxifen hepatocarcinogenicity will not be a problem.

Chapter 7 highlights metastatic liver cancer which is about 20 times as common as primary liver cancer, and its treatment by surgery or conventional chemotherapy is still limited and most patients die. Thus, a broad spectrum of recent novel treatments, including innovative molecular therapies, such as gene and active immunotherapy or replication-competent viral therapeutic strategies, is under preclinical investigation, and numerous clinical trials are in progress in order to combat this lethal disease. Active immunotherapy, intended to induce antigen-specific T-lymphocyte responses to tumor-associated or tumor-specific antigens, has reemerged as a promising approach for the treatment of metastatic liver malignancies, combined with other therapies, and, moreover, as a modality to prevent cancer metastases or recurrence. Locoregional immunotherapy appears to be an attractive and rational approach for the management of metastatic liver disease, offering several advantages over systemic immunotherapy. Locoregional immunological strategies include intrahepatic infusion of anti-tumor cytokines combined with chemotherapy, adoptive immunotherapy by using lymphokine-activated killer cells or activated tumor-infiltrated lymphocytes, embolization of liver tumors with immunostimulants and gene immunotherapy. New-fangled strategies in the immunotherapy of metastatic liver disease, to further improve the outcome of locoregional chemo-immunotherapy, are reviewed briefly, such as the use of granulocyte-macrophage colony-stimulating factor, tumor growth factors-beta antagonists, various monoclonal antibodies including vascular endothelial growth factor antibodies, costimulatory molecules, vaccines, transfection of syngeneic major histocompatibility complex class II genes, a variety of immunotherapeutic strategies based on dendritic cell-induced T-cell mediated anti-tumor immunity, Newcastle Disease Virus, intralesional gene therapy and suicide genes. The authors present their challenge in estimating of the effectiveness of immunotherapeutic approaches and optimizing their application in clinical practice.

The author of Chapter 8 informs the reader that during the past 15 years, liver transplantation has emerged as an effective therapy for selected patients with end-stage liver disease. Early in the era of liver transplantation, long-term survival was uncommon and clinical efforts were focused on improving surgical techniques, immunosuppression protocols and patient selection. With greater experience, the technical aspects of liver transplantation have been refined and five-year survival rates have increased to 70 – 75 %. Consequently, the clinical care of transplant recipients is increasingly focused on the management of the long-term medical problems which occur after transplantation. Surveillance for gastrointestinal (GI) malignancy is perhaps the most important long-term management issue for the gastroenterologist attending the liver recipient. This chapter presents current data regarding the risk of GI cancer after liver transplantation and provides rational guidelines for cancer surveillance in this patient population.

Chapter 9 shows how angiogenesis is an essential process in many physiological and pathological conditions and has become the focus of researches in angiogenesis related diseases such as ischemic coronary or peripheral artery diseases and various tumors. Therapeutical angiogenesis for ischemic disease and anti-angiogenesis for tumors have partially achieved in many experimental studies and clinical trials. Hepatocellular carcinoma, as a hypervascular cancer, has been proved to be more related with angiogenesis. Vascular density and many angiogenesis related factors have been confirmed to be much involved in almost all the process of hepatocarcinogenesis, tumor growth, invasion and metastasis, recurrence and prognosis. These factors include vascular endothelial growth factor, angiopoietin-tie system, somatostatin, angiostatin and endostatin, matrix metalloproteinase, angiogenin and even nerve growth factor, macrophage migration inhibitory factor, ephrin, and rennin-angiotension system. Many strategies targeting these factors and angiogenesis process have been established and proved to be efficient in inhibiting HCC tumor growth, invasion, metastasis and recurrence and consequently promote the five-year survival rate. Anti-angiogenesis may be another effective therapy for HCC besides chemotherapy and immunotherapy and also be a great benefit for both unresectable HCC patients and those after surgical operation.

The last chapter, Chapter 10, discusses angiogenesis, which is the process by which new blood vessels are developed, and is known to be fundamental to tumor growth and metastasis. Neovascularization must occur to provide oxygen and nutrients to the tumor cells, and to remove catabolites and carbon dioxide. Furthermore, the immature neovessels enhance tumor cell dissemination into the circulation. Hepatocellular carcinoma (HCC) is a hypervascular tumor characterized by neovascularization, which plays an important role in the growth and progression of HCC. Angiogenesis provides a target for novel prognostic and therapeutic approaches to HCC. Assessment of microvessel density, which is the density of newly formed vessels, using immunohistochemical staining for specific endothelial cell markers has been shown to provide prognostic information independent of conventional pathological parameters in HCC patients. Assessment of expression of angiogenic factors like vascular endothelial growth factor (VEGF) provides an alternative way of evaluating angiogenic activity of HCC that is more objective compared with microvessel density. Tumor expression of VEGF has been shown to correlate with tumor invasiveness and intrahepatic metastasis in our previous studies. As most angiogenic factors are soluble factors, it is possible to measure the circulating angiogenic factors as an indirect measurement of tumor angiogenic factors. Our previous studies have demonstrated that serum VEGF level does correlate with tumor expression of VEGF, and serum VEGF level can be used as a novel prognostic marker in patients with HCC. Further studies have led to the discovery of new angiogenic factors such as tissue factor in HCC, which may serve as new target for antiangiogenic therapy.

Studies in animal models have also demonstrated the efficacy of antiangiogenic agents in suppressing hepatocarcinogenesis and growth of HCC. Antiangiogenic therapy has already entered clinical trials in HCC patients and holds the promise of providing an effective novel treatment for HCC, which is of great clinical significance because there is no existing effective systemic therapy for HCC. Antiangiogenic therapy also shows promise as an adjuvant or adjunctive therapy in combination with existing surgical or locoregional therapies for HCC.

In: Liver Cancer: New Research
Editor: Felix Lee, pp. 1-41
ISBN 1-59454-182-5


*Chapter I*

# Malignant Epithelial Liver Tumors in Children, Adolescents and Adults: Molecular Pathways of Cancerogenesis, Growth, and Spread

***Arthur Zimmermann***
Institute of Pathology of the University, Berne, Switzerland

## ABSTRACT

Malignant epithelial tumors of the liver involving the hepatocyte lineage comprise hepatocellular carcinoma (HCC) and its variants, fibrolamellar (hepatocellular) carcinoma (FL-HCC), several types of mixed tumors, hepatoblastoma (HBL), and a novel entity, transitional liver cell tumor (TLCT). Carcinogenic pathways, patterns of growth, invasion, and metastatic spread of these lesions display considerable differences. HCC is one of the most common malignancies worldwide, whereas HBL is a very rare pediatric tumor. HCC is frequently a terminal complication of chronic, mainly viral-induced inflammatory and fibrotic liver disease. In contrast, HBL, FL-HCC and TLCT typically develop in nonfibrotic livers, but HBL is more frequently associated with a broad array of malformations in other organs. Cancerogenesis in HCC involves several groups of altered genes (mainly the p53, RB1, TGF-beta, and APC/WNT pathways), whereas in HBL the WNT/beta-catenin signaling protein network seems to be predominantly involved. Growth, differentiation and expansion of these tumors depends on an altered expression of several growth factors/oncogenes modulated by distinct protease systems, and on angiogenesis/antiangiogenesis factors. Invasion and spread of HCC involves changes of cell adhesion molecules, cellular junction proteins, factors of cellular remodeling, proteins affecting cell polarity, proangiogenic proteins, and metalloproteinases acting on the extracellular matrix. Several factors have been identified that regulate the metastatic behavior of HCC, while less is still known about gene products affecting the metastatic spread of HBL and related tumors. The present overview aims at summarizing novel findings in this rapidly evolving field.

# MALIGNANT LIVER CELL TUMORS: THE PHENOTYPES

The pathobiologic features of epithelial liver tumors reflect disordered molecular mechanisms as a consequence of progressive genomic instability occurring along the carcinogenic pathways. The diverse established and emerging phenotypes recognized by pathologists are the visible result of genomic changes, and novel phenotypes may direct the focus of further molecular investigations to distinct pathways.In fact, most of the molecular informations obtained so far, have been accumulated by studying tumors with a "standard" phenotype, or the exact pathology has not been specified. Therefore, a brief introduction to the evolving spectrum of lesions is given before discussing genetic and molecular features of liver tumors. In what follows, emphasis is, with few exceptions, placed exclusively on neoplasms of the hepatocyte lineage.

## Hepatocellular Carcinoma (HCC) and its Variants

Adult-type HCC occurs in several established macroscopic and histologic morphotypes with distinct growth and invasion patterns (Anthony, 1973; Nakashima et al., 1983; Kishi et al., 1983; Sawabe et al., 1987; Ishak et al., 1994; Okuda, 1997; Zimmermann, 2000). Part of these distinct features have been shown to affect tumor biology and prognosis (Jwo et al., 1992; Ng et al., 1995; Hu et al., 1996; Chau et al., 1997; Takata et al., 2000; Nagasue et al., 2001; Hanazaki et al., 2002; Grazi et al., 2003; Chen et al., 2003). In addition, these tumors frequently exhibit a rather broad spectrum of characteristic cellular, tissual, and extracellular features, sometimes in a heterogeneous pattern within a given tumor, causing considerable sampling errors in histologic typing based on biopsies. However, apart from these and other features expressed by many HCCs otherwise showing a standard morphology, there are HCCs with a more characteristic histology, having led to the formulation of distinct entities.

*Clear cell variant of HCC* (Ishak et al., 1994) shows cells rich in glycogen and lipids with a distinct immunophenotype (Adamek et al., 1998). Some of these tumors show a histology compatible with a chromophobe cell subtype, similar to chromophobe cell renal carcinoma (Emile et al., 2001). The frequency of clear cell HCC among HCCs varies between 0.4 % and 37% in the largest published series (Lai et al., 1979; Kashala et al., 1990; Emile et al., 2001), the variable prevalence likely to be due to ill-defined diagnostic criteria. The male to female ratio is lower than in ordinary HCC, i.e. 2.3: 1, and the prevalence of associated cirrhosis is very high. The recognition of clear cell HCC has a certain clinical impact insofar as it can be associated with hypoglycemia and hypercholesterolemia (Sasaki et al., 1981), and sudden death from severe hypoglycemia has been reported (Ross and Kurian, 1985). Furthermore, spontaneous regression of metastases has been described for this tumor (McDermott and Khettry, 1994).

*Encapsulated HCC* is characterized by a grossly distinct capsule-like fibrous tissue surrounding the tumors. In an autopsy series, the prevalence of this type was 10.3% of HCCs, the mean age of the patients was significantly higher compared with that of non-encapsulated HCC, and the tumors were relatively well differentiated, with a protracted clinical course (Okuda et al., 1977; Ros et al., 1990; Ng et al., 1992). It has been observed that the formation of capsules or capsule-like structures depends on the presence and activity of alpha-SMA-positive mesenchymal cells (myofibroblasts) at the interface of the tumors (Ishizaki et al., 2001).

*Small HCCs*, i.e. with a diameter <= 3 cm, have been identified for a long time, and their morphology, growth patterns and clinical behavior have been extensively documented in the literature, particularly in Japanese investigations (Okuda et al., 1977; Kondo et al., 1983; Wakasa et al., 1985; Nakashima et al., 1995; Kim et al., 1995; Tomizawa et al., 1995; Suehiro et al., 1995; Sasaki et al., 1996; Yamasaki et al., 1996; Yamamoto et al., 1996; Kojiro, 1998; Nakashima et al., 1999; Kojiro and Nakashima, 1999; Nakashima et al., 1999; Maeda et al., 2000; An et al., 2001; Hu et al., 2003; Shimozawa and Hanazaki, 2004). Even smaller tumors, i.e. with a diameter smaller than 1 cm, have been termed, minute HCC, and their biology has been analyzed (Maeda et al., 2000).

*Sclerosing HCC (sclerosing hepatic carcinoma)* is characterized by a high stromal/matrix content (Omata et al., 1981; Ohtomo et al., 1984). Sclerosing HCCs can induce hormone-induced hypercalcemia (Polterauer et al., 1980; Oldenburg et al., 1982; Yamashita et al., 1992; Martinez et al., 1997;), sometimes leading to hypercalcemic coma (Leone et al., 1999), and caused by the secretion of parathyroid hormone-related peptide (PTHrP) (Oldenburg et al., 1982; Yen et al., 1993; Tamura et al., 1994), a peptide involved in several forms of paraneoplastic hypercalcemia (Dunbar et al., 1996). PTHrP has been detected in HCC cells either by use of immunohistochemistry (Albar et al., 1996) or mRNA in situ hybridization (Kitazawa et al., 1999). Hypercalcemia in HCC patients does not seem to always be related to PTHrP. E.g., an HCC producing intact PTH instead of PTHrP has been reported (Koyama et al., 1999). Furthermore, and similar to other tumors, hypercalcemia in HCC may also be caused by the production of prostaglandin E known to affect calcium metabolism (Seyberth et al., 1978; Ikeda et al., 1988).

*Combined hepatocellular/cholangiocellular carcinoma (cHCC-CC)* is an uncommon subtype of primary liver cancer characterized by the simultaneous presence of cells of a hepatocyte and cholangiocyte lineage within the same tumor. The criteria for the diagnosis and classification of cHCC-CC have to be more refined, because terms employed to denote such lesions still vary to a certain degree. Several phenotypes have been proposed, i.e. separated (HCC and CC are clearly separated), collision, and intermingled types. Furthermore, a HCC-predominant type (the tumor resembles HCC) and a CC-predominant type (the tumor resembles CC) have been described. Based on morphology, one study identified a type I (HCC and CC clearly distinguished), type II (HCC and CC contiguous, sharing transitional features), and type III cancer cells evaluated as either HCC or CC, considered to be an intermediate type; Taguchi et al., 1996). In another study, the tumors were divided into two classes by reference to the macroscopic appearance, i.e. single nodular (SN) vs. multinodular (MN) types, being clinically relevant insofar as the SN type behaved as HCC, and the MN type more like intrahepatic cholangiocarcinoma (Sasaki et al., 2001). The lesions consistently reveal areas morphologically intermediate between HCC and CC (so-called transitional-type tumors), and in a larger series such areas formed at least 25 % of the tumor (Tickoo et al., 2002). Clinically, a recent study has demonstrated that the cHCC-CC patients show greater similarity with HCC patients than with CC patients with regard to male/female ratio, status of hepatitis viral infection, serum AFP, and non-tumor liver histology (Tickoo et al., 2002; Lee et al., 2002; Yano et al., 2003).

*HCCs with sarcomatoid change* show a broad spectrum of heterologous features, including rhabdomyoblastic , chondroid, or osteosarcomatous components (Komada et al., 1997; Ikebe et al., 1998; Akasofu et al., 1999; Koda et al., 2003).

Immunohistochemical studies have surfaced that the sarcomatoid cells do not express AFP or alpha-1-antitrypsin (Haratake and Horie, 1991), while the ordinary HCC cells express the markers established for such cell lineages, including cytokeratin 8, albumin, fibrinogen, and alpha-1-antitrypsin (Oda et al., 1994). The hypothesis that a transformed (progenitor) cell not yet definitively primed for either an epithelial or a mesenchymal cell lineage is suggested by the observation that sarcomatoid cells concomitantly express cytokeratins and a mesenchymal cell marker, vimentin (Eriguchi et al., 2001).

### *Emerging Phenotypes*

*Steatosis* is rather frequent in HCCs of diverse types, but there are tumors where this feature predominates (HCC with fatty metamorphosis; fatty HCC; *steatotic HCC*) (Itai et al., 1987; Yoshikawa et al., 1988; Ueda et al., 1989). Similar degrees of fatty change have also been reported in small HCCs (Kutami et al., 2000). In contrast to the non-neoplastic liver (Harrison and Diehl, 2002), the genetic and metabolic factors inducing marked tumor steatosis have not been clarified, but altered pathways involved in triglyceride and lipoprotein metabolism may be involved. In small HCCs arising in HCV-infected patients and showing fatty change, insulin-like growth factor II (IGF-II)was detectable in 80%, suggesting that this factor plays a role in the tumors' steatotic reaction (Sohda et al., 1997). It is of interest to note that other HCCs can express IGF-II, sometimes associated with hypoglycemia (Ishida et al., 1995). The detection of fat in HCV-associated HCCs is of interest insofar as HCV (in particular genotype 3) seems to induce fatty change in non-neoplastic liver (Hui et al., 2002; Lonardo et al., 2004; Ratziu et al., 2004). Furthermore, a p53 protein-mediated pathway, frequently altered in HCC, may be involved in steatogenesis. p53 in the nuclei is induced in the liver from obese ob/ob and lean transgenic mice overexpressing an active form of sterol regulatory element-binding protein (SREBP)-1 in the liver (Yahagi et al., 2004). Triglyceride accumulation in hepatocytes as such may, on the other hand, promote abnormal liver cell growth, because genetically obese, leptin-deficient ob/ob mice exhibit, similar to obese, diabetic patients, an increased incidence of HCC and show hepatic hyperplasia in their non-cirrhotic fatty livers (Yang et al., 2001).

HCCs can express *neuroendocrine features* (Wang et al., 1991; Zhao et al., 1993; Zhao and Zimmermann, 1997; Reubi et al., 1999; Vora et al., 2000). Neuroendocrine differentiation is detectable in a fraction of HCC by immunohistochemical identification of several neuroendocrine markers, and neuroendocrine differentiation was related to distinct tumor cell types, but not to tumor grade (Zhao et al., 1993). By use of in vitro receptor autoradiography we have found that 41% and 47% of HCC expressed somatostatin and VIP receptors, respectively, but VIP receptors were always identified in non-neoplastic liver tissue. The somatostatin receptors showed high affinity for somatostatin and octreotide (Reubi et al., 1999). A neuroendocrine differentiation of HCC appears to be associated with altered patterns of programmed cell death (Zhao and Zimmermann, 1997). Elevated serum levels of chromogranin A, a neuroendocrine marker, have been detected in 9.2% within one series of tumors (Leone et al., 2002), and chromogranin A is expressed in the cells of some HCC (Nakajima et al., 2000). However, elevation of this protein in serum is found in other non-endocrine tumors and therefore may represent a non-specific reaction (Wu et al., 2000).

A further subgroup of HCCs is characterized by marked leukocytic infiltrates, probably reflecting a cellular immune reaction directed against tumor-associated antigens. In small HCCs with a dense lymphocytic infiltration, the recurrence rate was lower and the 5-year survival higher than in control HCCs (Wada et al., 1998). In small HCCs with a dense lymphoid stroma (lymphoepithelioma-like carcinoma; Szekely, 2001), survival after OLT was superior to HCCs without lymphoid stroma (Emile et al., 2000). Plasma cell rich HCC with a medullary phenotype (medullary HCC) has been reported to show signs of regression (Zimmermann et al., 2002), a phenomenon otherwise very rare in HCCs (Markovic et al., 1996; Li et al., 2003).

## Fibrolamellar Hepatocellular Carcinoma (FL-HCC; Fibrolamellar Carcinoma)

FL-HCC mainly occurs in young individuals without liver cirrhosis and normal serum AFP. It is rare in oriental populations (Hoshino et al., 1996; Sooklim et al., 2003; Chang et al., 2003). It has originally been defined as a liver tumor presenting as a single, expanding mass with typical imaging features, consisting of eosinophilic and large, hepatocyte-like cells embedded in an abundant collagenous stroma (Edmondson, 1956; Craig et al., 1980; McLarney et al, 1999). A clear cell variant has also been described (Cheuk and Chan, 2001). Modern imaging techniques allow a highly precise preoperative diagnosis of this lesion, particularly based on the development of characteristic central scars in these neoplasms (Blachar et al., 2002). The pathogenesis of FL-HCC , and its relationship with ordinary HCC, have not yet been clarified, although it can coexist together with adult-type HCC (Okada et al., 1993; Seitz et al., 2002).

In a recent US population-based retrospective study, remarkable differences in the epidemiology and prognosis of FL-HCC compared to ordinary HCC was observed. The age-adjusted incidence rate for FL-HCC was 0.02 per 100'000. A greater proportion of cases with FL-HCC had localized disease, or received potentially curative therapy, the 1- and 5-year observed and relative survival rates were significantly longer in patients with FL-HCC than HCC, and FL-HCC was independently associated with a 46 % reduction in risk of mortality within 5 years compared with ordinary HCC (El-Serag and Davila, 2004). In contrast to former reports, a recent investigation has shown that children with Fl-HCC do not have favorable prognosis and do not respond any differently to current therapeutic regimens that patients with adult-type HCC (Katzenstein et al., 2003).

### Transitional liver cell tumors (TLCT)

TLCT form a novel group of hepatocellular tumors found to develop in older children and young adolescents, typically presenting as large tumors, a very high serum AFP, an aggressive course, and a chemotherapy response pattern clearly different from hepatoblastomas (Prokurat et al., 2002). We have found that, histologically, the morphotype is neither typical for hepatoblastoma nor for adult-type HCC, and we therefore suggested that the cells of these intriguing neoplasms are situated somewhere between hepatoblasts and mature hepatocytes, thus holding an intermediate or transitional position (a differentiation window) in the hepatogenic pathway, or representing somewhat like an upper end of the developmental scale starting from hepatocyte progenitors and ending at the level of the mature hepatocyte (Prokurat et al., 2002; Zimmermann, 2003).

### Hepatoblastoma

In the liver of infants, children and adolescents, several types of malignant epithelial neoplasms are recognized, hepatoblastoma being the predominant tumor type (review: Perilongo et al., 2002). The classification of hepatoblastoma and the assessment of criteria for classifying these lesions have recently been reviewed (Rowland, 2002). Recently, other phenotypes of pediatric epithelial liver tumors, or tumors containing an epithelial/hepatocyte lineage, have started to emerge. They include several variants of hepatoblastoma, but also complex lesions awaiting definition. One group of tumors is characterized by a bimodal differentiation, with a contribution of bile duct cells (cholangioblastic hepatoblastoma; Zimmermann, 2002; Libbrecht et al., 2003) or the development of ductal plate-like structures ('ductal plate tumors'; Gornicka et al., 2001; Zimmermann, 2002).A further novel group of pediatric non-HBL liver tumors is characterized by a predominance of stromal elements (pediatric hepatic stromal tumors; PHST), sometimes with signs of ossification (ossifying hepatic tumor of infancy; OHTI; Zimmermann and the SIOPEL Group, 2003). Finally, apart from extrarenal rhabdoid tumor of the liver, few other and in part epithelial tumors of the liver in childhood may contain cell populations with rhabdoid features (Zimmermann and the SIOPEL Group, 2003).

## Molecular Pathogenesis of Epithelial Liver Tumors

In what follows, emphasis is placed mainly on hepatocellular carcinoma and hepatoblastoma. Relatively few data are available for the fibrolamellar carcinoma, and genetic or molecular informations for transitional liver cell tumors are so far lacking.

## Hepatocellular Carcinoma

### *Hepatocellular Carcinoma: A Malignant Liver Tumor with a Broad Spectrum of Etiologies*

Etiologic causes of HCC chiefly comprise liver cirrhosis, in particular chronic fibrosing liver disease induced by hepatitis viruses (HBV and HCV) and alcohol toxicity, other toxic agents (including aflatoxin B1), and metabolic liver disorders (including iron storage diseases and hepatic steatosis), but any chronic liver disease associated with increased hepatic cell turnover may be followed by liver carcinogenesis. The most detailed knowledge regarding etiology of HCC has been accumulated by studying chronic viral infection of the liver (reviews: Ren, 1996; Henkler and Koshy, 1996; Idilman et al., 1998; Chen and Chen, 1999; Reeves and DeMatteo, 2000; Arbuthnot and Kew, 2001; Bruix and Llovet, 2003; Block et al., 2003; Van Dekken et al., 2003). A detailed discussion of pathogenic pathways involved in viral-induced liver cancer is beyong the scope of this review, but, as an example of the pathogenic complexity, several newer aspects of the role of HBx gene product are briefly discussed.

## HBx Gene and Gene Product: a Multitarget Factor

HBx protein is thought to play a role in hepatic carcinogenic pathways, although the pathogenic mechanisms have not yet been fully clarified (Su et al., 1998; Murakami, 2001). Mutations at nucleotides 1762 and 1764 in HBV, within a sequence encoding both the core promoter gene and the X gene, have been found frequently in patients with HCC, and genomic integration of the mutational DNA region has been observed (Momosaki et al., 2003). The integrated Hbx frequently is truncated (Wang et al., 2004) or contains point mutations. HBx has the ability to bind p53 (see below), and alleviates p53-mediated repression of AFP gene expression (Ogden et al., 2000; Arima et al., 2002). The action of HBx modifies the expression of several other genes, including a subset of oncogenes (c-myc, c-myb), growth factors (such as Egr-1; Chen et al., 2000), and tumor suppressor genes (p53, APC, WAF1, WT1), suggesting that HBx may affect the regulation of hepatocyte proliferation (Wu et al., 2001). However, it has also been shown that HBx exerts a paracrine inhibitory effect on liver cell proliferation (Tralhao et al., 2002).

### *What is the Role of HBx in Cancerogenesis?*

Transgenic mice expressing HBx protein are susceptible to carcinogen-induced hepatocarcinogenesis, so that HBx gene expression alone may not suffice for hepatic carcinogenesis (Zhu et al., 2004). HBx downregulates the expression of PTEN (a known tumor suppressor and negative regulator of PI-3-kinase/Akt) and activates Akt via an effect on the p53-mediated transcription of PTEN (Chung et al., 2003), thus possibly abolishing the tumor-suppressive effect of PTEN. Akt-2 (but not Akt1) expression in human HCCs itself is correlated with prognosis, being a novel independent predictor for development and progression of HCC (Xu et al., 2004).

### *How Does HBx Affect Growth and Progression?*

HBx protein has been demonstrated to induce angiogenesis by increasing the transcriptional activity and protein level of hypoxia-inducible factor-1alpha (HIF-1alpha) under both normoxic and hypoxic conditions (Yoo et al., 2003; Moon et al., 2004), an enhancement mediated by activation of the mitogen-activated protein kinase pathway (Yoo et al., 2003). HBx protein decreases the binding of the von Hippel-Lindau protein (pVHL) to HIF-1alpha and prevents ubiquitin-dependent degradation of HIF-1alpha. In Hbx-transgenic mice, HIF-1alpha and VEGF are strongly expressed in dysplastic lesions, where HBx is also more markedly expressed (Moon et al., 2004). HBx mutants derived from human HCCs retain the ability to abrogate p53-induced apoptosis (Huo et al., 2001). HBx also affects apoptosis through the induced expression of the FasL upregulator, Nur77 (an orphan nuclear receptor; Lee et al., 2001).

## HCC and Chromosomal Aberrations: Visualizing Progressive Genomic Instability

A broad array of chromosomal and genetic changes have been identified in HCCs, reflecting progressive genomic instability along the carcinogenic pathways (reviews: Ozturk, 1999; Buendia, 2000; Kondoh et al., 2001; Tannapfel and Wittekind, 2002; Levy et al., 2002; Wang et al., 2002); only a selection of these findings are briefly discussed in the present overview.

Complex patterns of loss of heterozygosity (LOH) are a frequent finding in HCC. LOH sites include 1q, 1p36, 4q, 8p, 8q, 9q, 10q, 13q, 14q, 16q, 17p and 20q (selected references: Nagai et al., 1997; Chang et al., 2002; Nishida et al., 2003; Koshikawa et al., 2004). The methods employed to detect these alterations comprise allelotype studies by microsatellite analysis (MSA) and by comparative genomic hybridization (CGH). In some situations, a correlation between a given LOH and the clinical behavior of HCC was found. E.g., tumors with more allelic losses were significantly more likely to be histologically poorly differentiated, to be advanced in T classification, and to be un-infected by HCV (Tamura et al., 1997). LOH of chromosome 1p occurs at an early stage of hepatocarcinogenesis (Kuroki et al., 1995), while deletion of 9p21 was preferentially found in large (later stage) HCCs (Chung et al., 2000). Allelic losses on 8p (Chan et al., 2002) and 13q (Wong et al., 2002) are related to an aggressive phenotype. The presence of LOH on 16q, 17p, and the number of chromosomes with LOH, were negatively associated with metastasis-free survival (Nishida et al., 2002). There is strong evidence that chromosome 17p13 is the most common deletion region in several tumors, suggesting that 17p harbors one or more of the genes associated with development or progression of many cancers, including HCC (Kondoh et al., 2001; Li et al., 2001). An HBV integration event in chromosome 17p near the p53 gene identifies the region of a commonly deleted chromosome in virus-associated HCC (Slagle et al., 1991). The region 17p13 also contains a novel gene, HCCS1, mutated in HCCs (see below; Zhao et al., 2001). 4q is preferentially lost in in HCCs containing a p53 mutation; in one study, LOH of 4q was present in 75% of HCC with, but only 25% of HCC without, a p53 gene mutation (Rashid et al., 1999).

# Genes and Gene Products Involved in Hepatocellular Carcinoma

An increased number of altered genes have been identified in HCCs, and at least part of them are linked to chromosomal changes occurring in these tumors (reviews: Fujimoto et al., 1994; Ozturk, 1999; Buendia, 2000; Kondoh et al., 2001; Feitelson et al., 2002; Levy et al., 2002; Thorgeirsson and Grisham, 2002; Kern et al., 2002; Buendia, 2002; Coleman, 2003). A selection of these genes will briefly be discussed, with reference to chromosomal changes/LOH where this is known.

## p53 Gene: a Multifacetted Affector of Several Critical Events of Growth Control

p53 is a major tumor suppressor gene assigned to the short arm of chromosome 17. The gene product, p53 protein, is at crossroads for several features of normal and neoplastic cells, including the regulation of cell cycle checkpoints, DNA repair, apoptosis, and cellular senescence, and therefore holds a key position in several carcinogenic mechanisms (review; Staib et al. 2003). A role of altered p53 expression in HCC is documented by numerous investigations referring to HCCs observed in several geographic areas (Murakami et al., 1991; Oda et al., 1992; Debuire et al., 1993; Volkmann et al., 1994; Hayashi et al., 1995; Kang et al., 1998). P53 mutations involving a mutational hotspot, codon 249, have frequently been found in HCCs from endemic areas and are related to aflatoxin exposure, but codon 249 mutations do not play a role in most HCCs in the US (Kazachkov et al., 1996). Apart from its effects on growth, p53 affects apoptosis both in HCC and liver cell dysplasia (Zhao and Zimmermann, 1997). In one study, the rate of apoptosis in HCCs showed a significant correlation with the p53 status, but not with p21WAF1/CIP1 (Park et al., 2003). As the development of HCC from nodular precursor lesions procedes along several morphologically identifiable steps (Sakamoto et al., 1991), often ending up with so-called nodule-in-nodule (NIN) lesions probably reflecting the emergence of a more malignant cellular subline in a preexisting nodular lesion (Arakawa et al., 1986), it was of interest to test whether this progressive morphologic heterogeneity would also show up in genetic alterations. In fact, tumor progression in HCC may be mediated by p53 mutations (Tanaka et al., 1993; Choi et al., 2001), and p53 overexpression has been observed in liver cell dysplasia and in dysplastic nodules (Zhao et al., 1994), in particular high-grade dysplastic nodules (Kang et al., 1998). However, in small HCCs, that have been shown to be microheterogeneous with multiple grades within a single lesion (Kenmochi et al., 1987), p53 gene mutational patterns were the same in heterogeneous tumor subpopulations, whereas beta-catenin mutations were detected only in less differentiated lesions (An et al., 2001), suggesting that differential carcinogenic pathways are present for dedifferentiated cell lines within a given tumor.

A novel gene partly homologous to p53 is p73, assigned to chromosome 1p36 (a region harboring a putative tumor suppressor gene and showing LOH and overexpression in HCC (Tannapfel et al., 1999; Koshikawa et al., 2004), encoding a gene product showing functional similarities to p53 protein. p73 seems to be biallelically expressed in the liver. LOH on p73 was observed in 33% of informative HCCs, but no mutations of the gene were found; tumors with LOH p73 had more frequently developed in non-cirrhotic livers, and disese-free survival rates of patients with LOH at p73 were significantly poorer than those without (Aoki et al., 2004). LOH of p73 seems to occur in early stages of the HCC pathway (Peng et al., 2000).

## Other Established or Putative Liver Cancer Genes

The p21WAF1 and p16/retinoblastoma (Rb) protein pathways are disrupted in a considerable fraction of early HCCs (Murakami et al., 1991; Hsia et al., 1994; Naka et al., 1998; Hui et al., 1999; Azechi et al., 2001; Huang et al., 2003), whereas amplifications of the c-myc (8q24.1) and AIB1 (20q12) oncogenes are late genetic alterations in the progression of HCC and are correlated with poor prognosis (Wange et al., 2002). The tumor suppressor gene p16INK4A (chromosome 9p21-22) is an important component of the cell cycle regulation. p16INK4A acts as an inhibitor of the cyclin-dependent kinase 4 (Cdk4). In HCCs, p16INK4A is altered frequently and early in disease development. The most frequent inactivation mechanism was hyper-methylation of the promoter region, partly associated with LOH at the 9p21 region (Anzola et al., 2004). Aberrant p16 RNA transcripts have been described to encode key peptides (amino acids 84-103) involved in binding with cyclin-dependent kinase (CDK) 4. However, overexpression of these aberrant transcripts resulted in decreased cell proliferation rate, enlargement of target cells, and reduced levels of hyperphosphorylated forms of pRb, suggesting that aberrant transcripts have functions similar to those of wild-type p16 (Cho et al., 2003). Ets-mediated activation of p16INK4A is opposed by inhibitors of differentiation and DNA-binding-1 (Id-1) proteins, and overexpression of Id-1 in HCCs therefore induces cell proliferation (Lee et al., 2003).

A further tumor suppressor gene involved in HCC is LKB1/STK11, mapped to chromosome 19p13, a region exhibiting frequent allelic loss in HCC. LKB1 encodes a serine/threonine kinase mutated in Peutz-Jeghers syndrome; this master kinase activates 13 kinases of the AMPK subfamily (Lizcano et al., 2004; Shaw et al., 2004; Carling, 2004). The gene is homologous to the Par-4 polarity genes in Drosophila and Caenorhabditis elegans. In human epithelia, activated LKB1 and LKB1-specific adaptor protein (STRAD) induce complete polarization in the absence of junctional cell-cell contacts (Baas et al., 2004), a phenomenon that may play a role in the disordered cell polarity of cancer cells. An allelic loss of LKB1 was found in 22% of informative HCC cases (all of them being HBV-positive), and it was suggested that genetic LKB1 alterations may play a role in the protection of HCC cells from p53-mediated apoptosis (Kim et al., 2004). In heterozygous Lkb1 knockout mice, more than 70% of male and 20% of female animals have been demonstrated to develop HCCs of various types, suggesting that lack of LKB1 activity is a novel mechanism for HCC development (Nakau et al., 2002).

A novel candidate HCC tumor suppressor gene is DLC-1 (deleted in liver cancer-1; chromosome 8p21-22) encoding a regulator of the Rho family of small GTPases altered in several other cancers (Park et al., 2003; Wong et al., 2003). Restoration of DLC-1 expression inhibits cell growth and tumorigenicity in HCC cells and induces apoptosis (Zhou et al., 2004).

Platelet-derived growth factor receptor-beta-like tumor suppressor gene (PRLTS) is located to 8p21.3-p22, an LOH site typical for part of HCCs. Alterations at PRLTS seem to be related to an early genetic event of hepatocarcinogenesis, in particular the formation of dysplastic nodules (Kahng et al., 2003). At a neighboring site, 8p23, is located a novel liver-related putative tumor suppressor (LPTS), that has a growth-inhibitory function in HCC cell lines. LOH of the LPTS site was identified in HCCs, and only in samples from patients with HBV infection (Park et al., 2002).

On 4q21-22, frequently altered in HCC, a novel gene termed DRLM ('down-regulated in liver malignancy'), belonging to the class of nucleosome assemble protein (NAP), has been identified and shown to be decreased in HCC (Harada et al., 2002).

A novel potential marker of advanced human HCC is downregulated SAP-1 (stomach cancer-associated protein tyrosine phosphatase-1), a transmembrane-type protein tyrosine phosphatase implicated as a negative regulator of integrin-mediated signaling. SAP-1 was almost undetectable in more than 80% of poorly differentiated HCCs, while in well-differentiated tumors it was present similar to non-cancerous liver tissue, suggesting a role of SAP-1 in the dedifferentiation process and in progression of HCC (Nagano et al., 2003).

## THE WNT/BETA-CATENIN NETWORK: ALTERATIONS OF AN EVOLUTIONARILY CONSERVED SIGNALING PATHWAY AFFECT GROWTH AND PROGRESSION OF HCC

The chief signaling effector of the Wnt pathway is an intracellular protein network mainly containing beta-catenin, Axins I and II, glycogen synthase kinase-3beta, adenomatous polyposis coli (APC) protein, and dishevelled (Dvl/Dsh). The convergence of WNT, beta-catenin, and cadherin pathways has recently been reviewed (Nelson and Nusse, 2004). Mutations at the serine and/or threonine residues near the NH2 terminus in the beta-catenin gene prevent their phosphorylation by the APC-axin-glycogen synthase kinase 3beta complex and subsequent degradation through the ubiquitin-proteasome pathway. Upon its stabilization, beta-catenin translocates to nuclei, associates with Tcf/Lef transcription factors, and activates the transcription of several genes (Huber et al., 1996).

Somatic mutations of the beta-catenin gene (the CTNNB1 gene) in HCC (review: Buendia, 2002) are focused at a mutational hotspot in exon 3 in the region of the consensus glycogen synthase kinase (GSK) -3beta phosphorylation and ubiquitination target sites, likely to result in stabilization of free cytoplasmic beta-catenin. (Miyoshi et al., 1998; Devereux et al., 2001; Wong et al., 2001). In fact, a recent study has shown that the expression of phospho-GSK-3beta is related with the accumulation of beta-catenin in surrounding tissues (Ban et al., 2003). The reported prevalence of beta-catenin gene mutations in human HCC ranges from 12 % to 61.8% (De la Coste et al., 1998; Terris et al., 1999; Huang et al., 1999; Kondo et al., 1999; Legoix et al., 1999; Hsu et al., 2000; Wong et al., 2001; Cui et al., 2001; Taniguchi et al., 2002; Ban et al., 2003; Cui et al., 2003; Ban et al., 2003). In contrast to hepatoblastomas (see below), HCCs seem to preferentially show point mutations of CBNNB1

(Taniguchi et al., 2002). A high prevalence of beta-catenin gene alterations has also been observed in HCCs developing in association with HCV infection, beta-catenin mutations being more frequent in HCV-associated HCC than in HBV-associated ones (Huang et al., 1999; Hsu et al., 2000; Wong et al., 2001; Ueta et al., 2002), and with high aflatoxin B1 exposure (Devereux et al., 2001).

Mutations of the beta-catenin gene, and in particular of the mutational hot spot in exon 3, are frequently associated with nuclear accumulation of beta-catenin in the neoplastic cells, detectable by use of immunohistochemistry (De la Coste et al., 1998; Terris et al., 1999; Huang et al., 1999; Wong et al., 2001), although nuclear immunostaining has also been found in tumors without beta-catenin gene mutation, and a significant fraction of HCCs with mutated beta-catenin shows cytoplasmic and/or membrane staining suggesting that other mechanisms of accumulation may also operate in HCC (Kondo et al., 1999; Devereux et al., 2001; Wong et al., 2001). The distinct nuclear expression pattern is significantly correlated with the proliferative activity and dedifferentiation of HCC cells (Tran van Nhieu et al., 1999; An et al., 2001; Ueta et al., 2002) and with cyclin D1 expression (Ueta et al., 2002), but beta-catenin mutations in HCC were independently correlated with with c-Myc overexpression (Cui et al., 2003). It has been suggested that accumulated beta-catenin may bind to the lymphocyte enhancer binding factor-1 (LEF-1) , form the beta-catenin/LEF-1 complex, and stimulates promoters regulating the cell cycle such as the cyclin D1 gene (Ueta et al., 2002).

What is the experimental evidence that beta-catenin mutations confer hepatocarcinogenesis? Murine models of chemically induced altered hepatocellular foci and hepatic tumors (adenomas and carcinomas) suggest that mutation of the beta-catenin gene is an early event in carcinogenesis (Devreux et al., 1999; Ogawa et al., 1999). However, in a mouse strain containing a mutant beta-catenin allele of which exon 3 was sandwiched by loxPsequences (Catnb lox (ex3) numerous adenomatous intestinal polyps occurred, but no liver neoplasia (Harada et al., 1999; Harada et al., 2002), suggesting that additional gene mutations might be required. In a more recently studied murine model, H-ras mutation alone caused large cell dysplasia of the liver, while the simultaneous induction of an additional mutation in the beta-catenin gene caused a clonal expansion of such dysplastic cells, followed by nodules and HCC (Harada et al., 2004).

Is there a relationship between beta-catenin expression patterns and the biology of HCC? The data so far available are somewhat controversial. In a study of 60 patients with HCC, tumors with a non-nuclear type of beta-catenin overexpression were more frequently larger than 5 cm in diameters and had poorer differentiation, and the patients had a significantly shorter disease-free survival (Wong et al., 2001). Among 366 unifocal resected HCCs selected for clinicopathologic analysis, beta-catenin mutations with nuclear beta-catenin accumulation were significantly associated with grade I and stage I and II, and a better 5-year survival rate, suggesting that beta-catenin gene mutations are a favorable prognostic factor related to low stage (Hsu et al., 2000). Patients with unifocal HCCs with visible nuclear expression of beta-catenin correlated with beta-catenin gene mutation had significantly lower frequencies of HBV surface antigen carriers and lower AFP elevation, but more often had non-invasive (stage I) HCC, absence of portal vein spread, and better survival (Mao et al., 2001). On the other hand, overexpression of beta-catenin exon 3 was found to be correlated with an invasive phenotype and high metastatic potential of HCCs in Chinese patients (Cui et al., 2001).

Are other members of the Wnt/beta-catenin network altered in HCC? Among 73 HCCs studied, several types of AXIN1 mutations were found in seven tumors (9.6%), and AXIN2 mutations in two tumors (2.7%), with LOH at the AXIN1 locus being present in four of five informative HCCs with AXIN1 mutations, suggesting a tumor suppressor function of this gene (Taniguchi et al., 2002).

## GROWTH AND EXPANSION OF HCCS: THE ROLE OF GROWTH AND DIFFERENTIATION FACTORS

The complex interplay of genes encoding growth-promoting and apoptotic factors instrumental in the development and progression of HCC has been reviewed (Tannapfel and Wittekind, 2002).

### Insulin-Like Growth Factor Pathways

Recent studies have discovered changes in the insulin-like growth factor (IGF) pathways that affect the molecular pathogenesis of HCC, including the autocrine synthesis and secretion of IGFs, IGF receptors (IGFR), IGF-binding proteins (IGFBP), and IGF proteases. 60-70% of HBV-negative and -positive HCCs show LOH at the mannose 6-phosphate/ILGFR locus (Yang et al., 2003), and the gene was mutated in 55% of these patients with LOH. Critical events in HCCs seem to be the overexpression of IGF-II and the IGF-I-R, both for malignant transformation and tumor growth. A simultaneous decrease of IGFBP expression and an increase of the proteolytic degradation of IGFBP cause an increased availability of IGFs. Furthermore, functional derangements of the IGF-II/mannose 6-phosphate receptor affect the degradation of IGF-II, the activation of TGF-beta1, and the lysosomal targeting of cathepsin proteases degrading ECM proteins (review: Scharf and Braulke, 2003).

The autocrine/paracrine loops involving IGF and insulin-like growth factor-binding protein-3 (IGFBP-3) seem to be lost in part of HCCs, causing deregulated growth (Huynh et al., 2002). The role of the IGF system is supported by observations on transgenic mice; overexpression of IGFBP in such mice caused a marked inhibition of hepatic preneoplasia, possibly by decreasing the mitogenic activity of IGF-I and/or IGF-II (Lu and Archer, 2003).

### Hepatocyte Growth Factor (HGF) and its Receptor (c-met)

The regulation of the HGF/c-met system in HCCs is complex and is characterized by a coordinately enhanced expression of c-met and a downregulation of HGF (Luo et al., 1999; Tavian et al., 2000). As such, HGF is a potent mitogen for normal hepatocytes, but it inhibits HCC cell growth in vitro. In HCC growth responses, HGF may however have a regulatory role because IGF-I, upregulated in HCCs, is a comitogen for HGF (Price et al., 2002). Furthermore, studies on carcinogen-treated transgenic mice have elucidated that HGF can, via c-met autocrine activation, promote hepatocarcinogenesis, possibley also through its enhancement of angiogenic responses (Horiguchi et al., 2002). The hepatocyte growth factor activator inhibitor 2/placental bikunin (HAI-2/PB) gene is, in contrast to normal liver, frequently hypermethylated in HCC cells, therefore HAI-2/PB expression being inappropriately repressed by promoter hypermethylation in HCC (Fukai et al., 2003).

### Mechanisms Affecting the Local Availability of Growth Factors

The local bioavailability of growth factors involved in paracrine/autocrine loops is modulated by several factors. Heparan sulphate proteoglycans (HSPGs; synde-cans, glypican, perlecan and others) that are involved in cell-matrix adhesion processes and in the regulation of growth factor actions (e.g. as a co-receptor for hepatocyte growth factor) are consistently expressed in HCCs (mainly syndecan-1 and syndecan-4) in a membranous staining pattern, whereas a strong reactivity for syndecan-3 and perlecan was detected in the tumor stroma, suggesting a role of these factors in differential tumor cell adhesion, angiogenesis, and generation of a growth factor reservoir (Roskams et al., 1998). A further potent molecular system to affect the bioavailability of growth factors and factors involved in spread is the urokinase-type plasminogen activator (uPA), uPA receptor (uPAR), and plasminogen activator inhibitor type-1 (PAI-1) system (Zheng et al., 2000).

The handling and bioavailability of factors involved in the growth response of HCCs is influenced by chaperoning activities. HCCs have been shown to overexpress chaperonins such as Hsp110 and Apg-2, but not Apg-1 (Gotoh et al., 2004). The bioavailability of regulatory proteins in HCCs is furthermore modulated by the regulation of the ubiquitin-mediated proteosomal pathway. E.G., in HCCs associated with HCV infection, a transcript similar to ubiquitin-conjugating enzyme is overexpressed (El-Nady et al., 2003). Glucose-regulated protein (grp) 78 is a transformation-associated gene product in HCC, and is a molecular chaperone involved in the unfolded protein response; its expression can be regulated by the transcription factors, ATF6 and XBP1. It was observed that activation of these two transcription factors, together with grp78, occurs in human HCCs (Shuda et al., 2003), rendering the endoplasmic reticulum stress pathway mediated by ATF6 and XBP1 esssential for the transformation-associated expression of a critical chaperone.

## The Growth Response of HCCs is Modulated by Altered Patterns of Apoptosis.

The growth response of HCC is markedly modified by apoptosis, and a deregulation of programmed cell death is thought to play a major role in growth and progression of these tumors (Xiao et al., 2002; Osada et al., 2004; review: Kountouras et al., 2003). Numerous factors are operational in apoptosis, and several of them have been studied in HCCs, including the Fas/FasL system, TNF-related apoptosis-inducing ligand (TRAIL), low

FADD/high TRADD (Sun et al., 2000), and diverse caspases (Shin et al., 2002; Okano et al., 2003; Chen et al., 2003; Yano et al., 2003; Hsieh et al., 2003). The apoptotic response varies between tumors of distinct etiologies, e.g. between HBV-and HCV-related HCCs (Yano et al., 2003). Pathogenic mechanisms involved in such differential reactions include, e.g., an HBV-induced enhancement of TRAIL cytotoxicity by increasing TRAIL-R1/death receptor 4 expression (Janssen et al., 2003), and the induction of the Fas/FasL system by HBx causing reversing apoptosis in HCC (Wang et al., 2003). An apoptotic response in HCCs is also promoted by Notch1 signaling, which however also affects cell division cycle regulation in these cells (Qi et al., 2003). Resistance to apoptosis of HCC cells is promoted by down-regulation of hSulf1 sulfatase via enhancing heparin-binding growth factor signaling (Lai et al., 2004). Induced apoptosis is regulated by the activity of a tumor suppressor involved in HCC, i.e. p16INK4A, associated with downregulation of the proapoptotic Bax protein (Al-Mohanna et al., 2004).The anti-apoptosis protein, survivin, is translocated from cytoplasm into the nucleus of HCC cells, and nuclear localization is correlated with tumor cell dedifferentiation, is inversely associated with apoptosis, strongly associated with Fas expression (Moon and Tarnawski, 2003), and correlated with poor prognosis of HCC (Ikeguchi et al., 2002).

# Factors Operational in Progression and Spread of HCC

In the past years, mechanisms involved in the invasion and spread of human HCCs have been elucidated to a considerable detail (review: Zhou, 2002). Overall, factors positively related to invasiness comprise p16 and p53 mutations, H-ras, C-cerbB2, mdm2, TGF-beta, EGFR, MMP-2, uPA, uPAR, PAI-1, ICAM-1, VEGF, PDECGF, and basic FGF. Conversely, factors negatively related to spread are nm23-H1, KAI1, TIMP-2, integrin-5, and E-cadherin. In what follows, some of the factors affecting the invasion and metastasis of HCC are discussed.

## Growth and Spread of HCCs Depend on Angiogenesis.

As for other tumors, growth, invasion and spread of HCC and its precursors critically depend on angiogenesis (Sugimachi et al., 2002; Tanaka et al., 2003; Zhao et al., 2003). In tumor-bearing livers, VEGF is expressed in HCC cells, surrounding hepatocytes, and vascular endothelial cells, but several times more endothelial cells were positive for VEGF in the tumor areas than in in non-carcinoma areas, suggesting that this factor plays an important role for HCC growth (Shimoda et al., 1999; An et al., 2000). The angiogenic reaction to VEGF in these tumors requires VEGF receptor expression (Dhar et al., 2002; Tanaka et al., 2002). Overexpression of VEGF and angiopoietin-2 determine a highly vascular phenotype (Moon et al., 2003), and VEGF mRNA expression was positively correlated with tumor microvessel density (Yasuda et al., 2004). VEGF is also expressed in hepatic stellate cells in adjacent liver tissue (Torimura et al., 1998). The neovascularization response in HCCs is also regulated by other angiogenic factors, including ephrin-B1 (Sawai et al., 2003) and basic fibroblast growth factor (El-Assal et al., 2001).

The vascularization response in and around HCCs is modulated by a complex interplay between pro-and anti-angiogenic factors. Human macrophage metalloelastase (HME), a matrix metalloproteinase responsible for the generation of the potent angiogenesis inhibitor, angiostatin, is expressed in part of HCCs, and such tumors exhibit a hypovascular phenotype, whereas HME-negative tumors were hypervascular (Gorrin-Rivas et al., 2000). In a transgenic mouse model, abnormal angiogenesis in HCC was associated with platelet activation by tissue factor (TF) produced by endothelial cells and invading macrophages (Dupuy et al., 2003), illustrating the complexity of the cellular network involved. The angiogenic response in HCCs is furthermore affected by hypoxia (Kim et al., 2002) and may be modulated by the tumors' expression of angiotensin-I converting enzyme (CD143; Rocken et al., 2004). A distortion of the autocrine TGF-beta signaling pathway involving Smad3 and Smad4 enhances not only cell growth, but also the production of VEGF and PAI-1 (Sugano et al., 2003).

How does angiogenesis affect the biology of HCCs? An increased expression of VEGF (in particular the isoforms 121 and 165) in HCCs is associated with tumor dedifferentiation and a hypervascularity, suggesting a more aggressive phenotype (Torimura et al., 1998). VEGF, basic fibroblast growth factor, and angiogenin have been demonstrated to have prognostic significance in resectable HCCs (Chao et al., 2003). The survival time for patients in the high angiopoietin-2/1 mRNA ratio group was significantly poorer when compared with the low Ang-2/1 nRNA ratio group (Mitsuhashi et al., 2003). A reversal of the Angiopoietin-1 and – 2 expression is one of the key mechanisms for the dedifferentiation processs in HCCs (Sugimachi et al., 2003).

## Distinct Features of the Extracellular Matrix (ECM) Play a Significant Role in the Invasion Cascade of HCCs.

Progression and spread of HCCs is markedly affected by the turnover of the extracellular matrix (ECM) and factors influencing ECM composition. Specifically, increased ECM remodeling is associated with the differential expression of ECM proteins, the function of ECM receptors (integrins; Gianelli et al., 2002; Zhang et al., 2003), and matrix metalloproteinases (MMPs) in HCCs, forming a complex interaction network (Murakami et al., 1999; Theret et al., 2001; Kim et al., 2001; Torbenson et al., 2002; Hah and Lee, 2003; Schoedel et al., 2003; Ishii et al., 2003). Several factors are known to affect the invasion cascade in HCCs, including HGF and its receptor c-met, and the transcription factor Ets-1 (Jiang et al., 2001). Hepatic myofibroblasts, which contribute to stroma formation, can secrete HGF (Neaud et al., 1997), and HGF-induced HCC invasion involves MMP3 (Monvoisin et al., 2002). The induction mechanisms of MMP expression depends on Ets-1, that has been shown to induce matrilysin in HCC (Ozaki et al., 2000), to modulate multiple matrix metalloproteinase genes induced by HGF in human HCC (Ozaki et al., 2003), and to affect the angiogenic property of HGF (Tomita et al., 2003). Further transcription factors shown to upregulate constitutive MMP expression are c-Jun known to play a role in hepatic carcinogenesis (Sugioka et al. , 2004), and the E cadherin gene repressors, Snail and SIP1/Smad interacting protein 1 induced during hepatocarcinogenesis (Miyoshi et al., 2004). Important for HBV-associated HCCs is the obser-vation that HBx protein has been found to promote invasion by inducing MMP-1 in a COx-2-dependent manner (Lara-Pezzi et al., 2002).

## Telomeres and Telomerase in Progression of HCC

In addition to established HCC, telomere shortening and telomerase reactivation is found in HCC precursor lesions, i.e. dysplastic nodules (Oh et al., 2003).

Reactivation of telomerase significantly predicted the recurrence of HCC after hepatectomy, but did not correlate with p53 overexpression (Kobayashi et al., 2002). The human telomerase reverse transcriptase gene (hTERT) is a major determinant of the enzymatic activity of telomerase, and the hTERT promoter contains several c-Myc binding sites which mediate hTERT transcriptional activation. However, a recent study showed that c-Myc does not play a role in gene regulationof the catalytic subunit of hTERT in human HCC (Chen et al., 2004). There is a distinct pattern of telomere length maintenance/length variation between chromosomes with respect to the association of cancer progression and telomere length regulation, the dispersion being significantly larger in HCCs than in control liver tissue. In addition, Telomeric repeat binding factor-1 was upregulated in HCCs with elongated longer terminal restriction fragments (TRF-L), whereas expression of of human telomerase reverse transcriptase was greater in HCCs with shorter TRF-S, suggesting that telomere length variation may be a crucial code in telomere maintenance through hepatocarcinogenesis (Yokota et al., 2003).

An aggressive behavior of HCC has been shown to be associated with the overexpression of DNA topoisomerase II in the tumors (Watanuki et al., 2002).

## Metastasis Genes in HCC

Metastasis of HCC is, similar to other malignant tumors, a multistep process involving the (altered) functions of numerous genes (reviews: Nicolson and Moustafa, 1998; Cheung et al., 2002).

Early steps of the invasion/metastasis cascade in HCCs involve the loosening of cellular junctions, a deranged intercellular adhesion, the activity of metalloproteinases (MMPs) to degrade components of the ECM, and mechanisms to enter and penetrate blood and lymph vessels. Subsequently, cancer cells are transported in blood or lymph, where they interact with components of the coagulation system, with thrombocytes, and leukoyctes. Finally, dislocated cancer cells home to remote endothelial surfaces, transmigrate through the distant vessel walls, and start to grow at the new site, provided they are still viable and capable to proliferate. An early effect on adhesion is the loss of a critical adhesion molecule, E-cadherin, and the repression of transcription of the E-cadherin gene is mediated by two transcription factors, Snail and SIP1 (Smad interacting protein 1), binding the E-box on the the E-cadherin promoter. Snail and SIP1 also affect invasion by upregulating MMPs Miyoshi et al., 2004).

There are few genes that have been shown to modulate metastasis, and their altered expression in HCCs therefore changes metastatic spread. The metastasis-associated gene, Nm23-H1, that encodes a nucleoside diphosphate kinase, is expressed in cancer cells with a low metastatic potential. In HCCs, the abundance of nm23 expression has been reported to be a major predictor of intrahepatic metastasis (Iizuka et al., 1995), although not confirmed in some other studies (Shimada et al., 1998). Its expression is regulated by p53 (Chen et al., 2003).

KAI1 is a novel metastasis suppressor gene, and its transcription level has been reported to be related with metastasis in diverse kinds of tumors. In HCCs, the expression rate of KAI1 is higher in tumors without a metastatic phenotype (Guo et al., 1998; Sun et al., 1998). Similar to other cancers, the metastasis-associated gene, MTA1, has been shown to exhibit differential expression patterns in HCC, high MTA1 expression HCCs preferentially being high-grade and causing lower disease-free survival rates (Hamatsu et al., 2003). TIP30 (CC3; Htatip2) is a putative metastasis suppressor promoting apoptosis and inhibiting angiogenesis. Human TIP30 is a cofactor that specifically enhances HIV-1 Tat-activated transcription, is a novel serine/threonine kinase, phosphorylating the heptapeptide repeats of the C-terminal domain of the largest RNA polymerase II subunit in a Tat-dependent manner, and induces expression of a number of genes that include the apoptosis-related genes Bad and Siva, as well as the metastasis suppressor NM23-H2 (Xiao et al., 2000). About a third of human HCCs show decreased expression of TIP30, in part associated with missense mutations, and TIP30-deficient mice exhibit a high incidence of HCC and other tumors (Ito et al., 2003).

## Fibrolamellar Carcinoma

FL-HCC mostly develops as a solitary lesion not associated with other hepatic neoplasms. There are only few reported exceptions, e.g. FL-HCC occurring several years after liver cell adenoma (Terracciano et al., 2004), coexistence/synchronicity of FL-HCC and HCC (Okada et al., 1993; Seitz et al., 2002), mixed FL-HCC/HCC (Okano et al., 1998), and recurrence of FL-HCC in the form of HCC (Chang et al., 2003),

Four chromosomal alterations were more frequent in FL-HCC than in high-grade dysplastic nodules and HCC, i.e. 4q+, 9p-, 16p- and Xq-, whereas 8p-was hardly found in FL-HCC (Terraciano and Tornillo, 2003). In another study, amplification of 1q was detected in a primary FL-HCC, whereas recurrent and metastatic tumors revealed considerable genomic instability, with 18 aberrations covering eleven genes in recurrent FL-HCCs and up to ten aberrations covering seven genes. These cytogenetic changes in FL-HCCs were clearly different from those observed in HCC and were interpreted to reflect secondary events based on genetic instability (Wilkens et al., 2000).

What are the genetic and molecular differences between HCC and FL-HCC? In contrast to HCCs, FL-HCC appears to genomically homogeneous based on DNA fingerprinting , suggesting that the tumorigenic pathways and the degree of somatic genomic changes may be less complex than in HCC (Sirivatanausksorn et al., 2001).In contrast to HCC and to hepatoblastoma, mutations of the beta-catenin gene have not been detected in FL-HCC (Terris et al., 1999), and HGF receptor levels have been found to be normal in Fl-HCC, whereas MMP-2 was increased in this tumor (Schoedel et al., 2003).

## HEPATOBLASTOMA

Hepatoblastomas disclose a complex pattern of cytogenetic abnormalities; these anomalies have recently been reviewed (Perilongo et al., 2002). A major breakthrough in the elucidation of molecular pathways involved in hepatoblastoma was the recognition of the frequent involvement of an altered WNT/beta-catenin signaling pathway.

It has been shown that activating mutations of the beta-catenin gene occur in a large proprtion of hepatoblastomas, and more than 85% of these tumors exhibit accumulation of this protein as an indicator for an activated pathway (Koch et al., 1999; review: Buendia, 2002). More than half of HBL showed deletions of the beta-catenin gene, whereas point mutations of this gene prevail in HCC (Taniguchi et al., 2002). Activating mutations of the beta-catenin gene result , similar to the situation in HCCs, in nuclear accumulation of the protein, and it was shown that, in addition to neoplastic epithelia, aberrant beta-catenin expression is also detectable in heterologous components, including cells of osteoid and chondroid tissue in mixed hepatoblastomas (Wei et al., 2000). The frequent beta-catenin gene mutations were not correlated with the histologic subtype in one study (Udatsu et al., 2001), whereas other investigations uncovered an association of nuclear beta-catenin expression with a poorly differentiated phenotype (Takayasu et al., 2001), nuclear accumulation being typical for embryonal or poorly differentiated variants, and membranous expression for a fetal morphlogy. Nuclear beta-catenin expression has been correlated with shorter survival (Park et al., 2001).

Other proteins of the WNT signaling system are sometimes mutated in hepatoblastoma. One is axin, suggesting that this protein also has a tumorigenic function in a subset of hepatoblastomas (Taniguchi et al., 2002; Miao et al., 2003). AXIN1 and AXIN2 gene mutations were reported for HBL in 7.4% and 0%, respectively (Taniguchi et al., 2002). Hepatoblastomas are known to develop in families with adenomatous polyposis coli (FAP), and the familial adenomatous polyposis gene (APC) participates in the beta-catenin-containing signaling network (Thomas et al., 2003; Cetta et al., 2003). Nuclear accumulation of beta-catenin without beta-catenin and APC mutations can also occur and may be a possible mechanism for tumorigenesis of hepatoblastoma in FAP families (Inukai et al., 2004). Recently, a potent inhibitor of the WNT signaling pathway, human Dickkopf-1 (hDkk-1), was found to be overexpressed in hepatoblastomas, suggesting uncontrolled WNT signaling via a negative feedback mechanism (Wirths et al., 2003).

What is the evidence that the beta-catenin pathway affects the proliferative activity and the differentiation of the hepatocyte lineage?

Transgenic mice expressing an oncogenic form of beta-catenin in their hepatocytes exhibit rapidly developing hepatomegaly soon after birth, caused by hepatocyte hyperplasia with increased proliferation without compensatory apoptosis (Cadoret et al., 2001). It has been shown that the beta-catenin signaling pathway is one of the targets of the transduction pathwy controlled by the polycystins that are mutated in a differentiation disorder of early nephrons, autosomal dominant polycystic kidney disease (ADPKD). Transgenic mice overexpressing an activated mutant of beta-catenin in renal epithelial cells develop severe polycystic kidney lesions soon after birth, suggesting that beta-catenin signaling affects early renal cell differentiation and tissue construction (Saadi-Kheddouci et al., 2001).

Based on the complex cytogenetic features of hepatoblastoma, genes and gene products other than those of the WNT signaling pathway will have to be assessed in more detail. E.g., there is evidence that 8q amplification is associated with poor prognosis in hepatoblastoma, and one gene involved is PLAG1, an IHG2 regulator overexpressed in hepatoblastoma (Zatkova et al., 2004).

## REFERENCES

Adamek HE, Spiethoff A, Kaufmann V, Jakobs R, Riemann JF (1998). Primary clear cell carcinoma of noncirrhotic liver: immunohistochemical discrimination of hepatocellular and cholangiocellular origin. *Dig Dis Sci* 43, 33-38.

Akasofu M, Kawahara E, Kaji K, Nakanishi I (1999). Sarcomatoid hepatocellular-carcinoma showing rhabdomyoblastic differentiation in the adult cirrhotic liver. *Virchows Arch* 434, 511-515.

Albar JP, De Miguel F, Esbrit P, Miranda R, Fernandez-Flores A, Sarasa JL (1996). Immunohistochemical detection of parathyroid hormone-related protein in a rare variant of hepatic neoplasm (sclerosing hepatic carcinoma). *Hum Pathol* 27, 728-731.

Al-Mohanna MA, Manogaran PS, Al-Mukhalafi Z, Al-Hussein K, Aboussekhra A (2004). The tumor suppressor p16 (INK4a) gene is a regulator of apoptosis induced by ultraviolet light and cisplatin. *Oncogene* 23, 201-212.

An FQ, Matsuda M, Fuji H, Matsumoto Y (2000). Expression of vascular endothelial growth factor in surgical specimens of hepatocellular carcinoma. *J Cancer Res Clin Oncol* 126, 153-160.

An FQ, Matsuda M, Fujii H, Tang RF, Amemiya H, Dai YM, Matsumoto Y (2001). Tumor heterogeneity in small hepatocellular carcinoma: analysis of tumor cell proliferation, expression and mutation of p53 and β-catenin. *Int J Cancer* 93, 468-474.

Anthony PP (1973). Primary Carcinoma of the Liver: a Study of 282 Cases in Ugandan Africans. *J Pathol* 110, 37-48.

Anzola M, Cuevas N, Lopez-Martinez M, De Pancorbo MM, Burgos JJ 8 2004). p16INK4A Gene alterations are not a prognostic indicator for survival in patients with hepatocellular carcinoma undergoing curative hepatectomy. *J Gastroenterol Hepatol* 19, 397-405.

Aoki T, Miyamoto A, Marbashi S, Nagano H, Umeshita K, Fujiwara Y, Dono K, nakamori S, Sakon M, Monden M (2004). Clinical value of alterations in p73 gene, related to p53 at 1p36, in human hepatocellular carcinoma. *Int J Oncol* 24, 441-446.

Arakawa M, Kage M, Sugihara S, Nakashima T, Suenaga M, Okuda K (1986). Emergence of Malignant Lesions within an Adenomatous Hyperplastic Nodule in a Cirrhotic Liver: Observations in 5 Cases. *Gastroenterology* 91, 198-208.

Arase Y, Endo Y, Hara M, Kumada H, Ikeda K, Yoshiba A (1988). *Hepatic Y. Acta Pathol Jpn* 38, 643-650.

Arbuthnot P, Kew M (2001). Hepatitis B Y. *Int J Exp Pathol* 82, 77-100.

Arima T, Nakao K, Nakata K, Ishikawa H, Ichikawa T, Hamasaki K, Ishii N, Eguchi K (2002). Transcativation of human alpha-fetoprotein by X-gene product of hepatitis B virus in human hepatoma cells. *Int J Mol Med* 9, 397-400.

Azechi H, Nishida N, Fukuda Y, Nishimura T, Minata M, Katsuma H, Kuno M, Ito T, Komeda T, Kita R, Takahashi R, Nakao K (2001). Disruption of the p16/cyclin D1/retinoblastoma protein pathway in the majority of human hepatocellular carcinomas. *Oncology* 60, 346-354.

Baas AF, Kuipers J, Van Der Wel NN, Batlle E, Koerten HK, Peters PJ, Clevers HC (2004). Complete Polarization of Single Intestinal Epithelial Cells Upon Activation of LKB1 by STRAD. *Cell* 116, 457-466.

Ban KC, Singh H, Krishnan R, Seow HF (2003). GSK-3beta phosphorylation and alteration of beta-catenin in hepatocellular carcinoma. *Cancer Lett* 199, 201-208.

Blachar A, Federle MP, Ferris JV, Lacomis JM, Waltz JS, Armfield DR, Chu G., Almusa O, Grazioli L, Balzano E, Li W (2002). Radiologist's performance in the diagnosis of liver tumors with central scars by using specific CT criteria. *Radiology* 223, 532-539.

Block TM, Mehta AS, Fimmel CJ, Jordan R (2003). Molecular viral oncology of hepatocellular carcinoma. *Oncogene* 22, 5093-5107.

Briux J, Llovet JM (2003). Hepatitis B virus and hepatocellular carcinoma. *J Hepatol* 39 (suppl 1), S59-S63.

Buendia MA (2000). Genetics of hepatocellular carcinoma. *Semin Cancer Biol* 10, 185-200.

Buendia MA (2002). Genetic alterations in hepatoblastoma and hepatocellular carcinoma: common and distinctive aspects. *Med Pediatr Oncol* 39, 530-535.

Cadoret A, Ovejero C, Saadi-Kheddouci S, Souil E, Fabre M, Romagnolo B, Kahn A, Perret C (2001). Hepatomegaly in transgenic mice expressing an oncogenic form of beta-catenin. *Cancer Res* 61, 3245-3249.

Carling D (2004). The AMP-activated protein kinase cascade – a unifying system for energy control. *Trends Biochem Sci* 29, 18-24.

Cetta F, Mazzarella L, Bon G, Zuckermann M, Casorelli A, Nounga H (2003). genetic alterations in hepatoblastoma and hepatocellular carcinoma associated with familial adenomatous polyposis. *Med Pediatr Oncol* 41, 496-497.

Chan KL, Lee JM, Guan XY, Fan ST, Ng IO (2002). High-density allelotyping of chromosome 8p in hepatocellular carcinoma and clinicopathologic correlation. *Cancer* 94, 3179-3185.

Chang J, Kim NG, Piao Z, Park C, Park KS, Paik YK, Lee WJ, Kim BR, Kim H (2002). Assessment of chromosomal losses and gains in hepatocellular carcinoma. *Cancer Lett* 182, 193-202.

Chang YC, Dai YC, Chow NH (2003). Fibrolamellar hepatocellular carcinoma with recurrence of classic hepatocellular carcinoma: a case report and review of Oriental cases.

Chao Y, Li CP, Chau GY, Chen CP, King KL, Lui WY, Yen SH, Chang FY, Chan WK, Lee SD (2003). Prognostic significance of vascular endothelial growth factor, basic fibroblast gfrowth factor, and angiogenin in patients with resectable hepatocellular carcinoma after surgery. *Ann Surg Oncol* 10, 355-362.

Chau GY, Lui WY, Tsay SH, King KL, Loong CC, Chiu JH, Wu CW, P'eng FK (1997). Prognostic significance of surgical margin in hepatocellular carcinoma resection: an analysis of 165 Childs' A patients. *J Surg Oncol* 66, 122-126.

Chen PJ, Chen DS (1999). Hepatitis B virus infection and hepatocellular carcinoma: molecular genetics and clinical perspectives. *Semin Liver Dis* 19, 253-262.

Chen WN, Oon CJ, Leong AL, Koh S, Teng SW (2000). Expression of integrated hepatitis B virus X variants in human hepatocellular carcinomas and its significance. *Biochem Biophys Res Commun* 276, 885-892.

Chen MF, Tsai HP, Jeng LB, Lee WC, Yeh CN, Yu MC, Hung CM (2003). Prognostic factors after resection for hepatocellular carcinoma in noncirrhotic livers: univariate and multivariate analysis. *World J Surg* 27, 443-447.

Chen XP, He SQ, Wang HP, Zhao YZ, Zhang WG (2003). Expression of TNF-related apoptosis-inducing ligand receptors and antitumor tumor effects of TNF-related apoptosis-inducing ligand in human hepatocellular carcinoma. *World J Gastroenterol* 9, 2433-2440.

Chen SL, Wu YS, Shieh HY, Yen CC, Shen JJ, Lin KH (2003). P53 is a regulator of the metastasos suppressor gene Nm23-H1. *Mol Carcinog* 36, 204-214.

Chen CJ, Kyo S, Liu YC, Cheng YL, Hsieh CB, Chan DC, Yu JC, harn HJ (2004). Moldulation of human telomerase reverse transcriptase in hepatocellular carcinoma. *World J Gastroenterol* 10, 638-642.

Cheuk W, Chan JK (2001). Clear cell variant of fibrolamellar carcinoma of the liver. *Arch Pathol Lab Med* 125, 1235-1238.

Cheung ST, Chen X, Guan XY, Wong SY, Tai LS, Ng IO, So S, Fan ST (2002). Identify metastasis-associated genes in hepatocellular carcinoma through clonality delineation for multinodular tumor. *Cancer Res* 62, 4711-4721.

Cho JW, Jeong YW, Han SW, Park JB, Jang BC, Baek WK, Kwon TK, Park JW, Kim SP, Suh MH, Suh SI (2003). Aberrant p16INK4A RNA transcripts expressed in hepatocellular carcinoma cell lines eegulate pRb phosphorylation by binding with CDK4, resulting in delayed cell cycle progression. *Liver* 23, 194-200.

Choi YL, Park SH, Jang JJ, Park CK (2001). Expression of the G1-S modulators in hepatitis B virus-related hepatocellular carcinoma and dysplastic nodule: association of cyclin D1 and p53 proteins with the progression of hepatocellular carcinoma. *J Korean Med Sci* 16, 424-432.

Chung MY, Wu JC, Chau GY, Lui WY, Tsay SH, Chiang H (2000). Preferentially deleted chromosome region 9p21 in large hepatocellular carcinomas. *Int J Mol Med* 5, 521-524.

Chung TW, Lee YC, Ko JH, Kim CH (2003). Hepatitis B virus X protein modulates the expression of PTEN by inhibiting the function of p53, a transcriptional activator in liver cells. *Cancer Res* 63, 3453-3458.

Coleman WB (2003). Mechanisms of human hepatocarcinogenesis. *Curr Mol Med* 3, 573-588.

Craig JR, Peters RL, Edmondson HA, Omata M (1980). Fibrolamellar carcinoma of the liver: A tumor of adolescents and young adults with distinctive clinico-pathologic features. *Cancer* 46, 372-379.

Cui J, Zhou XD, Liu YK, Tang ZY, Zile MH (2001). Abnormal beta-catenin gene expression with invasiveness of primary hepatocellular carcinoma in China. *World J Gastroenterol* 7, 542-546.

Cui J, Zhou X, Liu Y, Tang Z, Romeih M (2003). Alterations of beta-catenin and Tcf-4 instead of GSK-3beta contribute to activation of Wnt pathway in hepatocellular carcinoma. *Chin med J* 116, 1885-1892.

Debuire B, Paterlini P, Pontisso P, Basso G, May E (1993). Analysis of the p53 gene in European hepatocellular carcinomas and hepatoblastomas. *Oncogene* 8, 2303-2306.

Devereux TR, Anna CH, Foley JF, White CM, Sills RC, Barrett JC (1999). Mutation of beta-catenin is an early event in chemically induced mouse hepatocellular carcinogenesis. *Oncogene* 18, 4726-4733.

Devereux TR, Stern MC, Flake GP, Yu MC, Zhang ZQ, London SJ, Taylor JA (2001). CTNNB1 mutations and beta-catenin protein accumulation in human hepatocellular carcinomas associated with high exposure to aflatoxin B1. *Mol Carcinog* 31, 68-73.

Dhar DK, Naora H, Yamanoi A, Ono T, Kohno H, Otani H, Nagasue N (2002). Requisite role of VEGF receptors in angiogenesis of hepatocellular carcinoma: a comparison with angiopoietin/Tie pathway. *Anticancer Res* 22, 379-386.

Dunbar ME, Wysolmerski JJ, Broadus AE (1996). Parathyroid hormone-related protein: from hypercalcemia of malignancy to developmental regulatory molecule. *Am J Med Sci* 312, 287-294.

Dupuy E, Hainaud P, Villemain A, Bodevin-Phedre E, Brouland JP, Briand P, Tobelem G (2003). Tumoral angiogenesis and tissue factor expression during hepatocellular carcinoma progression in a transgenic mouse model. *J Hepatol* 38, 793-802.

Edmondson HA (1956). Differential diagnosis of tumors and tumor-like lesions of liver in infancy and childhood. *Arch Dis Child* 1, 168-186.

El-Nady GM, Ling R, Harrison TJ (2003). Gene expression in HCV-associated hepatocellular carcinoma – upregulation of a gene encoding a protein related to the ubiquitin-conjugating enzyme. *Liver Int* 23, 329-337.

El-Serag HB, Davila JA (2004). Is fibrolamellar carcinoma different from hepatocellular carcinoma? A US population-based study. *Hepatology* 39, 798-803.

Emile JF, Adam R, Sebagh M, Marchadier E, Falissard B, Dussaix E, Bismuth H, Reynes M (2000). Hepatocellular carcinoma with lymphoid stroma: a tumour with good prognosis after liver transplantation. *Histopathology* 37, 523-529.

Emile JF, Lemoine A, Azoulay D, Debuire B, Bismuth H, Reynes M (2001). Histological, genomic and clinical heterogeneity of clear cell hepatocellular carcinoma. *Histopathology* 38, 225-231.

Eriguchi N, Aoyagi S, Hara M, Okuda K, Fukuda S, Tamae T, Kanazawa N (2001). Malignant sarcomatoid tumor of the liver: report of a case. *Surg Today* 31, 170-173.

Feitelson MA, Sun B, Satiroglu Tufan NL, Liu J, Pan J, Lian Z (2002). Genetic mechanisms of hepatocarcinogenesis. *Oncogene* 21, 2593-2604.

Fujimoto Y, Hampton LL, Wirth PJ, Wang NJ, Xie JP, Thorgeirsson SS (1994). Alterations of tumor suppressor genes and allelic losses in human hepatocellular carcinomas in China. *Cancer Res* 54, 281-285.

Fukai K, Yokosuka O, Chiba T, Hirasawa Y, Tada M, Imazeki F, Kataoka H, Saisho H (2003). Hepatocyte growth factor activator inhibitor 2/placental bikunin (HAI-2/PB) gene is frequently hypermethylated in human hepatocellular carcinoma. *Cancer Res* 63, 8674-8679.

Gianelli G, Fransvea E, Marinosci F, Bergamini C, Colucci S, Schiraldi O, Antonaci S (2002). Transforming growth factor-beta1 triggers hepatocellular carcinoma invasiveness via alpha3beta1 integrin. *Am J Pathol* 161, 183-193.

Gornicka B, Ziarkiewicz-Wroblewska B, Michalowicz B, Pawlak J, Wroblewski T, Kracyk M, Wasiutynski A, Kappeler A, Zimmermann A (2001). Immature hepatic tumor of bimodal differentiation in a young adult patient: a novel lesion expressing β-catenin and mimicking a distinct pahse of hepatogenesis. *J Hepatol* 34, 955-961.

Gorrin-Rivas MJ, Arii S, Mori A, Takeda Y, Mizumoto M, Furutani M, Imamura M (2000). Implications of human macrophage metalloelastase and vascular endothelial growth factor gene expression in angiogenesis of hepatocellular carcinoma. *Ann Surg* 231, 67-73.

Gotoh K, Nonoguchi K, Higashitsuji H, Kaneko Y, Sakurai T, Sumitomo Y, Itoh K, Subjeck JR, Fujita J (2004). Apg-2 has a chaperone-like activity similar to Hsp110 and is overexpressed in hepatocellular carcinomas. *FEBS Lett* 560, 19-24.

Grazi GL, Cescon M, Ravaioli M, Ercolani G, Gardini A, Del Gaudio M, Vetrone G, Cavallari A (2003). Liver resection for hepatocellular carcinoma in cirrhotics and noncirrhotics. Evaluation of clinicopathologic features and comparison of risk factors for long-term survival and tumour recurrence in a single center. *Aliment Pharmacol Ther* 17 (suppl 2), 119-129.

Guo XZ, Friess H, Di Mola FF, Heinicke JM, Abou-Shady M, Graber HU, Baer HU, Zimmermann A, Korc M, Buchler MW (1998). KAI1, a new metastasis suppressor gene, is reduced in metastatic hepatocellular carcinoma. *Hepatology* 28, 1481-1488.

Hah N, Lee ST (2003). An absolute role of the PKC-dependent NF-kappaB activation for induction of MMP-9 in hepatocellular carcinoma cells. *Biochem Biophys Res Commun* 305, 428-433.

Hamatsu T, Rikimaru T, Yamashita Y, Aishima S, Tanaka S, Shirabe K, Shimada M, Toh Y, Sugimachi K (2003). The role of MTA1 gene expression in human hepatocellular carcinoma. *Oncol Rep* 10, 599-604.

Hanazaki K, Kajikawa S, Shimozawa N, Shimada K, Hiraguri M, Koide N, Adachi W, Amano J (2002). Hepatic resection for hepatocellular carcinoma in diameter of > or = 10 cm. *Hepatogastroenterology* 49, 518-523.

Harada N, Tamai Y, Ishikawa T, Sauer B, Takaku K, Oshima M, Taketo MM (1999). Intestinal polyposis in mice with a dominant stable mutation of the β-catenin gene. *EMBO J* 18, 5931-5942.

Harada N, Miyoshi H, Murai N, Oshima H, Tamai Y, Oshima M, Taketo MM (2002). Lack of tumorigenesis in the mouse liver after adenovirus-mediated expression of a dominant stable mutant of β–catenin. *Cancer Res* 62, 1971-1977.

Harada H, Nagai H, Ezura Y, Yokota T, Ohsawa I, Yamaguchi K, Ohue C, Tsuneizumi M, Mikami I, Terada Y, Yabe A, Emi M (2002). Down-regulation of a novel gene, DRLM, in human liver malignancy from 4q22 that encodes a NAP-like protein. *Gene* 296, 171-177.

Harada N, Oshima H, Katoh M, Tamai Y, Oshima M, Taketo MM (2004). Hepatocarcinogenesis in mice with beta-catenin and Ha-ras gene mutations. *Cancer Res* 64, 48-54.

Haratake J, Horie A (1991). An immunohistochemical study of sarcomatoid liver carcinomas. *Cancer* 68, 93-97.

Harrison SA, Diehl AM (2002). Fat and the liver – a molecular overview. *Semin Gastrointest Dis* 13, 3-16.

Hayashi H, Sugio K, Matsumata T, Adachi E, Takenaka K, Sugimachi K (1995). The clinical significance of p53 gene mutation in hepatocellular carcinomas from Japan. *Hepatology* 22, 1702-1707.

Henkler FF, Koshy R (1996). Hepatitis B virus transcriptional activators: mechanisms and possible role in oncogenesis. *J Viral Hepat* 3, 109-121.

Horiguchi N, Takayama H, Toyoda M, Otsuka T, Fukusato T, Merlino G, Takagi H, Mori M (2002). Hepatocyte growth factor promotes hepatocarcinogenesis through c-Met autocrine activation and enhanced angiogenesis in transgenic mice treated with diethylnitrosamine. *Oncogene* 21, 1791-1799.

Hoshino H, Katada N, Nishimura D, Imada J, Morita K, Yoshida N, Sano H, Okamoto K, Kato K (1996). Case report: fibrolamellar hepatocellular carcinoma in a Japanese woman: a case report and review of Japanese cases. *J Gastroenterol Hepatol* 11, 551-555.

Hsia CC, Di Bisceglie AM, Kleiner DE, Farshid M, Tabor E (1994). RB tumor suppressor gene expression in hepatocellular carcinomas from patients infected with the hepatitis B virus. *J Med Virol* 44, 67-73.

Hsieh SY, Liaw SF, Lee SN, Hsieh PS, Lin KH, Chu CM, Liaw YF (2003). Aberrant caspase-activated DNase (CAD) transcripts in human hepatoma cells. *Br J Cancer* 88, 210-216.

Hsu HC, Jeng YM, Mao TL, Chu JS, Lai PL, Peng SY (2000). Beta-catenin mutations are associated with a subset of low-stage hepatocellular carcinoma negative for hepatitis B virus and with favorable prognosis. *Am J Pathol* 157, 763-770.

Hu RH, Lee PH, Yu SC, Dai HC, Sheu JC, Lai MY, Hsu HC, Chen DS (1996). Surgical resection for recurrent hepatocellular carcinoma: prognosis and analysis of risk factors. *Surgery* 120, 23-29.

Hu RH, Lee PH, Chang YC, Yu SC, Ho MC, Wu YM (2003). Prognostic factors for hepatocellular carcinoma < or = 3 cm in diameter. *Hepatogastroenterology* 50, 2043-2048.

Huang H, Fujii H, Sankila A, Mahler-Araujo BM, Matsuda M, Cathomas G, Ohgaki H (1999). Beta-catenin mutations are frequent in human hepatocellular carcinomas associated with hepatitis C virus infection. *Am J Pathol* 155, 1795-1801.

Huang JZ, Xia SS, Ye QF, Jiang HY, Chen ZH (2003). Effects of p16 gene on biological behaviours in hepatocellular carcinoma cells. *World J Gastroenterol* 9, 84-88.

Huber O, Korn R, McLaughlin J, Ohsugi M, Herrmann BG, Kemler R (1996). Nuclear localization of β-catenin by interaction with transcription factor LEF-1. *Mech Dev* 59, 3-10.

Hui AM, Li X, Makuuchi M, Takayama T, Kubota K (1999). Over-expression and lack of retinoblastoma protein are associated with tumor progression and metastasis in hepatocellular carcinoma. Int J *Cancer* 84, 604-608.

Hui JM, Kench J, Farrell GC, Lin R, Samarasinghe D, Liddle C, Byth K, George J (2002). Genotype-specific mechanisms for hepatic steatosis in chronic hepatitis C infection. *J Gastroenterol Hepatol* 17, 873-881.

Huo TI, Wang XW, Forgues M, Wu CG, Spillare EA, Giannini C, Brechot C, Harris CC (2001). Hepatitis B virus X mutants derived from human hepatocellular carcinoma retain the ability to abrogate p53-induced apoptosis. *Oncogene* 20, 3620-3628.

Huynh H, Chow PK, Ooi LL, Soo KC (2002). A possible role for insulin-like growth factor-binding protein-3 autocrine/paracrine loops in controlling hepatocellular carcinoma cell proliferation. *Cell Growth Differ* 13, 115-122.

Idilman R, De Maria N, Colantoni A, Van Thiel DH (1998). Pathogenesis of hepatitis B abd C-induced hepatocellular carcinoma. *J Viral Hepat* 5, 285-299.

Iizuka N, Oka M, Noma T, Nakazawa A, Hirose K, Suzuki T (1995). NM23-H1 and NM23-H2 messenger RNA abundance in human hepatocellular carcinoma. *Cancer Res* 55, 652-657.

Ikebe T, Wakasa K, Sasaki M, Hamba H, Kaneko M, Yamamoto T, Mikami S, Shuto T, Hirohashi K, Kinoshita H, Sakurai M (1998). Hepatocellular carcinoma with chondrosarcomatous variation: case report with immunohistochemical findings, and review of the literature. *J Hepatobiliary Pancreat Surg* 5, 217-220.

Ikeda T, Tozuka S, Hasumura Y, Takeuchi J (1988). Prostaglandin-E-producing hepatocellular carcinoma with hypercalcemia. *Cancer* 61, 1813-1814.

Ikeguchi M, Ueda T, Sakatani T, Hirooka Y, Kaibara N (2002). Expression of survivin messenger RNA correlates with poor prognosis in patients with hepatocellular carcinoma. *Diagn Mol Pathol* 11, 33-40.

Inukai T, Furuuchi K, Sugita K, Uno K, Ooi A, Sasaki F, Hamada J, Moriuchi T, Nakazawa S (2004). Nuclear accumulation of beta-catenin without an additional somatic mutation in coding region of the APC gene in hepatoblastoma from a familial adnomatous polyposis patient. *Oncol Rep* 11, 121-126.

Ishak KG, Anthony PP, Sobin LH (1994). Histological typing of tumours of the liver. Berlin, Heidelberg, Springer Verlag.

Ishida S, Noda M, Kuzuya N, Kubo F, Yamada S, Yamanaka T, Isozaki O, Hizuka N, Kanazawa Y (1995). Big insulin-like growth factor II-producing hepatocellular carcinoma associated with hypoglycemia. *Intern Med* 34, 1201-1206.

Ishii Y, Nakasato Y, Kobayashi S, Yamazaki Y, Aoki T (2003). A study on angiogenesis-related matrix metalloproteinase networks in primary hepatocellular carcinoma. *J exp Clin Cancer Res* 22, 461-470.

Ishizaki M, Ashida K, Higashi T, Nakatsukasa H, Kaneyoshi T, Fujiwara K, Nouso K, Kobayashi Y, Uemura M, Nakamura S, Tsuji T (2001). The formation of capsule and septum in human hepatocellular carcinoma. *Virchows Arch* 438, 574-580.

Itai Y, Ohtomo K, Kokubo T, Makita K, Okada Y, Machida T, Yashiro N (1987). CT and MR imaging of fatty tumors of the liver. *J Comput Assist Tomogr* 11, 253-257.

Ito M, Jiang C, Krumm K, Zhang X, Pecha J, Zhao J, Guo Y, Roeder RG, Xiao H (2003). TIP30 deficiency increases susceptibility to tumorigenesis. *Cancer Res* 63, 8763-8767.

Janssen HL, Higuchi H, Abdulkarim A, Gores GJ (2003). Hepatitis B virus enhances tumor necrosis factor-related apoptosis-inducing ligand (TRAIL) cytotoxicity by increasing TRAIL-R1/death receptor 4 expression. *J Hepatol* 39, 414-420.

Jiang Y, Xu W, Lu J, He F, Yang X (2001). Invasiveness of hepatocellular carcinoma cell lines: contribution of hepatocyte growth factor, c-met, and transcription factor Ets-1. *Biochem Biophys Res Commun* 286, 1123-1130.

Jwo SC, Chiu JH, Chau GY, Loong CC, Lui WY (1992). Risk factors linked to tumor recurrence of human hepatocellular carcinoma after hepatic resection. *Hepatology* 16, 1367-1371.

Kahng YS, Lee YS, Kim BK, Park WS, Lee JY, Kang CS (2003). Loss of heterozygosity of chromosome 8p and 11p in the dysplastic nodule and hepatocellular carcinoma. *J Gastroenterol Hepatol* 18, 430-436.

Kang YK, Kim CJ, Kim WH, Kim HO, Kang GH, Kim YI (1998). p53 mutation and overexpression in hepatocellular carcinoma and dysplastic nodules in the liver. *Virchows Arch* 432, 27-32.

Kashala LO, Conne B, Kalengayi MMR, Kapanci Y, Frei PC, Lambert PH (1990). Histopathologic features of hepatocellular carcinoma in Zaire. *Cancer* 65, 130-134.

Katzenstein HM, Krailo MD, Malogolowkin MH, Ortega JA, Qu W, Douglass EC, Feusner JH, Reynolds M, Quinn JJ, Newman K, Finegold MJ et al. (2003). Fibrolamellar hepatocellular carcinoma in children and adolescents. *Cancer* 97, 2006-2012.

Kazachkov Y, Khaoustov V, Yoffe B, Solomon H, Klintmalm GB, Tabor E (1996). p53 abnormalities in hepatocellular carcinoma from United States patients: analysis of all 11 exons. *Carcinogenesis* 17, 2207-2212.

Kenmochi K, Sugihara S, Kojiro M (1987). Relationship of histologic grade of hepatocellular carcinoma (HCC) to tumor size, and demonstration of tumor cells of multiple different grades in single small *HCC. Liver* 7, 18-26.

Kern MA, Breuhan K, Schirmacher P (2002). Molecular pathogenesis of human hepatocellular carcinoma. *Adv Cancer Res* 86, 67-112.

Kim SR, Kang KB, Soh CG, Kim JH, Hayashi Y, Hanioka K, Itoh H (1995). Clinicopathological study of minimum-sized hepatocellular carcinoma: an approach to the definition of early hepatocellular carcinoma. *J Gastroenterol Hepatol* 10, 498-508.

Kim JH, Kim TH, Jang JW, Jang YJ, Lee KH, Lee ST 8 2001). Analysis of matrix metalloproteinase mRNAs expressed in hepatocellular carcinoma cell lines. *Mol cells* 12, 32-40.

Kim KR, Moon HE, Kim KW (2002). hypoxia-induced angiogenesis in human hepatocellular carcinoma. *J Mol Med* 80, 703-714.

Kim CJ, Cho YG, Park JY, Kim TY, Lee JH, Kim HS, Lee JW, Song YH, Nam SW, Lee SH, Yoo NJ, Lee JY, Park WS (2004). Genetic analysis of the LKB1/STK11 gene in hepatocellular carcinomas. *Eur J Cancer* 40, 136-141.

Kishi K, Shikata T, Hirohashi S, Hasegawa H, Yamazaki S, Makuuchi M (1983). Hepatocellular carcinoma. A clinical and pathologic analysis of 57 hepatectomy cases. *Cancer* 51, 542-548.

Kitazawa R, Kitazawa S, Yoon S, Kasuga M, Maeda S (1999). In situ demonstration of parathyroid hormone-related protein mRNA in sclerosing hepatic carcinoma. *Virchows Arch* 435, 137-142.

Kobayashi T, Sugawara Y, Shi YZ, Makuuchi M (2002). Telomerase expression and p53 status in hepatocellular carcinoma. *Am J Gastroenterol* 97, 3166-3171.

Koch A, Denkhaus D, Albrecht S, Leuschner I, von Schweinitz D, Pietsch T (1999). Childhood hepatoblastomas frequently carry mutated degradation targeting box of the beta-catenin gene. *Cancer Res* 59, 269-273.

Koda M, Maeda Y, Matsunaga Y, Mimura K, Murawaki Y, Horie Y (2003). Hepatocellular carcinoma with sarcomatous change arising after radiofrequency ablation for well-differentiated hepatocellular carcinoma. *Hepatol Res* 27, 163-167.

Kojiro M (1998). Pathology of early hepatocellular carcinoma: progression from early to advanced. *Hepatogestroenterology* 45 (suppl 3), 1203-1205.

Komada N, Yamagata M, Komura K, Hayashi K, Maruyama T, Kataoka H, Koono M, Tsubouchi H (1997). Hepatocellular carcinoma with sarcomatous change arising in primary biliary cirrhosis. J *gastroenterol* 32, 95-101.

Kondo Y, Niwa Y, Akikusa B, Takazawa H, Okabayashi A (1983). A histopathologic study of early hepatocellular carcinoma. *Cancer* 52, 687-692.

Kondo Y, Kanai Y, Sakamoto M, Genda T, Mizokami M, Ueda R, Hirohashi S (1999). Beta-catenin accumulation and mutation of exon 3 of the beta-catenin gene in hepatocellular carcinoma. *Jpn J Cancer Res* 90, 1301-1309.

Kondoh N, Wakatsuki M, Hada A, Shuda M, Tanaka K, Arai M et al. (2001). Genetic and epigenetic events in human heaptocarcinogenesis. *Int J Oncol* 18, 1271-1278.

Koshikawa K, Nomoto S, Yamashita K, Ishigure K, Takeda S, Nakao A (2004). Allelic imbalance at 1p36 in the pathogenesis of human hepatocellular carcinoma. H*epatogastroenterology* 51, 186-191.

Kountouras J, Zavos C, Chatzopoulos D (2003). Apoptosis in hepatocellular carcinoma. *Hepatogastroenterology* 50, 242-249.

Koyama Y, Ishijima H, Ishibashi A, Katsuya T, Ishizaka H, Aoki J, Endo K (1999). Intact PTH-producing hepatocellular carcinoma treated by transcatheter arterial embolization. *Abdom Imaging* 24, 144-146.

Kuroki T, Fujiwara Y, Tsuchiya E, Nakamori S, Imaoka S, Kanematsu T, Nakamura Y (1995). Accumulation of genetic changes during development and progression of hepatocellular carcinoma: loss of heterozygosity of chromosome arm 1p occurs at an early stage of hepatocarcinogenesis. *Genes Chromosomes Cancer* 13, 163-167.

Kutami R, Nakashima Y, Nakashima O, Shiota K, Kojiro M (2000). Pathomorphologic study on the mechanism of fatty change in small hepatocellular carcinoma of humans. *J Hepatol* 33, 282-289.

Lai CL, Wu PC, Lam KC, Todd D (1979). Histologic prognostic indicators in hepatocellular carcinomas. *Cancer* 44, 1677-1683.

Lai JP, Chien JR, Moser DR, Staub JK, Aderca I, Montoya DP, Matthews TA, Nagorney DM, Cunningham JM et al. (2004). hSulf1 Sulfatase promotes apoptosis of hepatocellular cancer cells by decreasing heparin-binding growth factor signaling. *Gastroenterology* 126, 231-248.

Lara-Pezzi E, Gomez-Gaviro MV, Galvez BG, Mira E, Iniguez MA, Fresno M, Martinez AC, Arroyo AG, Lopez-Cabrera M (2002). The hepatitis B virus X protein promotes tumor cell invasion by inducing membrane-type matrix metalloproteinase-1 and cyclooxygenase-2 expression. *J Clin Invest* 110, 1831-1838.

Lee MO, Kang HJ, Cho H, Shin EC, Park JH, Kim SJ (2001). Hepatitis B virus X protein induced expression of the Nur77 gene. *Biochem Biophys Res Commun* 288, 1162-1168.

Lee CC, Wu CY, Chen JT, Chen GH (2002). Comparing combined hepatocellular-cholangiocarcinoma and cholangiocarcinoma: a clinicopathological study. *Hepatogastroenterology* 49, 1487-1490.

Lee TK, Man K, Ling MT, Wang XH, Wong YC, Lo CM, Poon RT, Ng IO, Fan ST (2003). Over-expression of Id-1 induces cell proliferation in hepatocellular carcinomna through inactivation of p16INK4a/RB pathway. carcinogenesis 24, 1729-1736.

Leone N, Debernardi-Venon W, Marzano A, Massari M, Rizzetto M (1999). Hypercalcemia secondary to hepatocellular carcinoma. *Ital J Gastroenterol Hepatol* 31, 604-606.

Leone N, Pellicano R, Brunello F, Rizzetto M, Ponzetto A (2002). Elevated serum chromogranin A in patients with hepatocellular carcinoma. *Clin Exp Med* 2, 119-123.

Levy L, Renard CA, Wie Y, Buendia MA (2002). Genetic alterations and oncogenic pathways in hepatocellular carcinoma. *Ann N Y Acad Sci* 963, 21-36.

Li SP, Wang HY, Li JQ, Zhang CQ, Feng QS, Huang P, Yu XJ, Huang LX, Liang QW, Zeng YX (2001). Genome-wide analysis on loss ofheterozygosity in hepatocellular carcinoma in Southern China. *J Hepatol* 34, 840-849.

Li AJ, Wu MC, Cong WM, Shen F, Yi B (2003). Spontaneous complete necrosis of hepatocellular carcinoma: a case report. *Hepatobiliary Pancreat Dis Int* 2, 152-154.

Libbrecht L, Desmet V, Roskams T (2003). Stages of normal and aberrant intrahepatic bile duct development in a mixed hepatoblastoma. *Histopathology* 42, 618-620.

Lizcano JM, Goransson O, Toth R, Deak M, Morrice NA, Boudeau J, Hawley SA, udd L, Makela TP, Hardie DG, Alessi DR (2004). LKB1 is a master kinse that activates 13 kinases of the AMPK subfamily, including MARK/PAR-1. *EMBO J* 23, 833-843.

Lonardo A, Adinolfi LE, Loria P, Carulli N, Ruggiero G, Day CP (2004). Steatosis and hepatitis C: mechanisms and significance for hepatic and extrahepatic disease. *Gastroenterology* 126, 586-597.

Lu S, Archer MC (2003). Insulin-like growth factor binding protein-1 over-expression in transgenic mice inhibits hepatic preneoplasia. *Mol Carcinog* 36, 142-146.

Luo YQ, Wu MC, Cong WM (1999). Gene expression of hepatocyte growth factor and its receptor in HCC and nontumorous liver tissues. *World J Gastroenterol* 5, 119-121.

Maeda T, Takenaka K, Taguchi K, Kajiyama K, Shirabe K, Shimada M, Tsuneyoshi M, Sugimachi K (2000). Clinicopathological characteristics of surgically resected minute hepatocellular carcinomas. *Hepatogastroenterology* 47, 498-503.

Mao TL, Chu JS, Jeng YM, Lai PL, Hsu HC (2001). Expression of mutant nuclear beta-catenin correlates with non-invasive hepatocellular carcinoma, absence of portal vein spread, and good prognosis. *J Pathol* 193, 95-101.

Markovic S, Ferlan-Marolt V, Hlebanja Z (1996). Spontaneous regression of hepatocellular carcinoma. *Am J Gastroenterol* 91, 392-393.

Martinez R, Sebastian JJ, Garcia S, Fuentes J, Navarro M, Alvarez R, Artigas JM, Herrero A (1997). Sclerosing hepatocarcinoma not associated with hypercalcemia (in Spanish). *Rev Esp Enferm Dig* 89, 718-720.

McDermott WV, Khettry U (1994). Clear cell carcinoma of the liver with spontaneous regression of metastases. *J Surg Oncol* 57, 206-209.

McLarney JK, Rucker PT, Bender GN, Goodman ZD, Kashitani N, Ros PR (1999). Fibrolamellar carcinoma of the liver: radiologic-pathologic correlation. *Radiographics* 19, 453-471.

Miao J, Kusafuka T, Udatsu Y, Okada A (2003). Sequence variants of the Axin gene in hepatoblastoma. *Hepatol Res* 25, 174-179.

Mitsuhashi N, Shimizu H, Ohtsuka M, Wakabayashi Y, ito H, Kimura F, Yoshidome H, Kato A, Nukui Y, Miyazaki M (2003). Angiopoietins and Tie-2 expression in angiogenesis and proliferation of human hepatocellular carcinoma. *Hepatology* 37, 1105-1113.

Miyoshi Y, Iwao K, Nagasawa Y, Aihara T, Sasaki Y, Imaoka S, Murata M, Shimano T, Nakamura Y (1998). Activation of the beta-catenin gene in primary hepatocellular carcinomas by somatic alterations involving exon 3. *Cancer Res* 58, 2524-2527.

Miyoshi A, Kitajima Y, Sumi K, Sato K, Hagiwara A, Koga Y, Miyazaki K (2004). Snail and SIP1 increase cancer invasion by upregulating MMP family in hepatocellular carcinoma cells. Br J Cancer 90, 1265-1273.

Momosaki S, hsia CC, nakashima Y, Kojiro M, Tabor E (2003). Integration of hepatitis B virus containing mutations in the core promoter/X gene in patients with hepatocellular carcinoma. *Dig Liver Dis* 35, 795-800.

Monvoisin A, Bisson C, Si-Tayeb K, Balabaud C, Desmouliere A, Rosenbaum J (2002). Involvement of matrix metalloproteinase type-3 in hepatocyte growth factor-induced invasion of human hepatocellular carcinoma. *Int J cancer* 97, 157-162.

Moon WS, Rhyu KH, Kang MJ, Lee DG, Yu HC, Yeum JH, Koh GY, Tarnawski AS (2003). Overexpression of VEGF and angiopoietin 2: a key to high vascularity of hepatocellular carcinoma? *Mod Pathol* 16, 552-557.

Moon WS, Tarnawski AS (2003). Nuclear translocation of survivin in hepatocellular carcinoma: a key to cancer cell growth? *Hum Pathol* 34, 1119-1126.

Moon EJ, jeong CH, jeong JW, Kim KR, Yu DY, Murakami S, Kim CW, Kim KW (2004). Hepatitis B virus X protein induces angiogenesis by stabilizing hypoxia-inducible factor-1alpha. *FASEB J* 18, 382-384.

Murakami Y, Hayashi K, Hirohashi S, Sekiya T (1991). Aberrations of the tumor suppressor p53 and retinoblastoma genes in human hepatocellular carcinomas. *Cancer Res* 51, 5520-5525.

Murikami K, Sakukawa R, Ikeda T, Matsuura T, Hasumura S, Nagamori S, Yamada Y, Saiki I (1999). Invasiveness of hepatocellular carcinoma cell lines: contribution of membaren-type 1 matrix metalloproteinase. *Neoplasia* 1, 424-430.

Murakami S (2001). Hepatitis B virus X protein: a multifunctional viral regulator. *J Gastroenterol* 36, 651-660.

Nagai H, Pineau P, Tiollais P, Buendia MA, Dejean A (1997). Comprehensive allelotyping of human hepatocellular carcinoma. *Oncogene* 14, 2927-2933.

Nagano H, Noguchi T, Inagaki K, Yoon S, Matozaki T, Itoh H, Kasuga M, Hayashi Y (2003). Downregulation of stomach cancer-associated protein tyrosine phoshatase-1 (SAP-1) in advanced human hepatocellular carcinoma. *Oncogene* 22, 4656-4663.

Nagasue N, Ono T, Yamanoi A, Kohno H, El-Assal ON, Taniura H, Uchida M (2001). Prognostic factors and survival after hepatic resection for hepatocellular carcinoma without cirrhosis. *Br J Surg* 88, 515-522.

Naka T, Toyota N, Kaneko T, Kaibara N (1998). Protein expression of p53, p21WAF1, and RB as prognostic indicators in patients with surgically treated hepatocellular carcinoma. *Anticancer res* 18, 555-564.

Nakajima K, Sakurai A, Katai M, Yajima H, Mori J, Katakura M, Tsuchiya S, Hashizume K (2000). Chromogranin A expression in hepatocellular carcinoma in a patient with germline MEN1 gene mutation. *Intern Med* 39, 20-24.

Nakashima O, Sugihara S, Kage M, Kojiro M (1995). Pathomorphologic characteristics of small hepatocellular carcinoma: a special reference to small hepatocellular carcinoma with indistinct margins. *Hepatology* 22, 101-105.

Nakashima Y, Nakashima O, Hsia CC, Kojiro M, Tabor E (1999). Vascularization of small hepatocellular carcinomas: correlation with differentiation. *Liver* 19, 12-18.

Nakau M, Miyoshi H, Seldin MF, Imamura M, Oshima M, Taketo MM (2002). Hepatocellular carcinoma caused by loss of heterozygosity in Lkb1 gene knockout mice. *Cancer Res* 62, 4549-4553.

Neaud V, Faouzi S, Guirouilh J, Le Bail B, Balabaud C, Bioulac-Sage P, Rosenbaum J (1997). Human hepatic myofibroblasts increase invasiveness of hepatocellular carcinoma cells: evidence for a role of hepatocyte growth factor. *Hepatology* 26, 1458-1466.

Nelson WJ, Nusse R (2004). Convergence of Wnt, β-catenin, and cadherin pathways. *Science* 303, 1483-1487.

Ng IO, Lai EC, Ng MM, Fan ST (1992). Tumor encapsulation in hepatocellular carcinoma. A pathologic study of 189 cases. *Cancer* 70, 45-49.

Ng IO, Lai EC, Fan ST, Ng MM, So MK (1995). Prognostic significance of pathologic features of hepatocellular carcinoma. A multivariate analysis of 278 patients. *Cancer* 76, 2443-2448.

Ng IO, Poon RT, Lee JM, Fan ST, Ng M, Tso WK (2001). Microvessel density, vascular endothelial growth factor and its receptors Flt-1 and Flk-1/KDR in hepatocellular carcinoma. *Am J Clin Pathol* 116, 838-845.

Nhieu JT, Renard CA, Wie Y, Cherqui D, Zafrani ES, Buendia MA (1999). Nuclear accumulation of mutated beta-catenin in hepatocellular carcinoma is associated with increased cell proliferation. *Am J Pathol* 155, 703-710.

Nicolson GL, Moustafa AS (1998). metastasis-associated genes and metastatic tumor progression. *In Vivo* 12, 579-588.

Nishida N, Fukuda Y, Komeda T, Ito T, Nishimura T, Minata M, Kuno M, Katsuma H, Ikai I, Yamaoka Y, Nakao K (2002). Prognostic impact of multiple allelic losses on metastatic recurrence in hepatocellular carcinoma after curative resection. *Oncology* 62, 141-148.

Nishida N, Nishimura T, Ito T, Komeda T, Fukuda Y, Nakao K (2003). Chromosomal instability and human hepatocarcinogenesis. *Histol Histopathol* 18, 897-909.

Oda T, Tsuda H, Scarpa A, Sakamoto M, Hirohashi S (1992). Mutation pattern of the p53 gene as a diagnostic marker for multiple hepatocellular carcinoma. *Cancer Res* 52, 3674-3678.

Oda Y, Katsuda S, Nakanishi I (1994). An autopsy case of hepatic sarcomatoid tumor: immunohistochemical comparison with a sarcomatous component of hepatocellular carcinoma. *Pathol Int* 44, 230-236.

Ogawa K, Yamada Y, Kishibe K, Ishizaki K, Tokusashi Y (1999). Beta-catenin mutations are frequent in hepatocellular carcinomas but absent in adenomas induced by diethylnitrosamine in B6C3F1 mice. *Cancer Res* 59, 1830-1833.

Ogden SK, Lee KC, Barton MC (2000). Hepatitis B viral transactivator HBx alleviates p53-mediated repression of alpha-fetoprotein gene expression. *J Biol Chem* 275, 27806-27814.

Oh BK, Jo Chae K, Park C, Kim K, Jung Lee W, Han KH, Nyun Parl Y (2003). telomere shoertening and telomerase reactivation in dysplastic nodules of human hepatocarcinogenesis. *J Hepatol* 39, 786-792.

Ohtomo K, Furui S, Iio M, Kanamori H, Ishikawa T, Takaku F (1984). Sclerosing hepatic carcinoma: a report of a case treated with a transcatheter arterial embolization. *Radiat Med* 2, 104-107.

Okada K, Kim YI, Nakashima K, Tada I, Yoshida T, Kobayashi M, Yokoyama S (1993). Fibrolamellar hepatocellular carcinoma coexistent with a hepatocellular carcinoma of common type: report of a case. *Surg Today* 23, 626-631.

Okano A, Hajiro K, Takakuwa H, Kobashi Y (1998). Fibrolamellar carcinoma of the liver with a mixture of ordinary hepatocellular carcinoma: a case report. *Am J Gastroenterol* 93, 1144-1145.

Okano H, Shiraki K, Inoue H, Kawakita T, Saitou Y, Enokimura N, Yamamoto N, Sugimoto K, Fujikawa K, Murata K, Nakano T (2003). Over-expression of Smac promotes TRAIL-induced cell death in human hepatocellular carcinoma. *Int J Mol Med* 12, 25-28.

Okuda K, Musha H, Nakajima Y, Kubo Y, Shimokawa Y, Nagasaki Y, Sawa Y, Jinnouchi S, Kaneko T, Obata H, Hisamitsu T, Motoike Y, Okazaki N, Kojiro M, Sakamoto K, Nakashima T (1977). Clinicopathologic features of encapsulated hepatocellular carcinoma: a study of 26 cases. *Cancer* 40, 1240-1245.

Okuda K, Nakashima T, Obata H, Kubo Y (1977). Clinicopathological studies of minute hepatocellular carcinoma. Analysis of 20 cases, including 4 with hepatic resection. *Gastroenterology* 73, 109-115.

Okuda K, Ohtsuki T, Obata H. et al. (1985). Natural history of hepatocellular carcinoma and prognosis in relation to treatment. Study of 850 patients. *Cancer* 56, 918-928.

Okuda K (1997). Hepatocellular carcinoma: clinicopathological aspects. *J Gastroenterol Hepatol* 12, S314-S318.

Oldenburg WA, van Heerden JA, Sizemore GW, Abboud CF, Sheedy PF (1982). hypercalcemia and primary hepatic tumors. *Arch Surg* 117, 1363-1366.

Omata M, Peters RL, Tatter D (1981). Sclerosing hepatic carcinoma: relationship to hypercalcemia. *Liver* 1, 33-49.

Osada S, Saji S, Kuno T (2004). Clinical significance of combination study of apoptotic factors and proliferating cell nuclear antigen in estimating the prognosis of hepatocellular carcinoma. *J Surg Oncol* 85, 48-54.

Ozaki I, Mizuta T, Zhao G, Yotsumoto H, Hara T, Kajihara S, Hisatomi A, Sakai T, yamamoto K (2000). Involvement of the Ets-1 gene in overexpression of matrilysin in human hepatocellular carcinoma. *Cancer Res* 60, 6519-6525.

Ozaki I, Mizuta T, Zhao G, Zhang H, Yoshimura T, Kawazoe S, Eguchi Y, Yasutake T, Hisatomi A, Sakai T, Yamamoto K (2003). Induction of multiple metalloproteinase genes in human hepatocellular carcinoma by hepatocyte growth factor via a transcription factor Ets-1. *Hepatol Res* 27, 289-301.

Ozturk M (1999). Genetic aspects of hepatocellular carcinogenesis. *Semin Liver Dis* 19, 235-242.

Park WS, Oh RR, Park JY, Kim PJ, Shin MS, Lee JH, Kim HS, Lee SH, Kim SY, Park YG et al. (2001). Nuclear localization of beta-catenin is an important prognostic factor in hepatoblastoma. *J Pathol* 193, 483-490.

Park WS, Lee JH, Park JY, Jeong SW, Shin MS, Kim HS, Lee SK, Lee SN, Lee SH, Park CG, Yoo NJ, Lee JY (2002). Genetic analysis of the liver putative tumor suppressor (LPTS) gene in hepatocellular carcinomas. *Cancer Lett* 178, 199-207.

Park YN, Chae KJ, Kwon KW, Oh BK, Lee KS, Lee WJ, Park C (2003). p53 and p21WAF1/CIP1 in hepatitis B virus related hepatocarcinogenesis. *Hepatogastroenterology* 50, 1292-1296.

Park SW, Durkin ME, Thorgeirsson SS, Popescu NC (2003). DNA variants of DLC-1, a candidate tumor suppressor gene in human hepatocellular carcinoma. *Int J Oncol* 23, 133-137.

Peng CY, Tsai SL, Yeh CT, Hung SP, Chen MF, Chen TC, Chu CM, Liaw YF (2000). genetic alterations of p73 are infrequent but may occur in early stage hepatocellular carcinoma. *Anticancer res* 20, 1487-1492.

Perilongo G, Plaschkes J, Zimmermann A (2002). Hepatic Tumours. In: Oxford Textbook of Oncology (Souhami RL, Tannock I, Hohenberger P and Horiot JC, eds), second edition, vol 2, Oxford University Press, Oxford, pp 2657-2668.

Polterauer P, Kovarik J, Ulrich W (1980). Hypercalcemia in liver tumors (in German). *Wien Klin Wochenschr* 92, 689-693.

Price JA, Kovach SJ, Johnson T, Koniaris LG, Cahill PA, Sitzmann JV, McKillop ICH (2002). Insulin-like growth factor I is a comitogen for hepatocyte growth factor in a rat model of hepatocellular carcinoma. *Hepatology* 36, 1089-1097.

Qi R, An H, Yu Y, Zhang M, Liu S, Xu H, Guo Z, Cheng T, Cao X (2003). Notch1 signaling inhibits growth of human hepatocellular carcinoma through induction of cell cycle arrest and apoptosis. *Cancer Res* 63, 8323-8329.

Rashid A, Wang JS, Qian GS, Lu BX, Hamilton SR, Groopman JD (1999). genetic alterations in hepatocellular carcinomas: association between loss of chromosome 4q and p53 gene mutations. *Br J Cancer* 80, 59-66.

Ratziu V, Trabut JB, Poynard T (2004). Fat, diabetes, and liver injury in chronic hepatitis C. *Curr Gastroenterol Rep* 6, 22-29.

Reeves ME, DeMatteo RP (2000). Genes and viruses in hepatobiliary neoplasia. *Semin Surg Oncol* 19, 84-93.

Ren EC (1996). Hepatitis B virus and hepatocellular carcinoma. *Ann Acad Med Singapore* 25, 17-21.

Reubi JC, Zimmermann A, Jonas S, Waser B, Neuhaus P, Läderach U, Wiedenmann B (1999). Regulatory peptide receptors in human hepatocellular carcinomas. *Gut* 45, 766-774.

Rocken C, Carl-McGrath S, Grantzdorffer I, Mantke R, Roessner A, Lendeckel U (2004). Ectopeptidases are differentially expressed in hepatocellular carcinomas. *Int J Oncol* 24, 487-495.

Ros PR, Murphy BJ, Buck JL, Olmedilla G, Goodman Z (1990). Encapsulated hepatocellular carcinoma: radiologic findings and pathologic correlation. *Gastrointest Radiuol* 15, 233-237.

Roskams T, De Vos R, David G, Van Damme B, Desmet V (1998). Heparan sulphate preoteoglycan expression in human primary liver tumors. *J Pathol* 185, 290-297.

Ross JS, Kurian S (1985). Clear cell hepatocellular carcinoma: sudden death from severe hypoglycemia. *Am J Gastroenterol* 80, 188-194.

Rowland JM (2002). Hepatoblastoma: assessment of criteria for histologic classification. *Med Pediatr Oncol* 39, 478-483.

Saadi-Kheddouci S, Berrebi D, Romagnolo B, Cluzeaud F, Peuchmaur M, Kahn A, vandewalle A, Perret C (2001). Early development of polycystic kidney disease in transgenic mice expressing an activated mutant of the beta-catenin gene. *Oncogene* 20, 5972-5981.

Sakamoto M, Hirohashi S, Shimosato Y (1991). Early stages of multistep hepatocarcinogenesis: adenomatous hyperplasia and early hepatocellular carcinoma. *Hum Pathol* 22, 172-178.

Sasaki K, Okuda S, Takahashi M, Sasaki M (1981). Hepatic clear cell carcinoma associated with hypoglycemia and hypercholesterolemia. *Cancer* 47, 820-822.

Sasaki Y, Imaoka S, Ishiguro S, Nakano H, Kasugai H, Fujita M, Inoue E, Ishikawa O, Furukawa H, Nakamori S, Kuroda C, Iwanaga T (1996). Clinical features of small hepatocellular carcinomas as assessed by histologic grades. *Surgery* 119, 252-260.

Sasaki A, Kawano K, Aramaki M, Ohno T, Tahara K, Takeuchi Y, Yoshida T, Kitano S (2001). Clinicopathologic study of mixed hepatocellular and cholangiocellular carcinoma: modes of spreading and choice of surgical treatment by reference to macroscopic type. *J Surg Oncol* 76, 37-46.

Sawabe M, Nakamura T, Kanno J, Kasuga T (1987). Analysis of morphological factors of hepatocellular carcinoma in 98 autopsy cases with respect to pulmonary metastasis. *Acta Pathol Jpn* 37, 1389-1404.

Sawai Y, Tamura S, Fukui K, Ito N, Imanaka K, Saeki A, Sakuda S, Kiso S, Matsuzawa Y (2003). Expression of ephrin-B1 in hepatocellular carcinoma: possible involvement in neovascularization. *J Hepatol* 39, 991-996.

Scharf JG, Braulke T (2003). the role of the IGF axis in hepatocarcinogenesis. *Horm Metab Res* 35, 685-693.

Schoedel KE, Tyner VZ, Kim TH, Michalopoulos GK, Mars WM (2003). HGF, MET, and matrix-related proteases in hepatocellular carcinoma, fibrolamellar variant, cirrhotic and normal liver. *Mod Pathol* 16, 14-21.

Seitz G, Zimmermann A, Friess H, Buchler MW (2002). Adult-type hepatocellular carcinoma in the center of a fibrolamellar hepatocellular carcinoma. *Hum Pathol* 33, 765-769.

Seyberth HW, Raisz LG, Oates JA (1978). Prostaglandins and hypercalcemic states. *Annu Rev Med* 29, 23-29.

Shaw RJ, Kosmatka M, Bardeesy N, Hurley RL, Witters LA, DePinho RA, Cantley LC (2004). Inaugural article: The tumor suppressor LKB1 kinase directly activates AMP-activated kinase and regulates apoptosis in response to energy stress. *Proc Natl Acad Sci USA* 101, 3329-3335.

Shimada M, Taguchi K, Hasegawa H, Gion T, Shirabe K, tsuneyoshi M, Sugimachi K (1998). Nm23-H1 expression in intraheptic or extrahepatic metastases of hepatocellular carcinoma. *Liver* 18, 337-342.

Shimoda K, Mori M, Shibuta K, Banner BF, Barnard GF (1999). Vascular endothelial growth factor/vascular permeability factor mRNA expression in patients with chronic hepatitis C and hepatocellular carcinoma. *Int J Oncol* 14, 353-359.

Shimozawa N, Hanazaki K (2004). Longterm prognosis after hepatic resection for small hepatocellular carcinoma. *J Am Coll Surg* 198, 356-365.

Shin EC, Seong YR, Kim CH, Kim H, Ahn YS, Kim K, Kim SJ, Hong SS, Park JH (2002). Human hepatocellular carcinoma cells resist to TRAIL-induced apoptosis, and the resistance is abloshed by cisplatin. *Exp Mol Med* 34, 114-122.

Shuda M, Kondoh N, Imazeki N, Tanaka K, Okada T, Mori K, Hada A, Arai M, Wakatsuki T, Matsubara O, Yamamoto N, Yamamoto M (2003). Activation of teh ATF6, XBP1 and grp78 genes in human hepatocellular carcinoma: a possible involvement of the ER stress pathway in hepatocarcinogenesis. *J Hepatol* 38, 605-614.

Sinivatanauksorn Y, Sinivatanauksorn V, Lemoine NR, Williamson RC, Davidson BR (2001). Genomic homogeneity in fibrolamellar carcinomas. *Gut* 49, 82-86.

Slagle BL, Zhou YZ, Butel JS (1991). Hepatitis B virus integration event in human chromosome 17p near the p53 gene identifies the region of the chromosome commonly deleted in virus-positive hepatocellular carcinomas. *Cancer Res* 51, 49-54.

Sohda T, Kamimura S, Iwata K, Shijo H, Okumura M (1997). Immunohistochemical evidence of insulin-like growth factor II in human small hepatocellular carcinoma with hepatitis C virus infection: relationship to fatty change in carcinoma cells. *J Gastroenterol Hepatol* 12, 224-228.

Sooklim K., Sriplung H, Piratvisuth T (2003). Histologic subtypes of hepatocellular carcinoma in the southern Thai population. *Asian Pac J Cancer Prev* 4, 302-306.

Taguchi J, Nakashima O, Tanaka M, Hisaka T, Takazawa T, Kojiro M (1996). A clinicopathological study on combined hepatocellular and cholangiocarcinoma. *J Gastroenterol Hepatol* 11, 758-764.

Staib F, Hussain SP, Hofseth LJ, Wang XW, Harris CC (2003). TP53 and liver carcinogenesis. *Hum Mutat* 21, 201-216.

Su Q, Schroder CH, Hofmann WJ, Otto G, Pichlmayr R, Bannasch P (1998). Expression of hepatitis B virus X protein in HBV-infected human livers and hepatocellular carcinomas. *Hepatology* 27, 1109-1120.

Suehiro T, Matsumata T, Itasaka H, Yamamoto K, Kawahara N, Sugimachi K (1995). Clinicopathologic features and prognosis of resected hepatocellular carcinomas of varied sizes with special reference to proliferating cell nuclear antigen. *Cancer* 76, 399-405.

Sugano Y, Matsuzaki K, Tahashi Y, Furukawa F, Mori S, Yamagata H, Yoshida K, Matsushita M, Nishizawa M, Fujisawa J, Inoue K (2003). Distortion of autocrine transforming growth factor beta signal accelerates malignant potential by enhancing cell growth as well as PAI-1 and VEGF production in human hepatocellular carcinoma cells. *Oncogene* 22, 2309-2321.

Sugimachi K, Tanaka S, Terashi T, Taguchi K, Rikimaru T, Sugimachi K (2002). The mechanisms of angiogenesis in hepatocellular carcinoma: angiogenic switch during tumor rpogression. *Surgery* 131 (suppl), S135-S141.

Sugimachi K, Tanaka S, Taguchi K, Aishima S, Shimada M, Tsuneyoshi M (2003). Angiopoietin switching regulates angiogenesis and progression of human hepatocellular carcinoma. *J Clin Pathol* 56, 854-860.

Sugioka Y, Watanabe T, Inagaki Y, Kushida M, Niioka M, Endo H, Higashiyama R, Okazaki I (2003). c-jun NH2-terminal kinase pathway is involved in constitutive matrix metalloproteinase-1 expression in a hepatocellular carcinoma-derived cell line. *Int J Cancer* 109, 867-874.

Sun BH, Zhao XP, Wang BJ, Yang DL, Hao LJ (2000). FADD and TRADD expression and apoptosis in primary hepatocellular carcinoma. *World J Gastroenterol* 6, 223-227.

Sun HC, Tang ZY, Zhou G, Li XM (1998). KAI1 gene expression in hepatocellular carcinoma and its relationship with intrahepatic metastases. J *Exp Clin Cancer Res* 17, 307-311.

Szekely E (2001). Hepatocellular carcinoma with lymphoid stroma: ' lymphoepithelioma-like carcinoma '? *Histopathology* 39, 540.

Takata M, Yamanaka N, Tanaka T, Yamanaka J, Maeda S, Okamoto E, Yasojima H, Uematsu K, Watanabe H, Uragari Y (2000). What patients can survive disease free after complete resection for hepatocellular carcinoma? A multivariate analysis. *Jpn J Clin Oncol* 30, 75-81.

Tamura K, Kubota K, Take H, Kurabayashi H, Shirakura T (1994). Parathyroid hormone-related peptide as a possible cause of hypercalcemia in a hepatocellular carcinoma patient. *Am J Gastroenterol* 89, 644-645.

Tamura S, Nakamori S, Kuroki T, Sasaki Y, Furukawa H, Ishikawa O, Imaoka S, Nakamura Y (1997). Association of cumulative allelic losses with tumor aggressiveness in hepatocellular carcinoma. J *Hepatol* 27, 669-676.

Tanaka S, Toh Y, Adachi E, Matsumata T, Mori R, Sugimachi K (1993). Tumor progression in hepatocellular carcinoma may be mediated by p53 mutation. *Cancer Res* 53, 2884-2887.

Tanaka S, Sugimachi K, Yamashita Yi Y, Ohga T, Shirabe K, Shimada M, Wands JR, Sugimachi K (2002). Tie2 vascular endothelial receptor expression and function in hepatocellular carcinoma. *Hepatology* 35, 861-867.

Tanaka S, Sugimachi K, Yamashita Y, Shirabe K, Shimada M, Wands JR, Sugimachi K (2003). Angiogenic switch as a molecular target of malignant tumors. *J Gastroenterol* 38 (suppl 15), 93-97.

Taniguchi K, Roberts LR, Aderca IN, Dong X, Qian C, Murphy LM, Nagorney DM, Burgart LJ, Roche PC, Smith DI, Ross JA, Liu W (2002). Mutational spectrum of beta-catenin, AXIN1, and AXIN2 in hepatocellular carcinomas and hepatoblastomas. *Oncogene* 21, 4863-4871.

Tannapfel A, Wittekind C (2002). Genes involved in hepatocellular carcinoma: deregulation in cell cycling and apoptosis. *Virchows Arch* 440, 345-352.

Tannapfel A, Wasner M, Krause K, Geissler F, Katalinic A, Hauss J, Mossner J, Engeland K, Wittekind C (1999). Expression of p73 and its relation to histopathology and prognosis in hepatocellular carcinoma. *J Natl Cancer Inst* 91, 1154-1158.

Tavian D, de Petro G, Benetti A, Portolani N, Giulini SM, Barlati S (2000). u-PA and c-MET mRNA expression is co-ordinately enhanced while hepatocyte growth factor mRNA is down-regulated in human hepatocellular carcinoma. *Int J Cancer* 87, 644-649.

Terracian L, Tornillo L (2003). Cytogenetic alterations in liver cell tumors as detected by comparative genomic hybridization. *Pathologica* 95, 71-82.

Terracciano LM, Tornilio L, Avoledo P, Von Schweinitz D, Kuhne T, Bruder E (2004). Fibrolamellar hepatocellular carcinoma occurring 5 years after hepatocellular adenoma in a 14-year-old girl: a case report with comparative genomic hybridization analysis. *Arch. Pathol. Lab. Med.* 128, 222-226.

Terris B, Pineau P, Bregeaud L, Valla D, Belghiti J, Tiollais P, Degott C, Dejean A (1999). Close correlation between beta-catenin gene alterations and nuclear accumulation of the protein in human hepatocellular carcinomas. *Oncogene* 18, 6583-6588.

Theret N, Musso O, Turlin B, Lotrian D, Bioulac-Sage P, Campion JP, Boudjema K, Clement B (2001). Increased extracellular matrix remodeling is associated with tumor progression in human hepatocellular carcinomas. *Hepatology* 34, 82-88.

Thomas D, Pritchard J, Davidson R, McKiernan P, Grundy RG, de Ville de Goyet J (2003). Familial hepatoblastoma and APC gene mutations: renewed call for molecular research. *Eur J Cancer* 39, 220-2204.

Thorgeirsson SS, Grisham JW (2002). Molecular pathogenesis of human hepatocellular carcinoma. *Nat Genet* 31, 339-346.

Tickoo SK, Zee SY, Obiekwe S, Xiao H, Koea J, Robiou C, Blumgart LH, Jarnagin W, Ladanyi M, Klimstra DS (2002). Combined hepatocellular-cholangiocarcinoma: a histopathologic, immunohistochemical, and in situ hybridization study. *Am J Surg Pathol* 26, 989-997.

Tomita N, Morishita R, Taniyama Y, Koike H, Aoki M, Shimizu H, Matsumoto K, Nakamura T, Kaneda Y, Ogihara T (2003). Angiogenic property of hepatocyte growth factor is dependent on upregulation of essential transcription for angiogenesis, ets-1. *Circulation* 107, 1411-1417.

Tomizawa M, Kondo F, Kondo Y (1995). Growth patterns and interstitial invasion of small hepatocellular carcinoma. *Pathol Int* 45, 352-358.

Torbenson M, Wang J, Choti M, Ashfaq R, Maitra A, Wilentz RE, Boitnott J (2002). hepatocellular carcinomas show abnormal expression of fibronectin protein. *Mod Pathol* 15, 826-830.

Torimura T, Sata M, Ueno T, Kin M, Tsuji R, Suzaku K, Hashimoto O, Sugawara H, Tanikawa K (1998). Increased expression of vascular endothelial growth factor is associated with tumor progression in hepatocellular carcinoma. *Hum Pathol* 29, 986-991.

Tralhao JG, Roudier J, Morosan S, Giannini C, Tu H, Goulenok C, Carnot F, Zavala F, Joulin V, Kremsdorf D, Brechot C (2002). Paracrine in vivo inhibitotry effects of hepatitis B virus X protein (HBx) on liver cell proliferation: an alternative mechanism of HBx-related pathogenesis. *Proc Natl Acad Sci USA* 99, 6991-6996.

Tran van Nhieu J, Renard CA, Wei Y, Cherqui D, Zafrani ES, Buendia MA (1999). Nuclear accumulation of mutated β-catenin in hepatocellular carcinoma is associated with increased cell proliferation. *Am J Pathol* 155, 703-710.

Udatsu Y, Kusafuka T, Kuroda S, Miao J, Okada A (2001). High frequence of beta-catenin mutations in hepatoblastoma. *Pediatr Surg Int* 17, 508-512.

Ueda E, Hirota S, Fujii M, Tanaka K, Shimizu M, Kono M, Hase M, Sako M (1989). Three cases of hepatocellular carcinoma with remarkable fatty metamorphosis (in Japanese). *Rinsho Hoshasen* 34, 921-924.

Ueta T, Ikeguchi M, Hirooka Y, Kaibara N, Terada T (2002). Beta-catenin and cyclin D1 expression in human hepatocellular carcinoma. *Oncol Rep* 9, 1197-1203.

van Dekken H, Wink J, Alers JC, de Man RA, Ijzermans JN, Zondervan PE (2003). genetic evaluation of the dysplasia-carcinoma sequence in chronic viiral liver disease: a detailed analysis of two cases and review of the literature. *Acta Histochem* 105, 29-41.

Volkmann M, Hofmann WJ, Muller M, Rath U, otto G, Zentgraf H, Galle PR (1994). p53 overexpression is freuqnt in European hepatocellular carcinoma and largely independent of the codon 249 hot spot mutation. *Oncogene* 9, 195-204.

Vora IM, Amarapurkar AD, Rege JD, Mathur SK (2000). Neuroendocrine differentiation in hepatocellular carcinoma. *Indian J Gastroenterol* 19, 37-38.

Wada Y, Nakashima O, Kutami R, Yamamoto O, Kojiro M (1998). Clinicopathological study on hepatocellular carcinoma with lymphocytic infiltration. *Hepatology* 27, 407-414.

Wakasa K, Sakurai M, Okamura J, Kuroda C (1985). Pathological study of small hepatocellular carcinoma: frequency of their invasion. *Virchows Arch A Pathol Anat Histopathol* 407, 259-270.

Wang JH, Dhillon AP, Sankey EA, Wightman AK, Lewin JF, Scheuer PJ (1991). ' Neuroendocrine ' differentiation in primary neoplasms of the liver. *J Pathol* 163, 61-67.

Wang XW, Hussain SP, Huo TI, Wu CG, Forgues M, Hofseth LJ, Brechot C, Harris CC (2002). Molecular pathogenesis of human hepatocellular carcinoma. *Toxicology* 181-182, 43-47.

Wang Y, Wu MC, Sham JS, Zhag W, Wu WQ, Guan XY (2002). prognostic significance of c-myc and AIB1 amplification in hepatocellular carcinoma. A broad survey using high-throughput tissue microarray. *Cancer* 95, 2346-2352.

Wang XZ, Chen XC, Chen YX, Zhang LJ, Li D, Chen FL, Chen ZX, Chen HY, Tao QM (2003). Overexpression of HBxAg in hepatocellular carcinoma and its relationship with Fas/FasL system. *World J Gastroenterol* 9, 2671-2675.

Wang Y, Lau SH, Sham JS, Wu MC, Wang T, Guan XY (2004). Characterization of HBV integrants in 14 hepatocellular carcinomas: association of truncated X gene and hepatocellular carcinogenesis. *Oncogene* 23, 142-148.

Watanuki A, Ohwada S, Fukusato T, Makita F, Yamada T, Kikuchi A, Morishita Y (2002). Prognostic significance of DNA topoisomerase IIalpha expression in human hepatocellular carcinoma. *Anticancer Res* 22 (2B), 1113-1119.

Wei Y, Fabre M, Brancherau S, Gauthier F, Perilongo G, Buendia MA (2000). Activation of beta-catenin in epithelial and mesenchymal hepatoblastomas. *Oncogene* 19, 498-504.

Wilkins L, Bredt M, Flemming P, Kubicka S, Klempnauer J, Kreipe H (2000). Cytogenetic aberrations in primary and recurrent fibrolamellar hepatocellular carcinoma detected by comparative genomic hybridization. Am J *Clin Pathol* 114, 867-874.

Wirths O, Waha A, Weggen S, Schirmacher P, Kuhne T, Goodyer CG, Albrecht S, Von Schweinitz D, Pietsch T (2003). Overexpression of human Dickkopf-1, an antagonist of wingless/WNT signaling, in human hepatoblastoma and Wilms' tumor. *Lab Invest* 83, 429-434.

Wong CM, Fan ST, Ng IO (2001). Beta-catenin mutation and overexpression in hepatocellular carcinoma: clinicopathologic and prognostic significance. *Cancer* 92, 136-145.

Wong CM, Lee JM, Lau TC, Fan ST, Ng IO (2002). Clinicopathological significance of loss of heterozygosity on chromosome 13q in hepatocellular carcinoma. *Clin Cancer Res* 8, 2266-2272.

Wong CM, Lee JM, Ching YP, Jin DY, Ng IO (2003). Genetic and epigenetic alterations of DLC-1 gene in hepatocellular carcinoma. *Cancer Res* 63, 7646-7651.

Wu JT, Erickson AJ, Tsao KC, Wu TL, Sun CF (2000). Elevated serum chromogranin A is detectable in patients with carcinomas at advanced disease stages. *Ann Clin Lab Sci* 30, 175-178.

Wu CG, Salvay DM, Forgues M, Valerie K, Farnsworth J, Markin RS, Wang XW (2001). Distinctive gene expression profiles associated with Hepatitis B virus x protein. *Oncogene* 20, 3674-3682.

Xiao H, Palhan V, Yang Y, Roeder RG (2000). TIP30 has an intrinsic kinase activity required for up-regulation of a subset of apoptotic genes. *EMBO J* 19, 956-963.

Xiao EH, Hu GD, Li JQ (2002). Relationship between apoptosis and invasive and metastatic potential of hepatocellular carcinoma. *Hepatobiliary Pancreat Dis Int* 1, 574-576.

Xu X, Sakon M, Nagano H, Hiraoka N, Yamamoto H, Hayashi N, Dono K, Nakamori S, Umeshita K, Ito Y, Matsuura N, Monden M (2004). Akt2 expression correlates with prognosis of human hepatocellular carcinoma. *Oncol Rep* 11, 25-32.

Yahagi N, Shimano H, Matsuzaka T, Sekyia M, Najima Y, Okazaki S, Okazaki H, Tamura Y, Iizuka Y, Inoue N, Nakagawa Y, Takeuchi Y et al. (2004). p53 involvement in the pathogenesis of fatty liver disease. J *Biol Chem* ........

Yamamoto T, Ikebe T, Mikami S, Shuto T, Hirohashi K, Kinoshita H, Sakurai M (1996). Immunohistochemistry and angiography in adenomatous hyperplasia and small hepatocellular carcinoma. *Pathol Int* 46, 364-371.

Yamasaki T, Kurokawa F, Kato A, Irie K, Yutoku K, Terai S, Matsuzaki Y, Yasunaga M, Okita K (1996). Clinicopathologic features of early hepatocellular carcinoma. *Hepatogastroenterology* 43, 926-931.

Yamashita F, Iwao T, Torimura T, Tanaka M, Hirai K, Abe M, Toyonaga A, Sugihara S, Kojiro M, Tanikawa K (1992). Sclerosing hepatocellular carcinoma with hypercalcemia - a case report. *Kurume Med* J 39, 113-116.

Yang S, Lin HZ, Hwang J, Chacko VP, Diehl AM (2001). hepatic hyperplasia in noncirrhotic fatty livers: is obesity-related hepatic steatosis a premalignant condition? *Cancer Res* 61, 5016-5023.

Yang EB, Qin LL, Zhao YN, Zhang K, Chow P (2003). Genetic changes and expression of the mannose 6-phosphate/insulin-like growth factor II receptor gene in human hepatitis B virus-associated hepatocellular carcinoma. *Int J Mol Med* 11, 773-778.

Yano Y, Yamamoto J, Kosuge T, Sakamoto Y, Yamasaki S, Shimada K, Ojima H, Sakamoto M, Takayama T, Makuuchi M (2003). Combined hepatocellular and cholangiocarcinoma: a clinicopathologic study of 26 resected cases. *Jpn J Clin Oncol* 33, 283-287.

Yano Y, Hayashi Y, Nakji M, Nagano H, Seo Y, Ninomiya T, Yoon S, Wada A, Hirai M, Kim SR, Yokozaki H, Kasuga M (2003). Different apoptotic regulation of TRAIL-caspase pathway in HBV-and HCV-related hepatocellular carcinoma. *Int J Mol Med* 11, 499-504.

Yen TC, Hwang SJ, Wang CC, Lee SD, Yeh SH (1993). Hypercalcemia and parathyroid hormone-related protein in hepatocellular carcinoma. *Liver* 13, 311-315.

Yokota T, Suda T, Igarashi M, Kuroiwa T, Waguri N, Kawai H, Mita Y, Aoyagi Y (2003). Telomere length variation and maintenance in hepatocarcinogenesis. *Cancer* 98, 110-118.

Yoo YG, Oh SH, Park ES, Cho H, Lee N, Park H, Kim DK, Yu DY, Seong JK, Lee MO (2003). Hepatitis B virus X protein enhances transcriptional activity of hypoxia-inducible factor-1alpha through activation of mitogen-activated protein kinase pathway. *J Biol Chem* 278, 39076-39084.

Yoshikawa J, Matsui O, Takashima T, Ida M, Takanaka T, Kawamura I, Kakuda K, Miyata S (1988). Fatty metamorphosis in hepatocellular carcinoma: radiologic features in 10 cases. *AJR Am J Roentgenol* 151, 717-720.

Zatkova A, Rouillard JM, Hartmann W, Lamb BJ, Kuick R, Eckart M, von Schweinitz D, Koch A, Fonatsch C et al. (2004). Amplification and overexpression of the IGF2 regulator PLAG1 in hepatoblastoma. Genes Chromosomes cancer 39, 126-137.

Zhang H, Ozaki I, Mizuta T, Yoshimura T, Matsuhashi S, Hisatomi A, Tadano J, Sakai T, Yamamoto K (2003). Mechanism of beta 1-integrin-mediated hepatoma cell growth involves p27 and S-phase kinase-associated protein 2. *Hepatology* 38, 305-313.

Zhao M, Laissue JA, Zimmermann A (1993). " Neuroendocrine " differentiation in hepatocellular carcinomas (HCCs): immunohistochemical reactivity is related to distinct tumor cell types, but not to tumor grade. *Histol Histopathol* 8, 617-626.

Zhao M, Zhang NX, Laissue JA, Zimmermann A (1994). Immunohistochemical analysis of p53 protein overexpression in liver cell dysplasia and in hepatocelullar carcinoma. *Virchows Arch* 424, 613-621.

Zhao M, Zimmermann A (1997). Apoptosis in hepatocellular carcinomas with neuroendocrine differentiation. *Histol Histopathol* 12, 973-980.

Zhao M, Zimmermann A (1997). Apoptosis in human hepatocellular carcinoma and liver cell dysplasia is correlated with p53 protein immunoreactivity. *J Clin Pathol* 50, 394-400.

Zhao X, Li J, He Y, Lan F, Fu L, Guo J, Zhao R, Ye Y, He M, Chong W, Chen J, Zhang L, Yang N, Xu B, Wu M, Wan D, Gu J (2001). A novel growth suppressor gene on chromosome 17p13.3 with a high frequency of mutation in human hepatocellular carcinoma. *Cancer Res* 61, 7383-7387.

Zhao ZC, Zheng SS, Wan YL, Jia CK, Xie HY (2003). The molecular mechanism underlying angiogenesis in hepatocellular carcinoma: the imbalance activation of signaling pathways. *Hepatobiliary Pancreat Dis Int* 2, 529-536.

Zheng Q, Tang ZY, Xue Q, Shi DR, Song HY, Tang HB (2000). Invasion and metastasis of hepatocellular carcinoma in relation to urokinase-type plasminogen activator, its receptor and inhibitor. *J Cancer Res Clin Oncol* 126, 641-646.

Zhou XD (2002). Recurrence and metastasis of hepatocellular carcinoma: progress and prospects. *Hepatobiliary Pancreat Dis Int* 1, 35-41.

Zhou X, Thorgeirsson SS, Popescu NC (2004). Restoration of DLC-1 gene expression induces apoptosis and inhibits both cell growth and tumorigenicity in human hepatocellular carcinoma cells. *Oncogene* 23, 1308-1313.

Zhu H, Wang Y, Chen J, Cheng G, Xue J (2004). Transgenic mice expressing hepatitis B virus X protein are more susceptible to carcinogen induced hepatocarcinogenesis. *Exp Mol Pathol* 76, 44-50.

Zimmermann A (2000). Tumors of the liver – pathologic aspects. In: Surgery of the Liver and Biliary Tract, (eds. Blumgart LH, Fong Y), 3rd ed., Vol. II, *WB Saunders, London*, 1343-1396.

Zimmermann A, Kappeler A, Friess H, Buchler MW (2002). Hepatocellular carcinoma with an unusual medullary-like histology and signs of regression (" medullary-like hepatocellular carcinoma "). *Dig Liver Dis* 34, 748-753.

Zimmermann A (2002). Hepatoblastoma with cholangioblastic features (' cholangioblastic hepatoblastoma ') and other liver tumors with bimodal differentiation in young patients. *Med Pediatr Oncol* 39, 487-491.

Zimmermann A (2003). Hepatocellular carcinoma: From molecular hepatogenesis to novel entities. Proceedings of the 7th Biennial ASHBPS Congress, Chennai (ed Rau BK), *Monduzzi Editore*, pp 121-128.

Zimmermann A and the SIOPEL Group (2003). Liver cell tumors in childhood and adolescence: an expanding spectrum of intriguing lesions. *Bangladesh J Child Health* 27 (suppl), S36-S55.

In: Liver Cancer: New Research
Editor: Felix Lee, pp. 43-57

ISBN 1-59454-182-5


*Chapter II*

# Tumor Biology of Colorectal Liver Metastases

***Curtis J. Wray*, Russell S. Berman+,1 and Syed A. Ahmad*,2***

*Department of Surgery, University of Cincinnati College of Medicine, Cincinnati, OH

+Department of Surgery, New York University School of Medicine, New York, NY

## ABSTRACT

Metastatic development is the primary cause of cancer treatment failure and is responsible for nearly all deaths from colorectal cancer. For the majority of patients, by the time primary colorectal cancers are diagnosed, sub-clinical or clinically relevant liver metastases have already occurred. The formation of liver metastases represents a highly selective sequence in which a subpopulation of cells within a tumor express genes that allow them to progress through distinct steps and spread to distant organs. Modification of gene expression in these cells leads to transformation, growth, angiogenesis, invasion, dissemination, survival in systemic circulation and attachment in the organ of metastases. Existing therapies directed at metastatic disease of the liver have had minimal impact on outcome. Contemporary treatment regimens are not likely to appreciably alter the natural history of liver metastases. Consequently, understanding the molecular and biologic

[1]Co-authors addresses: Russell S. Berman, MD, Division of Surgical Oncology, New York University School of Medicine, NBV 1515N-1, 530 First Avenue, New York, New York 10016

[2] Address for Correspondence and Reprint: Syed A. Ahmad, MD, Division of Surgical Oncology, Department of Surgery, University of Cincinnati College of Medicine, 234 Goodman Street ML 0772, Cincinnati, Ohio 45219, Phone: 513-584-1992, Fax: 513-584-0499, Email: syed.ahmad@ucphysicians.com

mechanisms of liver metastases may allow for the development of therapeutic strategies designed to prevent and treat liver metastases. This review focuses on the molecular and biologic mechanisms that transpire during the development of colorectal liver metastases. In addition, this report will evaluate novel therapeutic strategies targeting liver metastases, angiogenesis and apoptosis.

**Keywords:** Colon cancer, Angiogenesis, Anti-Angiogenic therapy

# INTRODUCTION

## Colorectal Hepatic Metastases Formation

The development of metastases is an inefficient progression. Primary tumor masses shed enormous quantities of cells into the vasculature; yet, only 0.001% of these cells form tumor foci [1]. Colorectal cancer (CRC) evolution is recognized to be a complex, multistage progression in which the transformation from normal cells to cancer cells involves genetic changes that lead to many phenotypic alterations. The characteristics and capabilities of cells following malignant transformation include the following: [1] self sufficiency in growth signaling; autocrine loop of growth factors; [2] resistance to inhibitory factors such as transforming growth factor-beta; [3] resistance to apoptosis (avoidance of destruction by immune mechanisms); [4] unlimited replication potential; [5) sustained angiogenesis (recruitment of nutritional supply to the tumor mass); [6] tissue invasion and metastasis. In this review, we will focus on the latter events of this sequence.

# ALTERATION OF CELL-CELL AND CELL-MATRIX INTERACTIONS

Adhesion molecules play a fundamental role in tumor progression and metastases formation. First, after the initial transformation and growth, subpopulations of cells develop genetic modifications leading to multiple degrees of a metastatic phenotype. These new clones down-regulate cell-cell adhesion and cell-extracellular matrix (ECM) adhesion, which in turn increases cell motility and the capacity for these clones to detach from the primary tumor. Assortments of cell surface receptors mediate these interactions; they include integrins, cadherins, selectins, and immunoglobulin-like proteins.

The integrin family of adhesion molecules acts as cell surface receptors to bind to the laminin, fibronectin, and collagen components of the ECM. Many integrins are expressed on the surface of human CRC cells. For example, CRC cells express the $\alpha6\beta4$ integrin, an adhesion molecule that is thought to facilitate tumor cell motility and progression [2]. An additional integrin, $\alpha V\beta3$, directly binds to matrix metalloproteinase (MMP). MMPs are a family of zinc-dependent endopeptidases that have been characterized as proteases crucial to cancer dissemination. Expression of $\alpha V\beta3$ aids invading cells localize MMP-2 on the surface of the endothelial cells, which in turn enables the metastatic cells to degrade type IV collagen and remodel the ECM during invasion. Once tumor cells adhere to the ECM and basement membrane (BM), and produce degradable substances, the tumor cells must then detach to migrate into the stroma. Consequently, decreased integrin expression promotes detachment from the primary tumor, which in turn correlates with tumor progression [3].

Another protein family involved in cellular adhesion is the cadherins, which are a large family of single-pass transmembrane glycoproteins. E-cadherin is the proto-type molecule of this superfamily, it binds to the intracellular actin cytoskeleton, which is facilitated by cytoplasmic proteins called *catenins*. In contrast to normal colonic mucosa where the levels of free cytosolic β-catenin are low, high levels of β-catenin accumulate in various types of cancer. Tyrosine phosphorylation of β-catenin has been suggested to enhance the metastaic potential of and invasiveness by stabilizing β-catenin and promoting its binding to proliferative transcription factors [4]. Decreased expression of the E-cadherin/β-catenin/α-catenin cell-cell adhesion complex promotes separation of metastatic phenotypes from primary tumors and correlates with a higher metastatic potential, poor differentiation, and worse prognosis in CRC [5].

Cell-cell adhesion interactions may actually promote metastatic formation during tumor cell arrest in the distant organ. Embolized tumor cells usually circulate as clusters of cells adherent to other tumor cells or platelets. This ability to cluster during tumor cell embolization may augment trapping of tumor cells in the microcirculation of distant organs. Immunoglobulin and selectin molecules may mediate these "trapped" cell-cell interactions in distant organs. Molecules in the immunoglobulin superfamily mediate signal transduction, cellular immunity and cell adhesion [6]. Carcinoembryonic antigen (CEA), an additional component of the immunoglobulin superfamily, may facilitate adhesion of CRC cells to other tumor or host organ cells [7]. Jessup *et al.* have demonstrated that CEA injected intravenously into athymic nude mice increases the ability of weakly metastatic CRC to develop liver metastases [8]. Once a metastatic cell has traveled to a distant site, it must attach to hepatic or other remote organ endothelial cells or ECM components through expression of specific adhesion molecules. For CRC, these adhesion molecules include CD44, the ganglioside GM2 and the sialyl-$Le^x$ carbohydrate antigen [9-11].

## INVASION AND METASTASIS

For a tumor cell to invade and metastasize to the liver or another distant organ, it must be able to invade and traverse the BM and the ECM. Countless mechanisms of tumor cell invasion of the BM have been characterized [12]. These consist of mechanical pressure forcing tumor cells along the path of least resistance, amplified cell motility and degradation of the BM and the ECM. This latter theory has been the focal point of numerous preclinical and clinical research projects aimed at preventing the formation of liver metastases.

CRC cells produce an assortment of proteases. The family of proteases that has received the most attention has been the matrix metalloproteinases (MMPs). MMPs play a crucial role in normal homeostatic physiology because the ECM and BM is a dynamic matrix of structural proteins, growth factors and enzymes, which is continually being remodeled.

MMPs function to cleave and activate growth factors, regulate apoptosis, cell migration, and cell-cell communication [13]. MMPs are collectively able to degrade virtually all ECM components, i.e. collagens, laminins, fibronectin, vibronectin, enactin, and proteoglycans [14]. There are at least 20 MMPs that are historically divided into four subfamilies based upon ECM substrate specificity and homology to other MMPs. MMPS are grouped into the following families: the collagenases, the gelatinases, the stromelysins and the metalloelastases [15].

CRC produces increased levels of matrilysin and stromelysin-1, -2, and –3, compared to normal colorectal mucosa [15]. The expression of the proteases correlated with an invasive phenotype and tumor progression. Other MMPs are important in CRC liver metastases formation. Masaki et al have shown that increased expression of MMP-7 is associated with CRC liver metastases [16]. There has been almost unanimous agreement that enhanced expression of MMP-7 in CRC (as measured by immunohistochemistry and *in situ* hybridization) correlates with the presence of nodal or distant metastases. Experimental studies have provided confirmation of the role MMP-7 in CRC development and progression. MMP-7 has been shown to be important in the growth of early colonic adenomas and their progression to an invasive phenotype [17].

There are also four naturally occurring MMP inhibitors, known as tissue inhibitors of metalloproteinases (TIMPs) [18]. The TIMPs (TIMP1-4) are capable of reversible inhibition of activated MMPs with varying affinities and specificities. TIMP levels have been evaluated in CRC. TMIP-1 is the primary inhibitor of MMP-9 and an imbalance in the MMP-7/TIMP-1 ratio has been proposed to be a potential reason for the transformation of adenomas to invasive carcinomas [19]. Ogata *et al.* have also demonstrated that an imbalance of MMP-7 and TIMP-1 is associated with liver metastases from CRC [20]. TIMP-1 and -2 expression have been localized to peri-cancer stromal cells, while malignant and normal mucosa cells were weak or negative in *in situ* hybridization studies of CRC [21].

Another cellular mechanism involved in the process of invasion and metastases are the proteins of the plasminogen activation system. These proteins are closely related to enzymes that degrade the ECM, either directly or through their ability to activate prometalloproteases. Urokinase-type plasminogen activator (uPA) converts enzymatically inactive plasminogen into serine plasmin, which degrades proteins in the ECM. The proteolytic action of uPA is controlled by its inhibitors, plasminogen activator inhibitor-1 and -2, which bind to the cell surface-associated uPA receptor (uPAR) forming an inactive trimeric receptor-protease-inhibitor complex [22].

More recently, scientists have concentrated on uPAR, which facilitates a proteolytic cascade located on the cell surface. uPAR has been acknowledged as a multifunctional protein that interacts with integrins and initiates signaling events that modify cell adhesion, migration, tumor proliferation, and angiogenesis. uPAR has also been implicated in the formation of liver metastases from CRC [23]. The uPAR molecules are expressed at the invasive front of colonic adenocarcinomas; elevated levels of uPAR protein expression are associated with both reduced survival (<5 years) and liver metastases formation in CRC patients [23]. Lastly, transfection of CRC cells with antisense uPAR cDNA diminishes their ability to form metastases [23]. The MMP and uPAR family of proteases undoubtedly are involved with tumor cells' capacity to form metastases. Drugs targeting these systems are at this time being investigated in clinical trials.

## Migration and Motility

Cell migration is required for tumor cells to gain access to the microcirculation. Cell migration requires interaction of the tumor cells' cytoskeleton, forming membrane ruffles, filopodia and pseudopodia, and the ECM. This complex interaction is stimulated by cytokines such as hepatocyte growth factor (HGF) and transforming growth factor β (TGF-β).

HGF is a naturally occurring peptide secreted by mesodermal cells. The receptor for HGF, c-met, is a transmembrane receptor tyrosine kinase that is expressed primarily in epithelial tissues. C-met has been shown to play a significant role in the development of human colorectal carcinoma. *In vitro* experiments have demonstrated treatment of primary CRC cell lines with HGF leads to c-met activation and induces human colorectal carcinoma cell motility [24]. Endogenous activation of HGF/c-met in highly metastatic KM12SM CRC cells results in increased survival and growth in anchorage independent conditions, as well as increased *in vitro* migration [25]. In human pathology specimens, concentrations of c-met m RNA have been demonstrated to be higher in hepatic metastases than in primary colorectal tumors [26]. About 50% of primary CRCs overexpress c-met [27]. Approximately 70% of liver metastases overexpress c-met compared with the primary colorectal tumor. These studies imply that overexpression of the c-met protein and HGF may be essential to promoting the development of CRC liver metastases.

TGF-β is a dimeric polypeptide that belongs to a large family of structurally related proteins. TGF-β has also been implicated in the augmentation of colon cancer cell migration and motility. TGF-β is a powerful negative regulator of epithelial cell growth and can cause total inhibition of nontransformed colon cells growth. In comparison, colon cancer is frequently associated with the acquisition of resistance to TGF-β. Markowitz *et al.* demonstated malignant evolution of colon adenoma cell lines correlates with the acquisition of both TGF-β resistance and TGF-β receptor mutations [28].

## Growth Factors and Growth Factor Receptors

Once a tumor cell becomes fixed into the hepatic parenchyma, it must be able to interact appropriately with the new microenvironment. Proliferation, which is a crucial step in the expansion of clinically relevant metastases, may occur secondary to constitutively activated oncogenes or other microenvironmental stimuli, such as growth factors. Growth factors act by binding to specific tyrosine kinase receptors. It is the activation of these receptors that leads to the transcription of genes that regulate metastatic tumor growth. Growth factor ligands thought to be involved the growth of colorectal liver metastases includes epidermal growth factor (EGF), insulin-like growth factor (IGF) and HGF.

The EGF axis is composed of the EGF receptor (EGFR) and its ligands, EGF and transforming growth factor-α. These ligands are involved with the growth, proliferation and metastases of CRC cells [28]. *In vitro* cell migration assay studies have shown that treatment of HT29 CRC cells with EGF induces a vigorous chemomigratory response [29]. Levels of EGFR expression in primary cultures of established human CRC cell lines are significantly higher in cell lines from patients with Duke's stage D lesions than in cell lines established from Duke's stage B lesions. Certain *in vivo* studies demonstrate that increased expression of EGFR correlate directly with the ability to produce hepatic metastases [25].

Parker et al have shown that increased EGFR gene expression and functional protein levels correlate with metastatic potential of human colon carcinoma cell in nude mice [26]. In this experiment, using monoclonal antibodies specific for the phosphorylated EGFR, increased immunoreactivity was observed in metastatic lesions growing in the liver when compared to primary tumors growing orthotopically in the cecum or ectopically in the subcutis of nude mice. This implies that colorectal liver metastases growth is dependent upon response to organ-derived growth factors and activation of cell-surface tyrosine kinase receptors.

Another growth factor implicated in the progression and metastases of CRC is IGF. The IGF system is composed of three ligands (IGF-I, IGF-II and insulin), three receptors (IGF-IR, IGF-IIR and insulin receptor), and at least six structurally and functionally distinct IGF binding proteins [32]. IGFs circulate in the plasma complexed to a family of binding proteins (BP). The function of the IGF-BPs appears to be diverse, however, at this time they remain poorly understood. IGF-BP3, the most abundant systemic IGF-BP, alters the action of IGF-I by binding to it and transporting it from the circulatory system to the cell surface receptor. As long as IGF-I is bound to IGF-BP3, it is inactive, but after dissociation from IGF-BP3, IGF-I can bind to and activate IGF-IR.

Increased expression of IGF-I and its receptor has been demonstrated in CRC [33]. IGF-I functions as a survival factor for human colon carcinoma cells. The highest source of IGF-I is the liver, which is also the most frequent site of CRC metastasis. Studies have also shown that IGF-I and insulin protect CRC cells from IFN-γ/TNF-α-induced apoptosis [34]. Therefore, blocking IGF-IR signaling may sensitize CRC cells to DNA-damaging agents. IGF-IR and insulin have also been implicated in liver metastatic formation [35]. Koenuma *et al.* demonstated that IGF-I and insulin stimulated growth of highly metastatic colon cancer cell lines, compared to low-metastatic cell lines, suggesting a role for IGF-I-induced liver metastatic formation. Reinmuth *et al.* transfected HT29 CRC cells with a truncated IGF-IR lacking the cytosolic tyrosine kinase domain. This led to a decreased tumor growth, angiogenesis, increased apoptosis, decreased tumorgenicity and growth in the liver [36]. These IGF-mediated pathways all appear to be fundamentally involved in the metastatic formation.

## Liver Metastases and Tumor Angiogenesis

Once a tumor ascertains an invasive phenotype in the organ of metastasis, it must establish its own neovascular blood supply. Amplified vascularity may allow not only an increase in tumor growth but also a better chance of hematogenous tumor embolization. Preliminary work in this field was based on a simple model in which a tumor cell would secrete a soluble factor that would bind to an endothelial cell receptor and induce proliferation. Current models suggest that angiogenesis is dependent upon the balance among stimulatory and inhibitory molecules (Table 1). Numerous angiogenic growth factors contributing to metastases formation have been identified in colon cancer.

**Table 1: Endogenous Stimulatory and Inhibitory Angiogenic Factors.**

| Stimulatory | Inhibitory |
|---|---|
| • Acidic FGF | Angiostatin |
| • Basic FGF | Endostatin |
| • Angiogenin | Vasculostatin |
| • Hepatocyte growth factor | Interferon α, β, γ |
| • IL-8 | IP-10 |
| • Placenta growth factor | Platelet factor 4 |
| • Platelet-derived endothelial cell growth factor | Prolactin fragment |
| • Transforming growth factor-α, β | Thrombospondin-1,2 |
| • Tumor necrosis factor-α | TIMP |
| • Vascular endothelial growth factor/Vascular permeability factor | Others |
| • Others | |

## Vascular Endothelial Growth Factor

Vascular endothelial growth factor (VEGF) is the best-characterized angiogenic effector molecule. VEGF is known to be upregulated in CRC, and the relationship of VEGF level with the metastatic potential of primary colon cancers and with overall patient survival has been well documented. Takahashi *et al.* used immunohistochemical techniques to analyze human colon cancer and adenoma specimens for Factor VIII (blood vessel counts), VEGF and basic fibroblast growth factor levels [37]. VEGF and VEGF-receptors were present in greater amounts in metastatic than nonmetastatic tumors, and correlated directly with the extent of neovascularization and degree of proliferation. Vessel counts were higher in metastatic tumors than non-metastatic tumors.

In a subsequent paper, VEGF and vessels counts were assessed for their ability to serve as prognostic markers in patients with node-negative colon cancer [38]. Patients in this study were not given adjuvant chemotherapy and were observed for a minimum of 5 years. Relatively low vessel counts correlated with a more favorable prognosis and high vessels counts were associated with disease recurrence. Patients whose tumors had low VEGF expression had a significantly improved survival rate than did patients with elevated VEGF expression. These and other studies support the importance of vessel counts and VEGF expression in colorectal metastases [39].

## Thrombospondin

Thrombospondin (TSP), a high molecular weight (450kDa) multifunctional glycoprotein, and is an anti-angiogenic protein that regulates cell-cell and cell-substratum interactions. TSP was initially characterized as a product of platelets released in response to thrombin activation. TSP is present in the ECM of a wide assortment of tissues and contains binding sites for numerous ECM- and cell-associated molecules. TSP is synthesized and secreted by endothelial cells, fibroblasts, smooth muscle cells, monocytes, macrophages, megakaryocytes, in addition to neoplastic cells. TSP, under defined conditions, can inhibit endothelial cell growth and adhesion on a fibronectin matrix.

Of the 5 subtypes of TSP (TSP-1 to -5), TSP-1 and TSP-2 have been implicated in the *inhibition* of angiogenesis. The intact TSP-1 molecule has been shown to induce apoptosis in endothelial cells [40]. Tomii *et al.* cloned and transfected human TSP-2 cDNA into the SW-480 CRC cell line [41]. Over-expression of TSP-2 cDNA did not affect proliferation of SW-480 cells. However, these TSP-2-transfectants were subsequently added to culture containing bovine pulmonary microvascular endothelial cells (BPMEC), the BPMEC proliferation was significantly inhibited. Tomii's results suggest that TSP-2 is a potential inhibitor of angiogenesis. Tokunaga *et al.* used reverse-transcriptase polymerase chain reaction and immunohistochemical techniques to investigate the significance of TSP-1, TSP-2, $VEGF_{189}$ and CD34 in colon cancer [42]. Among 61 CRC specimens, 38 were positive for TSP-2 expression; the incidence of hepatic metastasis in these patients was much lower than that in patients whose tumors did not express TSP-2. These results suggest that primary tumors expressing TSP may have a better prognosis and that an equilibrium between pro- and anti-angiogenic factors may determine whether primary tumors are able to form liver metastases.

## Angiopoietins

Angiopoietins (Ang's) comprise a novel family of angiogenic factors that are ligands for the endothelium specific tyrosine kinase receptor Tie-2 [43]. Of the four currently known Ang's (Ang-1 to Ang-4), Ang-1 and Ang-2 are the best characterized. Ang-1 helps to maintain and stabilize mature vessels by promoting interaction between endothelial cells and surrounding support cells [43]. It is likely that Ang-1 works in combination with VEGF to help stabilize the neovascular networks. Ang-2 is expressed at sites of vascular remodeling and is believed to antagonize the stabilizing action of Ang-1. In the presence of VEGF, vessel destabilization by Ang-2 has been hypothesized to induce an angiogenic response; however, in the absence of VEGF, Ang-2 leads to vessel regression and endothelial cell apoptosis.

Angiopoietins have also been implicated in facilitating hepatic metastases formation. In contrast to the prevailing view that tumors and metastases begin as an avascular mass, Holash *et al.* have performed studies to suggest that metastases initially grow by co-opting existing vasculature [44]. This co-opted host vasculature does not immediately undergo angiogenesis to support the tumor but instead regresses, leading to a secondarily avascular tumor and massive tumor cell loss. Ultimately, the remaining tumor is rescued by robust angiogenesis at the tumor margin secondary to increased VEGF expression due to hypoxia. The secretions patterns of Ang-1 and Ang-2 help mediate this balance between vascular regression and growth.

Ahmad *et al.* also demonstrated the expression of Ang-1 and Ang-2 by colorectal hepatic metastases [43]. Immunofluorescent staining of colorectal hepatic metastases revealed the presence of Ang-2 protein in cancer epithelium, but Ang-1 was not expressed in tumors. This suggests that the net gain of Ang-2 activity is possibly an initiating factor for tumor angiogenesis and may aid in hepatic metastases formation.

## LIVER METASTASES AND APOPTOSIS

Another mechanism by which colorectal liver metastases survive in the new microenvironment is by avoiding the process of apoptosis. Apoptosis was initially described as a physiologic process of cellular suicide or "programmed cell death." Apoptosis is vital for normal homeostasis and the apoptotic machinery is present in almost all eukaryotic cells. The activation of death-inducing factors or the withdrawal of surviving factors can trigger apoptosis. A complex balance of pro- and anti-apoptotic factors regulates this process. Colorectal liver metastases cells can exploit these factors to bypass the normal pathways that would trigger defective cells to undergo apoptosis. The up-regulation of anti-apoptotic genes and the down-regulation of proapoptotic genes are mechanisms to avoid apoptosis. An alteration in the Bcl-2 family of proteins, a major apoptosis-regulatory protein family, often occurs in cancers.

During the adenoma to carcinoma transition, decreased levels of apoptosis have been associated with expression of mutant p53, demonstating a lack of function of this protein believed to be involved in the regulation of apoptosis and cell cycle arrest. Numerous groups have studied the expression of Bcl-2 family members during colon tumorigenesis. Bcl-$X_L$ overexpression has been observed in colon adenocarcinoma and in some adenomas, implying that up-regulation of Bcl-$X_L$ is a relatively early event in adenoma to carcinoma transition. Bcl-2 expression, however, decreases during progression [45]. Decreased expression of the pro-apoptotic gene Bak also may be associated with tumor progression.

Once colon cancer cells gain access to the circulation, they must be able to survive until they arrest in the liver or other distant organs. This requires the establishment of extracellular matrix-independent survival and resistance to anoikis. Anoikis, or detachment-induced apoptosis, is a normal physiologic mechanism discovered in epithelial cells that were experimentally dissociated from their ECM [46]. The physiologic process prevents normal cells from colonizing at ectopic sites. Resistance to anoikis is required for metastatic formation. Berman *et al.* have evaluated rates of anoikis in paired colon cancer cell lines SW620 and SW480 [47]. The metastatic cell line SW620 had significantly increased anchorage-independent survival after 24, 48 and 72 hours when contrasted to the nonmetastatic cell line SW480. The resistance to anoikis in detachment conditions suggests a survival advantage for potentially malignant cells.

# Biologically Based Treatment of Liver Metastases

## Anti-VEGF therapy

It is clear that angiogenesis is vital for both tumor growth and metastases formation. This fact has led to an enormous research effort in an attempt to discover anti-angiogenesis compounds. However, angiogenesis is not only a pathologic process, but is also crucial for homeostasis. Physiologic angiogenesis is important in reproduction, wound healing, menses, as well as a compensatory response to ischemia in coronary artery and peripheral vascular disease. Thus, therapeutic efficacy of anti-angiogenic therapy requires equilibrium where angiogenesis in tumors is inhibited without interrupting physiologic angiogenesis.

Warren *et al.* first reported on the effects of VEGF monoclonal antibody (mAb) on the growth of colorectal hepatic metastases [48]. Treatment with these mAbs significantly decreased the growth of several human colon cancer cell lines in the livers of nude mice, when compared to mice treated with isotopic control antibody. An analogous strategy may be utilized for anti-VEGF receptor antibodies. DC101 (Imclone, Brooklyn, NY), a monoclonal antibody directed against VEGFR-2 (KDR) has been shown to inhibit angiogenesis, EC survival and VEGF-mediated ascites formation in a murine model of colon cancer carcinomatosis [49].

This same antibody, Bevacizumab (Genentech, San Francisco, CA) has also been involved in clinical trials. Kabbinavar *et al.* reported intriguing results from a phase II trial comparing bevacizumab plus 5-FU/leucovorin versus 5FU/leucovorin alone in the treatment of metastatic CRC [50]. Compared with the control arm, treatment with bevacizumab plus 5-FU/leucovorin resulted in higher response rates, longer median time to disease progression and longer median survival. In a subsequent phase III trial, bevacizumab plus irinotecan/5-FU/leucovorin (IFL) was demonstrated to be more effective than a standard IFL chemotherapy regimen [51]. In this report, Hurwitz *et al.* documented median survival of 20.3 months in the patients given bevacizumab/IFL compared to 15.6 months in the control group. In the experimental group, the median time to disease progression was longer (10.6 months versus 6.2 months, p value<0.00001). Those patients receiving bevacizumab/IFL demonstrated a better response to treatment (44.9%) than IFL chemotherapy alone (34.7%) (Table 2).

**Table 2: Summary of Bevacizumab Plus Standard Chemotherapy Compared to Standard Chemotherapy Only.**

| Survival and Response rates | IFL/Placebo (n=412) | IFL/BV (n=403) | P value |
|---|---|---|---|
| Median Survival (months) | 15.6 | 20.3 | 0.00003 |
| Progression-free survival | 6.24 | 10.6 | <0.00001 |
| Objective response | 35% | 45% | 0.0029 |
| Duration of response (months) | 7.1 | 10.4 | 0.0014 |

## Tissue Inhibitors of Metalloproteinases

TIMPs serve to balance MMP activity in physiologic processes. The synthetic MMP inhibitor, BB-94 (British Biotech, Oxford, UK), is an example of a peptidomimetic and has been used to study the effects in colon cancer. BB-94 (Batimastat) is a pseudopeptide derivative that mimics the MMP substrate. In experimental studies, human CRC lines were injected systemically or into the peritoneal cavity of nude mice followed by treatment with Batimastat. Batimastat significantly reduced the number of liver tumors compared with control vehicle treatment [44]. Results of early clinical trials using MMP inhibitors have been disappointing; however, these trials were conducted in patients with advanced disease when metastases and invasion had already occurred [45]. It may, however, prove more useful for patients in the adjuvant setting.

## Inhibitors of Epidermal Growth Factor

Clinical phase I/II trials using anti-EGFR strategies have also shown promising results. Saltz *et al.* have reported on the use of IMC-C225, a chimeric monoclonal antibody that binds selectively to EGFR with high affinity, competes for ligand binding, and down-regulates receptor expression on the cell-surface. In this particular study, IMC-C225 was used in combination with CPT-11 (Irinotecan) chemotherapy in patients with refractory and advanced CRCs, many of whom had liver metastases [54]. Dose limiting toxicities attributable to IMC-C225 were minor. Twenty-one patients (17%) achieved a partial response, and an additional 37 patients (31%) had stable disease or minor responses.

## Inhibitors of Cyclooxygenase

Another biologic strategy that has received considerable attention has been inhibition of the cyclooxygenase-2 (COX-2) enzyme. Several previous studies suggest that nonsteroidal anti-inflammatory drugs (NSAIDS) can prevent the development of colorectal cacrcinoma in humans. One of the targets of NSAIDS is the COX-2 enzyme, which catalyzes the conversion of arachidonic acid to prostaglandin $H_2$ ($PGH_2$). $PGH_2$ may in turn upregulate the expression of VEGF. Preclinical studies have demonstrated the role of COX-2 in CRC growth, angiogenesis and liver metastases formation. Chen *et al.* studied COX-2 expression in primary CRC, metastatic hepatic lesions and corresponding adjacent normal mucosa [55]. Immunoblot-detectable COX-2 expression was significantly higher in metastatic liver lesions when compared with the corresponding primary colon cancer. Other researchers have found similar results [56]. These results suggest that investigation of the effect of selective COX-2 inhibition on metastatic growth may be indicated. Clinical trials using COX-2 inhibition for the treatment of liver metastases are currently on-going.

## Summary

The elucidation of the interaction of the tumor and its microenvironment has increased surgeons' understanding of the biologic mechanisms regulating metastases development. The capability to develop effective biologic therapies will depend on understanding the complex interactions among endothelial and tumor cells. Biologic therapies must be directed to both the primary site and metastatic focus. By the time metastases form, most steps in the metastatic cascade have been completed. Therapy to down-regulate or interrupt the last stages of metastases, proliferation, angiogenesis and other mechanisms to disrupt cell survival appear to be the most promising areas of clinical research.

## References

[1] Butler TP and Gullino P. Quantitation of cell shedding into efferent blood vessels of mammary adenocarcinoma. *Cancer Res.* **1975**;35:512.

[2] Koretz K, Schlag P, Boumsell L, et al. Expression of VLA-alpha 2, VLA-alpha 6, and VLA-beta 1 chains in normal mucosa and adenomas of the colon, and in colon carcinomas and their liver metastases. *Am J Pathol.* **1991**;138:741-5.

[3] Pignatelli M, Smith ME and Bodnar WF. Low expression of collagen receptors in moderate and poorly differentiated colorectal adenocarcinomas. *Br J Cancer.* **1990**;61:636-8.

[4] Wong NA and Pignatelli M. Beta-catenin—a linchpin for colorectal carcinogenesis. *Am J Pathol.* **2002**;160:389-401.

[5] Raftopoulos I, Davaris P, Karatzas G, et al. Levels of α-catenin expression in colorectal cancer correlates with invasiveness, metastatic potential and survival. *J Surg Oncol.* **1998**;68:92-9.

[6] St-Pierre Y. Dissemination of T-cell lymphoma to target ogans: a post-homing event implicating ICAM-1 and matrix metalloproteinases. *Leuk Lymphoma.* **1999**;34:53.

[7] Benchimol S, Fuks A, Jothy S, et al. Carcinoembryonic antigen, a human tumor marker, functions as an intracellular adhesion molecule. *Cell.* **1989**;57:327-34.

[8] Jessup JM, Ishii S, Mitzoi T, et al. Carcinoembryonic antigen facilitates experimental metastasis through a mechanism that does not involve adhesion to liver cells. *Clin Exp Metastasis.* **1999**;17:481-8.

[9] Tanabe KK, Ellis LM and Saya H. Expression of CD44R1 adhesion molecule in colon carcinomas and metastases. *Lancet.* **1993**;341:725-6.

[10] Coulombe J and Pelletier G. Gangliosides and organ-specific metastatic colonization. *Int J Cancer.* **1993**;53:104-9.

[11] Irimura T, Nakamori S, Matsushita Y, et al. Colorectal cancer metastasiis determined by carbohydrate-mediated cell adhesion: role of sialyl-Le$^x$ antigens. *Semin Cancer Biol.* **1993**;4:319-24.

[12] Gutman M and Fidler IJ. Biology of human colon cancer metastasis. *World J Surg.* **1995**;19:226-34.

[13] McCawley LJ and Matrisian LM. Matrix metalloproteinases: they're not just for matrix anymore. *Curr Opin Cell Biol.* **2001**;13:534-40.

[14] Zucker S and Vacirca J. Role of matrix metalloproteinases (MMPs) in colorectal cancer. *Cancer and Met Rev.* **2004**;23:101-17.

[15] Matrisian LM, Wright J, Newell K, et al. Matrix-degrading metalloproteinases in tumor progression. *Princess Takamatsu Symp.* **1994**;24:153-61.

[16] Masaki T, Matsuoka H, Sugiyama H, et al. Matrilysin (MMP-7) as a significant determinant of malignant potential of early invasive colorectal carcinomas. *Br J Cancer.* **2001**;10:1317-21.

[17] Wilson CL, Heppner KJ, Labonsky PA, et al. Intestinal tumorigenesis is suppressed in mice lacking the metalloproteinase matrilysin. *PNAS.* **1997**;94:1402-7.

[18] Kleiner DE and Stetler-Stevenson G. Matix metalloproteinases and metastasis. *Cancer Chemother Pharmacol.* **1999**;43:S42.

[19] Roeb D, Dietrich CG, Winograd R, et al. Activity and cellular origin of gelatinases in patients with colon and rectal carcinoma differential activity of matrix metalloproteinase-9. *Cancer.* **2001**;92:2680-2691.

[20] Ogata Y, Miura K, Ohkita A, et al. Imbalance between matrix metalloproteinase-9 aand tissue inhibitor of metalloproteinase-1 expression by tumor cells implicated in liver metastases from colorectal carcinoma. *Kurume Med J.* **2001**;48:211-8.

[21] Joo YE, Seo KS, Kim HS, et al. Role of tissue inhibitors of metalloproteinases (TIMPs) in colorectal carcinoma. *J Korean Med Sci.* **1999**;14:417-23.

[22] Fujii T, Obara T, Tanno S, et al. Urokinase-type plasminogen activator and plasminogen activator inhibitor-1 as a prognostic factor in human colorectal carcinomas. *Hepatogastroenterology.* **1999**;46:2299-308.

[23] Wang Y, Liang X, Wu S, et al. Inhibition of colon cancer metastases by a 3'-end antisense urokinase receptor mRNA in a nude mouse model. *Int J Cancer.* **2001**;92:257-62.

[24] Hiscox SE, Hallett MB, Puntis MCA, et al. Expression of the HGF/SF receptor, c-met, and its ligand in human colorectal cancers. *Cancer Invest.* **1997**;15:513-21.

[25] Herynk MH, Tsan R, Radinsky R and Gallick GE. Activation of c-met in colorectal carcinoma cells leads to constitutive association of tyrosine-phosphorylated β-catenin. *Clin Exp Met.* **2003**;20:291-300.

[26] Fujita S and Sugano K. Expression of c-met proto-oncogene in primary colorectal cancer and liver metastases. *Jpn J Clin Oncol.* **1997**;27:378-83.

[27] DiRenzo MF, Olivero M, Giacomini A, et al. Overexpression and amplification of the Met/HGF receptor gene during the progression of colorectal cancer. *Clin Cancer Res.* **1995**;1:147-54.

[28] Markowitz SD, Molkentin K, Gerbic C, et al. Growth stimulation by coexpression of transforming growth factor-α and epidermal growth factor receptor in normal and adenomatous human colon epithelium. *J Clin Invest.* **1990**;86:356.

[29] Suzuki E, Ota T, Tsukuda K, et al. *nm23-H1* reduces *in vitro* cell migration and the liver metastatic potential of colon cancer cells by regulating myosin light chain phosphorylation. *Int J Cancer.* **2004**;108:207-11.

[30] Radinsky R, Risin S, Fan D, et al. Level and function of epidermal growth factor receptor predict the metastatic potential of human colon carcinoma cells. *Cancer Res.* **1998**;58:3101-4.

[31] Parker C, Roseman BJ, Bucana CD, et al. Preferential activation of the epidermal growth receptor in human colon carcinoma liver metastases in nude mice. *J Histochem Cytochem*. **1998**;46:595-602.

[32] Singh P and Rubin N. Insulin like growth factors and binding proteins in colon cancer. *Gastroenterology*. **1993**;105:1218-37.

[33] Feier S, Weiss O, Eran M, et al. Expression of the insulin-like growth factors and their receptors in adenocarcinoma of the colon. *Gut*. **1999**;44:704-8.

[34] Remacle-Bonnet MM, Garrouste FL, Heller S, et al. Insulin-like growth factor-I protects colon cancer cells from death-induced apoptosis by potentiating tumor necrosis factor alpha-induced mitogen-activated protein kinase and nuclear factor kappaB signaling pathways. *Cancer Res*. **2000**;60:2007-17.

[35] Koenuma M, Yamori T and Tsuruo T. Insulin and insulin-like growth factor-I stimulate proliferation of metastatic variants of colon carcinoma. *Jpn J Cancer Res*. **1989**;80:51-8.

[36] Reinmuth N, Liu W, Fan F, et al. Blockade of insulin-like growth factor receptor-I function inhibits growth and angiogenesis of colon cancer. *Clin Cancer Res*. **2002**;10:3259-69.

[37] Takahasi Y, Kitadai Y, Bucana CD, Cleary KR, Ellis LM: Expression of vascular endothelial growth factor and its receptor, KDR, correlates with vascularity, metastasis and proliferation of human colon cancer. *Cancer Res.* **1995**;55:3964-8.

[38] Takahashi Y, Tucker SI, Kitadai Y, et al. Vessel counts and expression of vaqscular endothelial growth factor as a prognostic factor in node negative colon cancer. *Arch. Surg*. **1997**;132:541-6.

[39] Kang SM, Maeda K, Chung YS, et al. Vascular endothelial growth factor expression correlates with hematogenous metastasis and prognosis in colorectal carcinoma. *Oncol Rep*. **1997**;4:381-4.

[40] Guo N, Krutzsch HC, Inman JK and Roberts DD. Thrombospondin-1 and type I repeat peptides of thrombospondin-1 specifically induce apoptosis of endothelial cells. *Cancer Res*. **1997**;57:1735-42..

[41] Tomii Y, Kamochi J, Yamazaki H, et al. Human thrombospondin-2 inhibits proliferation of microvascular endothelial cells. *Int J Onc*. **2002**;20:339-42.

[42] Tokunaga T, Nakamura M, Oshika Y et al. Thrombospondin 2 expression is correlated with inhibition of angiogenesis and metastasis of colon cancer. *Br J Cancer* **1999**;79:354-9.

[43] Ahmad SA, Wenbiao L, Jung YD et al. Differential expression of angiopoietin-1 and angiopoietin-2 in colon carcinoma: a possible mechanism for the initiation of angiogenesis. *Cancer* **2001**;92:1138-43.

[44] Holash J, Masonpierre PC, Compton D, et al. Vessel co-option, regression, and growth in tumors mediated by angiopoietins and VEGF. *Science*. **1999**;2841994-1998.

[45] Berman RS, Portera CA and Ellis LM. Biology of liver metastases. In: Talamonti M, editor. Liver-directed therapy for primary and metastatic lung tumors. **2001**. p. 1-29.

[46] Frisch SM and Francis H. Disruption of epithelial cell-matrix interactions induces apoptosis. *J Cell Biol.* **1994**;124:619-26.

[47] Berman RS, Sweeney B and McConkey DJ. Metatstatic colorectal cells are resistant to anoikis, inducing Akt phosphorylation (A2162). Proceedinga of the 90th annual meeting of the American Association for Cancer Research. *New Orleans (LA):Annual Cancer Society*; **1999**;40:326.

[48] Warren RS, Yuan H, Malti MR, et al. Regulation by vascular endothelial growth factor of human colon cancer tumorigenesis in a mouse model of experimental liver metastasis. *J Clin Invest.* **1995**;95:1789-97.

[49] Shaheen RM, Ahmad SA, Liu W, et al. Inhibited growth of colon cancer carcinomatosis by antibodies to vascular endothelial and epidermal growth factor receptors. *Br J Cancer.* **2001**;85:584-9.

[50] Kabbinavar F, Hurwitz HI, Fehrenberger L, et al. Phase II, randomized trial comparing bevacizumab plus fluoruracil (FU)/leucovorin (LV) with FU/LV alone in patients with metastatic colorectal cancer. *J Clin Oncol.* **2003**;21:60-5.

[51] Hurwitz H, Fehrenbacher L, Cartwright T *et al.*: Bevacizumab (a monoclonal antibody to VEGF) prolongs survival in first-line colorectal cancer (CRC): Results of a phase III trial of bevacizumab in combination with bolus IFL (irinotecan, 5-fluorouracil, leucovorin) as first-line therapy in subjects with metastatic CRC. *Am Soc Clin Oncol.* (2003) **22**:3646 (Abstract).

[52] Watson SA, Morris TM, Robinson G, et al. Inhibition of organ invasion by the matrix metalloproteinase inhibitor batimastat (BB-94) in two human colon carcinoma metastasis models. *Cancer Res.* **1995**;55:3629-33.

[53] Bramhall SR, Rosemurgy A, Brown C, et al. Marimastat as firstline therapy for patients with unresectable pancreatic cancer: a randomized trial. *J Clin Oncol.* **2001**;19:3447-55.

[54] Saltz LB, Cox JV, Blanke C, et al. Irinotecan plus fluorouracil and leucovorin for metastatic colorectal cancer. Irinotecan study group. *New Eng J Med.* **2000**;343:905-14.

[55] Chen WS, Wei SJ, Liu JM, et al. Tumor invasivenss and liver metastasis of colon cancer cells correlated with cyclooxygenase-2 (COX-2) expression and inhibited by a COX-2-selective inhibitor, etodolac. *Int J Cancer.* **2001**;91:894-9.

[56] Hull MA, Fenwick SW, Chapple KS, et al. Cyclooxygease-2 expression in colorectal cancer liver metastases. *Clin Exp Metastasis.* **2000**;1821-7.

In: Liver Cancer: New Research
Editor: Felix Lee, pp. 59-78

ISBN 1-59454-182-5


*Chapter III*

# Colorectal Cancer Liver Metastases Destruction or Resection?

***Salvatore Gruttadauria[1] and Zakiyah Kadry[2]***
(1) University of Pittsburgh Medical Center European Medical Division
(IsMeTT-UPMC) Istituto Mediterraneo per i Trapianti e Terapie ad Alta Specializzazione
(2) Thomas E Starzl Transplantation Institute
University of Pittsburgh Medical Center

## Abstract

Treatment of metastatic colorectal cancer to the liver has evolved over the past decade. Although surgical resection remains the gold standard, only 15% to 20% of newly diagnosed patients are candidates for curative resection [1]. To extend indications for curative treatment of 'unresectable' colorectal liver metastases, other therapeutic modalities are being developed such as loco regional chemotherapy with tumor 'down staging', two stage liver resections after portal vein embolization and the use of loco-regional ablative therapy. Within the latter category, radio frequency thermal ablation (RFA) has recently gained popularity with reported early survival results equivalent to liver resection in selected cases using either percutaneous image-guided, laparoscopic or open radio frequency thermo ablation techniques. Published reports have shown an overall survival in the range of 67% at 2 years and 33% at 3 years respectively [2]. These results however, are hampered by the short follow up period in the majority of cases and are generally reported in conjunction with RFA of other tumor types.

In patients with 'operable' colorectal cancer liver metastases, there are no randomized clinical trials that demonstrate improvement in survival after thermal ablation. In patients with resectable disease, liver resection survival rates at one–, two-, three- and four-years are 90%, 62%, 48% and 40% respectively [3], and with improved patient selection using preoperative tests such as PET scan the actuarial survival rate after liver resection has been reported to be 77% at 3 years [4]. Although radio frequency thermal ablation of colorectal liver metastases has many advantages, primarily related to decreased morbidity and reduced costs using a laparoscopic or percutaneous approach compared to surgical resection, there are few reports of 5-year survivors as compared to 30% to 40% 5-year survival after surgical resection. A critical appraisal of the reported data in the English literature does not at present suggest a role for radio frequency thermal ablation in the treatment of resectable hepatic metastases from colorectal cancer. There does appear to be an indication however for its use in specific situations such as in combination with hepatic resection in patients with marginal liver function or small residual liver volume precluding a complete R0 resection, in unresectable multiple bilateral liver only metastases within a multimodal clinical research protocol, with unresectable local liver only tumor recurrences after resection, and in patients judged to carry too high a risk to undergo a surgical resection.

The purpose of this review is to underline the role of liver resection as the first line therapy in the management of hepatic metastatic colorectal cancer within the context of an increasing utilization of new treatment modalities such as the thermal ablative therapy, which has not yet been completely evaluated in the long term. A review of the published literature as well as a discussion on the effect of RFA on liver function, per operative lactate production and the impact on residual liver functional reserve are presented [5].

## List of Abbreviations

| | |
|---|---|
| RFA: | Radiofrequency thermal ablation |
| FDG-PET: | 18 Fluoro-2-deoxy-D-glucose Positron Emission Tomography |
| IOUS: | Intra-operative Ultrasound |
| MRI: | Magnetic Resonance Imaging |

## Introduction

Colorectal carcinoma is the fourth most common tumor worldwide [6-7]. In the United States there are approximately 150,000 new cases diagnosed annually of which 30,000 progress to develop hepatic metastases [8]. In Italy there are 28,000 new cases with 18,000 deaths per year from colorectal tumors [9]. It is estimated that 8-10% of tumor deaths world wide are attributable to colorectal cancer, many of which have hepatic involvement [3, 7].

The liver, after lymph node involvement, is the most frequent site of distant metastases from colorectal cancer [10-11]. It is the first major organ cancer cells reach through the splanchnic circulation. Such metastases are classified by the AJCC staging system as stage IV disease [12] and their surgical treatment was previously considered not feasible [13]. Autopsy studies however have since demonstrated that the liver is often the only metastatic site from primary colorectal cancer [14]. This subsequently led to the development of surgical resection as a viable and potentially curative treatment option in isolated hepatic metastases [3]. In general, the prognosis of patients with untreated colorectal liver metastases is poor, with a 5 year survival rate of 0-2% [15-16]. Although the median survival time of a patient with untreated colorectal liver metastases is generally quoted as being less than 1 year, the overall survival is dependant on several prognostic factors [17]. Extent of extra hepatic disease, the total number of liver metastases and the degree of liver involvement seem to be particularly important. For unresected single liver lesions the median survival is approximately 15 to 20 months as compared to only 3 months in widespread bilobar disease [19]. Synchronous liver metastases are present in 15%-25% percent of patients when colorectal cancer is initially diagnosed. Metachronous development of liver metastases occurs in approximately 40% per cent of patients after diagnosis of the primary tumor [18]. Synchronous liver metastases are frequently quoted as being a worse prognostic factor after liver resection as compared to metachronous hepatic lesions [3]. Median survival in patients with untreated synchronous liver metastases is reported to range between 6.6 to 11 months [19].

In the last two decades there have been numerous studies showing long-term survival of up to 20 years after liver resection of colorectal liver metastases [20-36]. More than 23 single institutions have reported in the past 25 years individual series exceeding 100 patients who underwent liver resection for this disease [37] with 5 year survivals ranging from 18% to 46%. At present no equally successful treatment exists as an alternative to liver resection, which represents the gold standard to which any other treatment modality needs to be compared. [3].Unfortunately, a major limitation is the fact that few patients with colorectal liver metastases are candidates for liver resection. Only 15% to 20% of patients are resectable either due to unfavorable tumor biology, lesion number and location or patient co-morbidities. Moreover, despite careful patient selection and improvements in surgical expertise, with emphasis being placed on achieving adequate negative resection margins, approximately two thirds of these patients subsequently develop cancer relapse, which in 30% to 50% is limited to the residual liver. In such cases of local liver recurrence, repeat resections have been advocated, however more recently there has been a shift towards the use of loco regional ablative therapy as only 25% to 30% are amenable to surgery [38]. There are two multi-institutional series reporting 32% and 16% 5 year survival respectively after re-resection in patients with isolated intra-hepatic recurrence [39,13] and up to 74% 5 year survival in a single institution report [40]. Despite these results however, there has been a trend towards the implementation of local ablative therapy using thermal energy especially when re-resection is technically difficult or evaluated as not possible [2, 7, 17, 38].

In the treatment of unresectable hepatic colorectal metastases, several interstitial ablative techniques have shown promising results. Of these methods the most experience has been accumulated with radiofrequency and cryotherapy. Radiofrequency however is associated with fewer complications hence the increasing interest in this technique. Radio frequency thermal ablation (RFA) is a localized thermal treatment technique designed to destroy tumor cells by heating the tissue to temperatures that exceed 50° C. Its mechanism of action involves the conversion of a radio frequency alternating electrical current into thermal energy which is localized to the targeted tissue [5]. RFA has recently gained popularity with reports of early survival equivalent to liver resection in selected cases using either percutaneous image-guided, laparoscopic or open techniques. The overall survival in one report being in the range of 67% at 2 years and 33% at 3 years respectively [2]. These results however are still early and are hampered by the short follow up period quoted in many other publications, variable patient selection criteria relating to the inability to perform a resection, and have generally involved grouping of RFA of several tumor types including colorectal liver metastases in spite of differing disease natural histories [17].

The purpose of this review is to present the basic principles of RFA with an assessment of its role in the treatment of metastatic colorectal cancer to the liver. The literature relating to its application in the treatment of unresectable liver lesions, and its reported effectiveness in comparison with liver resection for the treatment of the resectable lesions will be discussed.

## Indications for Radiofrequency Thermal Ablation in Colorectal Liver Metastases

Although RFA is being widely implemented for the ablation of liver tumors there are at present no clear cut clinical indications for its use in the treatment of colorectal cancer hepatic metastases. Its curative role remains unproven and as such it should be reserved for patients with unresectable disease or patients with severe co morbidities that preclude a liver resection. Definition of non resectability includes multifocal bilateral liver lobe lesions, proximity to major vascular and/or biliary strictures, or large lesions where the required extent of the resection is not compatible with patient survival. Within these categories, large diameter lesions and proximity to major vascular &/or biliary structures can also be a limitation for RFA. The combination of RFA and formal hepatic resection however may allow an extension of the indications for surgery in patients with extensive metastatic disease who would not otherwise be candidates for resection. Another approach in situations where surgical options are limited is either systemic or intrahepatic regional chemotherapy with the aim of downstaging the tumor mass to a volume where resection with or without RFA can be performed [44-47].

Although like other ablative modalities, RFA has been mainly used for unresectable colorectal hepatic metastases, the ideal lesions for thermal ablation are smaller then 5 cm in diameter and preferably smaller then 3 cm in diameter [48]. The size limitation is based on the diameter of the thermal injury that can be produced by a single ablation although larger lesions have been treated with multiple ablations with an increased risk of incomplete ablation and tumor recurrence [49]. The saline perfused electrode produced by RITA systems is also reportedly able to produce ablation of lesions up to 7 cm [50]. Published series of percutaneous RFA in colorectal liver metastases have included a very heterogeneous patient population ranging from extensive hepatic tumor involvement to single or two lesions of less than 5 cm diameter confined to one liver lobe [49]. This heterogeneity in tumor types has made evaluation of local recurrence rates and overall survival after RFA difficult to interpret.

Margin negative resections of metastatic colorectal cancer to the liver may not be possible due to proximity to major blood vessels and bile ducts. This however is also a limitation in RFA because of the 'heat sink'effect [51]. Blood flow away from the area of ablation can result in ineffective ablation with a zone of spared tumor close to larger blood vessels, hence blood vessels can be considered to act as a 'heat sink'. This effect was studied by Lu et al who noted that vessels smaller than 3 mm near the area of ablation thrombosed whereas those greater than 3 mm were not injured and maintained flow during RFA [52] As a method of overcoming this heat sink effect, several studies in animals have demonstrated that coagulative necrosis is enhanced when inflow occlusion is performed [50-51, 53-56]. On the other hand, the potential for thrombosis and injury to adjacent vessels is increased when a concomitant inflow occlusion is performed. Acute thrombosis with cavernomatous transformation of the portal vein has been reported after percutaneous thermoablation of a liver metastasis emphasizing that RFA can cause thermally mediated damage of vascular structures even without inflow occlusion [57]. For large bile ducts RFA can also cause severe injury, consequently RFA of centrally located large metastases near the hilum should be avoided. Dominique et al have recently described intraductal cooling during RFA in 3 patients to prevent biliary injury or strictures [58]. This experience is of course limited and raises questions as to the adequacy of tumor ablation close to the biliary tree during intraductal cooling. No follow up is available on this limited series hence the efficacy of this manouever requires further study and follow up.

RFA has been implemented in special situations of marginal liver function where it may or may not be combined with a limited hepatic resection, as well as in situations where the future residual liver volume may preclude a complete R0 resection. Other appropriate indications for RFA include its use within a multimodal clinical research protocol involving 'unresectable' colorectal liver metastases, and in technically difficult local liver only tumor recurrences after resection. Patients judged to carry too high a risk to undergo a surgical resection may also be good candidates for percutaneous RFA and there is also the subcategory of patients who refuse surgery in spite of the data available on outcomes after surgical resection. Recently Elias et al reported their results of hepatic resection for colorectal liver metastases in the presence of extra hepatic disease [59], which may also impact on the indications to perform RFA within this context.

Whole body positron emission tomography or FDG PET has been reported to increase the sensitivity of the preoperative diagnosis of colorectal metastases from 70% up to 95% [4]. This has been shown to improve the long term outcome after liver resection for colorectal liver metastases where the actuarial survival rate has been reported to reach 77% at 3 years [4]. There appears to be a better preoperative detection of extrahepatic disease not seen on standard radiological examination [4]. This could also potentially play an important role in the future in RFA where many patients already have extensive intra hepatic tumor involvement and are at high risk for occult extra hepatic disease.

## Methods of Radiofrequency Thermal Ablation in Colorectal Liver Metastasis

Percutaneous RFA has the advantage of avoiding the risks and complications associated with an open operative or laparoscopic procedure, and allows RFA to be performed on an outpatient basis [54]. On the other hand, in selected cases, the surgical approach, whether open or laparoscopic, permits the management of larger lesions, including particularly difficult ones located adjacent to the diaphragm, bowel, or gallbladder [60]. The open or laparoscopic approach also allows a detailed intraoperative ultrasound thus increasing the chance of potential detection of small lesions not previously described in the preoperative CT scan or MRI [61, 65]. In fact complete mobilization of the liver associated with intraoperative ultrasound and, in the case of open surgery, bimanual palpation of the liver have been advocated as methods of reducing the risk of missing smaller liver lesions. It has been clearly shown that the association of conventional imaging plus intraoperative ultrasound is superior to traditional preoperative imaging alone in the detection of occult liver metastases and liver lesions in general. A figure of up to 35% more new lesions has been quoted to have been discovered through intraoperative ultrasound [62, 63]. The rate however of patients operated on for hepatic metastases in whom the operative strategy was modified by intraoperative ultrasound is variable, although the sensitivity of intraoperative ultrasound in the detection of occult liver metastases has been emphasized in several reports (Table1) [64]. With the present literature, it is impossible to evaluate the impact of intraoperative ultrasound when comparing percutaneous versus laparoscopic or open RFA due to the heterogeneity in tumor size and types.

**Table1: Sensitivity of Intraoperative and Preoperative Techniques and Impact of Intraoperative Ultrasound on Hepatectomies.**

| Author | No. Patients | Preoperative CT/MRI % | IOUS % | Surgical Strategy Changes % |
|---|---|---|---|---|
| **Gozzetti et al. 1986 [66]** | 37 | 74 | 98 | 51 |
| **Castaing et al 1986 [67]** | 56 | 66 | 79 | 32 |
| **Parker et al 1989 [68]** | 42 | 77 | 98 | 49 |
| **Staren et al 1997 [69]** | 59 | 67 | 98 | 34 |
| **Conlon et al 2003 [65]** | 80 | NR | * NR+47% | 18 |

* NR=not reported; the authors reported that IOUS gave additional information compared to MRI in 47% of the patients.

Open RFA compared with the laparoscopic approach allows a greater freedom in placement of the ultrasound probe and the radio frequency needle [71]. It also permits the treatment of large unresectable metastases located close to major vessels and biliary structures, and in other anatomical conditions not safely managed through a laparoscopic approach. Inflow occlusion can be used in both open and laparoscopic RFA, which has been shown to enhance the ablative process by minimizing the heat sink effect [72]. It carries however the theoretical risk of large vessel damage and thrombosis and should be implemented with prudence. The percutaneous approach on the other hand has the advantage of reduced cost and is a less invasive procedure although experimental studies do show a better ability to achieve tumor free margins with an open surgical approach [73].

When comparing a percutaneous versus laparoscopic versus open RFA, there is so far no evidence in the literature of any difference in survival outcome using one approach over another, and in the majority of publications the outcomes using these three techniques are reported together. Of course patients with a high co-morbidity who are unable to undergo an open or laparoscopic approach could benefit from a percutaneous RFA technique.

For percutaneous RFA [49,74-75] the patient is sedated or intubated and the thermal probe is inserted into the lesion using a Seldinger method under radiological control, whilst concomitantly avoiding major hepatic vessels. Ultrasound is the most frequently used radiological technique, although CT scan and MRI provide greater tumor delineation and multiplane guidance [17].

Despite the debate over the choice of RFA administration, in situ thermal ablation with radio frequency energy is still achieved in all 3 techniques through the use of electrodes. In the case of a unipolar system, the active electrode is placed through image guidance into the metastasis to be ablated while the second passive electrode is a large electrically conductive pad placed on the thigh of the patient. A radio frequency generator uses an oscillator that converts an alternating current to the appropriate frequency which is emitted from the exposed tip of the active electrode, passing through the intervening tissue to the ground pad. This leads to an ionic agitation, which is then converted by friction into heat and ultimately induces irreparable cellular damage and coagulation necrosis [74]. The ionic agitation and the subsequent heat are directly related to the intensity and duration of the alternating current. The devices which are currently in use are the RITA Medical System, Radiotherapeutics (RITA, Radiotherapeutics/Boston Scientific, Mountain View, CA) and Radionics (Radionics/Valleylab, Boulder, CO). The RITA Medical System and Radiotherapeutics systems use single active electrodes with deployable tines while Radionics uses a triangular array of internally cooled electrodes. The RITA system also has a saline perfusion electrode which projects 9 tines, 5 of which are active and allow saline perfusion. This system is theoretically capable of ablating lesions of up to 7 cm in diameter.

Regardless of the system used, the diameter of the ablation must be 2 cm greater than the tumor sphere in order to achieve at least a 1 cm margin of ablation. The RITA system produces a spherical ablation while the Radiotherapeutics electrode results in a more cylindrical spheroid and the Radionics system causes an elongated sphere. The principles relating to therapeutic curative margins which apply in a liver resection are also implemented in RFA since a 1 cm margin of ablation is recommended. Thus a lesion of 3 cm would require a 5 cm RFA ablation in order to achieve this result, and in lesions greater than 5 cm multiple electrode deployments have been used [50]. For metastases which require several RFA applications, the risk of electrode placement error and recurrence rate are higher [76, 77].

## Impact of Radiofrequency Thermal Ablation on Liver Function

Liver metastasis from colorectal cancer rarely present in cirrhotic liver although very often the surgeon, the interventional radiologist or the oncologist have to deal with a relatively large tumor lesion in a steatotic liver or in liver already damaged by several sessions of systemic chemotherapy. This can be a problem when deciding on a liver resection if the estimated future remnant liver is too small or the overall liver function is marginal or compromised. Liver dysfunction has been reported as a complication of RFA, mainly after treatment of primary tumor on chronically diseased liver [79] and death has occasionally been reported in patients with metastatic disease treated by RFA associated with liver resection [80]. RFA performed concomitantly with liver resection has expanded the number of potentially surgically treatable patients by 20% to 25% [70] although the same authors have reported 3 transient hepatic failures following this combined treatment. As an estimate of the functional hepatic reserve during open RFA, intra operative serum lactate levels were measured in our institution in a group of 10 patients who underwent open RFA for the treatment of unresectable metastatic colorectal liver cancer [5]. The liver plays an important role in lactate clearance and utilization [81,82]. Moreover, in the liver transplant literature, in both cadaveric and living donor procedures, it has been demonstrated that the rate of lactate elimination after reperfusion of the transplanted liver, represents a very sensitive and reliable indicator of liver function [83-85].

**Table 2. Open RFA: Patient Population And Treatment Data in Patients Where Serial Serum Lactate Levels Were Measured. Degree of Tumor Necrosis After RFA (RITA Systems) Was Estimated on CT Scan Performed 2 Days After Surgery.**

| Diagnosis | Age | Sex | N. of lesions | Size of the lesions (cm) | n. of RITA applications | Tumor necrosis after RITA (%) |
|---|---|---|---|---|---|---|
| **CRC Liver Mets** | 76 | M | 1 | 3.6 | 2 | 80 |
| **CRC Liver Mets** | 60 | M | 1 | 11 | 11 | 80 |
| **CRC Liver Mets** | 65 | F | 2 | 6.5; 3 | 7;1 | 80 |
| **CRC Liver Mets** | 55 | M | 7 | 1 | 1 | 100 |
| **CRC Liver Mets** | 67 | F | 3 | 6;3;2 | 5 | 100 |
| **CRC Liver Mets** | 73 | M | 1 | 10 | 18 | 90 |
| **CRC Liver Mets** | 76 | M | 2 | 1,5;5 | 6 | 100 |
| **CRC Liver Mets** | 75 | F | 1 | 5 | 8 | 100 |
| **CRC Liver Mets** | 59 | F | 1 | 4.2 | 3 | 100 |
| **CRC Liver Mets** | 73 | M | 1 | 3 | 3 | 85 |

In the 10 patients suffering from colorectal hepatic metastases in non cirrhotic liver, with an age ranging between 55 and 76 years, arterial lactate levels (mmol/L) were measured prior to probe insertion into the tumor (T0), at the end of open-RFA ablation (T1), after wound closure (T2) and 24 hrs after surgery (T3). Tumor size and number as well as total number of RFA ablations performed are listed in Table 2. Hemodynamic parameters including mean arterial pressure, and central venous pressure, at T0, T1, T2, T3 and the perioperative rate of lactate production were also analyzed. Total bilirubin, transaminases and the international normalized ratio for prothrombin activity (INR) were measured preoperatively and on postoperative days 1, 2, 3 and 7. Data was expressed as mean +/- SD and ANOVA as well as the Duncan post hoc test were used for multiple comparisons of the differences in mean values. A p-value <0.05 was considered significant.

Lactate levels did not increase significantly at the time points specified above (P = NS). Similarly, hemodynamic parameters analyzed did not show any significant change at the different time points (P = NS). Total bilirubin and INR did not demonstrate statistically significant changes at the aforementioned time points. Serum transaminases peaked during the immediate postoperative period and normalized to preoperative values by one-week post surgery. These results were felt to demonstrate that open-RFA does not induce hyperlactatemia and did not significantly reduce the functional residual liver parenchyma in these patients. Within a total group of 141 liver resections performed in the same period in our institution, forty-five were liver resections performed for metastases from colorectal cancer [86] and five of these were performed in association with intraoperative RFA in order to achieve an R0 resection. In the latter group, one patient has since died from recurrent disease at 2.5 years follow up. This approach follows larger series which have been published using RFA in combination with liver resection for the treatment of extensive colorectal metastatic disease in order to achieve radical therapy in patients previously considered inoperable [70,99].

## MONITORING THE EFFECTIVENESS OF RFA TREATMENT FOLLOW-UP AND COMPLICATIONS

No reliable visible signs of the ablated zone are apparent at the time of RFA, in fact the so called "out gassing" sign which is the result of the micro bubble formation visualized as an expanding echogenic blush is not a reliable marker of complete ablation [50] despite its being advocated as such by some groups [88]. Doppler Ultrasound after injection of intravenous contrast medium has recently been reported as being useful for the monitoring of the effectiveness of the RFA ablation [88]. Intra-operative MRI has also been described in the monitoring of the ablation necrosis, although due to the cost and the limited facilities few can acquire the proper expertise [89, 90].

While pathological examination of tumor margins can judge the effectiveness of a liver resection by defining the exact resection margin, the clinical evaluation of the ability to achieve an 'R0 ablation' with RFA is dependant on the absence of local recurrence on long term follow up. As a result a regular radiological follow-up is mandatory and is of paramount importance.

In examining the literature, the majority of centers involved in RFA of hepatic metastases from colorectal cancer perform CT scan with intravenous contrast injection. CT scan performed immediately after ablation is the preferred method of assessment although lately even MRI has been advocated [17]. Zones of residual contrast enhancement correspond to portions of persistent viable tumor. Periodic imaging is mandatory every 3 months in order to detect any signs of recurrence. There are no studies that correlate trends of tumor markers and relapse of disease after ablation of hepatic metastases from colorectal cancer, although a drop in CEA level has been reported in this specific condition [60]. Recently FDG-PET has been described as an effective imaging technique in the surveillance of patients treated with RFA for malignancies of the liver [91].

In the setting of non imaging methods to assess the completeness of intraoperative RFA, several studies have shown that reaching a given target temperature in a predefined period of time can be a good predictor of successful ablation [80, 87]. This concept is used by both RITA and Radiotherapeutics systems, where the temperature of active tines is measured 30 seconds after ablation in the former, and 'roll off' of impedance is used in the latter.

In terms of complications, Solbiati et al. published in 2001 the largest series of patients treated with percutaneous RFA for colorectal liver metastases in which they describe one right colon perforation requiring surgery after treatment with RFA [49]. The reported complication rates after percutaneous, laparoscopic or open RFA for the treatment of liver only metastatic colorectal cancer vary widely within the published literature. Death, hepatic abscess, liver dysfunction, pleural effusion, biliary strictures, bleeding, biliary peritonitis, segmental infarct and grounding pad burn have all been described [92,93].

## Clinical Results of Radiofrequency Ablation

The fact that the major part of published literature on patient series who have undergone RFA treatment pool together primary and secondary hepatic tumors associated with the relatively short-term follow-up make it impossible to evaluate the merits of this technique in the treatment of hepatic colorectal metastases. In fact RFA of hepatocellular carcinoma, neuroendocrine liver metastases, colorectal liver metastases and miscellaneous other liver metastases have been considered and reported together in the early and late publications on this therapy [50].

A study in 2001, by Solbiati et al, reported the long-term results in their series of 117 patients who underwent percutaneous RFA ablation for hepatic colorectal metastases [49]. Two Italian tertiary medical centers were involved in this study and a total of 179 hepatic colorectal tumors were treated. The estimated 1, 2 and 3-year survival rates were 93%, 69%, and 46%, respectively. The percentage of patients with no new metastases after initial treatment at 1 and 2 years were 49% and 35% respectively, while in 39% of the lesions a local recurrence developed after treatment. Frequency and time to local recurrence appeared to be related to tumor size. Their conclusion was that RFA is an effective treatment for hepatic metastases from colorectal carcinoma, and could be considered as an alternative to metastasectomy due to the lower morbidity and cost. Although these results are encouraging, a drawback of this study relates to tumor size and number, with 74 patients (63.2%) presenting a single liver lesion which could potentially have been amenable to liver resection and could have ultimately played a role in the results of this study. The mean diameter of the lesions in this study was 2.8 cm with a 1 cm distance from major biliary & vascular structures.

There are no randomized trials published comparing RFA with other established therapeutic modalities such as liver resection or systemic chemotherapy in unresectable colorectal liver metastases. Furthermore the determination of resectability or non resectability is a subjective judgment dependent on center experience in liver surgery, making it difficult to evaluate results of RFA as the tumor size and number in most series are very heterogeneous [50].

**Table 3:Patient Outcomes After RFA for Non Resectable Colorectal Metastases. NR= not reported. DFS=disease free survival (not specified in Jiao study).**

| Author | N. | RFA Approach | Mean Follow-up duration (months) | One Year Survival Disease Free |
|---|---|---|---|---|
| **Rossi 1996-1998 [75,93]** | 25 | Perc. | 12 | 18% |
| **Lencioni 1998 [119]** | 29 | Perc. | 6.5 | 48% |
| **Solbiati 1997 [110,112]** | 24 | Perc. | 10.3 | 50% |
| **Livraghi 1997 [111]** | 11 | Perc. | 9 | NR |
| **Jiao 1999 [113]** | 27 | Perc (3); Open (24) | NR | 78% (no DFS) |
| **Siperstein 2000 [76]** | 18 | Laparosc. | 13.9 | NR |

Does RFA for colorectal metastases to the liver achieve local recurrence rates and overall survival rates similar to liver resection? Three reviews in the English literature on this specific topic have been published during 2003 [17, 38, 50], moreover a critical analysis of the same problem was published in 2002 [94]. The collective review published by Seidenfeld in the JACS in 2002 on RFA ablation for unresectable liver metastases examined the medical literature on the topic from January 1975 to February 2001. Inclusion criteria within this analysis required a minimum of 10 patients in any series as well as reporting on the percentage of treated lesions completely ablated, rates of hepatic recurrence, median survival or percent survival up to 5 years after treatment, disease-free or recurrence-free survival, and measures of palliation or quality of life. Only six articles met these selection criteria and reported outcomes for RFA used alone for unresectable hepatic metastases. The mean duration of follow up was $\leq$ 12 months in 4 of the studies; five studies reported survival at one year from 84% to 96% and only one study indicated survival data at 2 years or more. Local relapse in the liver ranged from 34% to 64% in four series. The conclusion of this meta-analysis was that the available evidence is insufficient to permit conclusions on survival after RFA compared to other alternative treatment modalities for patients with inoperable metastatic tumor. Moreover insufficient data is available comparing the outcome of percutaneous, laparoscopic or an open approach for unresectable liver metastases.

## Discussion

Colorectal carcinoma is the fourth most common tumor worldwide and approximately one third of patients who die from this disease have tumor limited to the liver [6, 7]. The prognosis of patients with colorectal liver metastases is poor, with a 5 year survival rate of 0-2% if left untreated [15-16]. Surgical resection remains the gold standard, even though only 15% to 20% of newly diagnosed patients are candidates for curative resection [1]. Numerous studies have focused on factors determining recurrence and survival rates after curative resection of colorectal metastases [99-107]. More then 4 liver metastases, tumor positive resection margin, advanced stage of primary colorectal cancer, larger diameter of the liver metastases, elevated serum CEA, time elapsed between diagnosis of liver metastases and primary colorectal cancer, bilateral location of liver metastases, the presence of satellite lesions, non anatomical liver resection and percentage of the hepatic parenchyma invasion have all been reported to be important factors in determining long term survival [99, 107]. New treatment modalities such as RFA ablation do not have the benefit of such long term data and no randomized controlled studies comparing RFA with resection or chemotherapy have been published to date.

The principles of hepatic resection for colorectal metastases are an important guide when considering patients for RFA ablation. According to the natural history of the disease, there is almost no survival after 5 years if colorectal liver metastases are left untreated while more than one-third of patients who have been completely resected with an adequate negative margin are alive after 5 years [108]. Survival rates have been reported to be even higher if whole-body positron emission tomography with FDG-PET is performed preoperatively due to improved patient selection [4, 109]. In spite of these results, RFA ablation is gaining in popularity due to its low morbidity, minimally invasive potential and low cost, ultimately resulting in its relatively wide application. The indications for RFA are still controversial but with its continued development and potential for complete tumor destruction, it has gained considerable appeal. One of the main limitations to surgical resection is the fact that only 15% to 20% of newly diagnosed patients are candidates for curative resection [1]. Loco regional ablative therapy such as RFA provides a means to treat patients previously considered unresectable and can even be combined with surgical resection. It also allows a relative sparing of liver parenchyma which can be especially important in situations of marginal liver function such as steatosis, viral hepatitis or post chemotherapy.

For RFA to rival surgery the same principles must be followed: complete destruction of the tumor with an adequate margin. The efficacy of RFA can only be measured through rigorous follow up with evaluation of local recurrence rates, overall- and disease free-survival. Such an evaluation requires time and to date the majority of published data are hampered by a short follow up. A recent meta analysis evaluating the medical literature on RFA indicates that controlled clinical series are required and that at present the data is still lacking and does not allow definite conclusions to be drawn as to the benefits of this treatment modality compared to established therapy such as resection or chemotherapy [94].

Lately there have been some positive reports showing improved tumor destruction when RFA is combined with neoadjuvant liposomal doxorubicin therapy [114]. Few studies reported improved survival in liver resection after giving neoadjuvant chemotherapy for previously unresectable liver metastases [115-117]. Unfortunately, as quoted by Seidenfeld et al in their meta-analysis on RFA in unresectable liver metastases, it is impossible to determinate if RFA is equal, inferior or superior to neoadjuvant hepatic artery infusion followed by liver resection due to the lack of controlled comparative studies [94].

RFA can have a role in the treatment of non-resectable liver only metastatic colorectal cancer as well as cases of difficult local tumor recurrences. Lesions should be smaller than 5 cm as larger lesions have been shown to have higher local recurrence rates reflecting the limitations in present RFA technology as well as the difficulty in accurate multiple probe deployments to achieve complete ablation of such lesions. At present RFA ablation should only be used in the context of: multimodal clinical trials, in cases of colorectal liver tumors evaluated as unresectable in a specialized hepatobiliary center [118], in patients where the functional residual liver volume is too limited to sustain a curative resection, in patients with severe co morbidities precluding a surgical resection, in situations of technically difficult liver tumor recurrences, and within prospective randomized trials comparing RFA to other recognized therapeutic modalities.

## REFERENCES

[1] Taylor I: Liver metastases from colorectal cancer: lessons from past and present clinical studies. *Br J Surg* 1996; 83: 456-460.

[2] Solbiati L, Ierace T, tanolino M, et al. Radio frequency thermal ablation of hepatic metastases. *Eur J ultrasound* 2001; 13: 149-158.

[3] Fong Y, Fortner J, Sun RL, et al. Clinical score for predicting recurrence after hepatic resection for metastatic colorectal cancer: analysis of 1001 consecutive cases. *Ann Surg* 1999; 230: 309-321.

[4] Strasberg SM, Dehdashti F, Siegel BA, et al. Survival of patients evaluated by FDG-PET before hepatic resection for metastatic colorectal carcinomas: a prospective database study. *Ann Surg* 2001, 233: 293–299.

[5] Gruttadauria S, Doria C, Luca A, et al. Lactate levels in open interstitial thermal ablation for liver tumors. J Exp *Clin Cancer Res* 2002; 21,2: 171-176.

[6] Wilmink ABM. Overview of the epidemiology of colorectal cancer. *Dis Colon Rectum* 1997; 40: 483493.

[7] Xin Liu, Wei Hui Zhang, Hong chi Jiang Current treatment for liver metastases from colorectal cancer. *World J Gastroenterol* 2003 feb 15; 9 (2):193-200.

[8] Landis Sh, Murray T, Bolden S, et al. Cancer statistics, 1999. *Ca Cancer J clin.* 1999;49:8.

[9] Consenso sugli screening in oncologia: indirizzo per la ricerca e raccomandazioni al Servizio sanitario Nazionale. CNR-AIRC. *Roma giugno* 1996: 53-68.

[10] Kemeny N, Fong Y. Treatment of liver metastases.In: Holland JF, Frei E, Bast RC, Kufe DW, Morton DL, Weichselbaum RR, eds. Cancer medicine. Baltimore: *Williams & Wilkins*; 1997: 1939-1954.

[11] Weiss L, Grundmann E, Torhorst J et al. Haematogenous metastatic patterns in colonic carcinoma: an analysis of 1541 necropsies. *J Pathol.* 1986; 150: 195-203

[12] Fong Y, Blumgart LH, Cohen A, Fortner J, Brennan MF. Repeat hepatic resections for metastatic colorectal cancer. *Ann Surg*. 1994; 220: 657-62.

[13] Fernandez Trigo V, Shamsa F, Sugarbaker PH, Repeat liver resections from colorectal metastasis. *Repeat Hepatic Metastases Registry. Surgery* 1995; 117: 296-304.

[14] Wagman LD, Kemeny MM, Leong L et al. A prospective, randomized evaluation of the treatment of colorectal cancer metastatic to the liver. *J. Clin: Oncol*. 1990; 8: 1885-93.

[15] Wilson SM, Adson MA, Surgical treatment of hepatic metastases from colorectal cancers. *Arch. Surg*. 1976; 111: 330-4.

[16] Wagner JS, Adson MA, van Heerden JA, Adson MH, Ilstrup DM. The natural history of hepatic metastases from colorectal cancer. A comparison with resective treatment. *Ann. Surg*. 1984; 199: 502-8.

[17] Erce C., Parks R.W. Interstitial ablative techniques for hepatic tumours. *British Journal of Surgery* 2003; 90:272-289.

[18] Wade TP, Virgo KS, Li MJ, Callander PW, Longo WE, Johnson FE. Outcomes after detection of metatstatic carcinoma of the colon and rectum in a national hospital system. *J Am Coll Surg* 1996; 182: 353-361.

[19] Porte R. "Epidemiology, Diagnosis, and Algorithms for Treatment."Chapter 2 In *Malignant Liver Tumors 2$^{nd}$ Edition* 2003

[20] Scheele J, Stang R, Altendorf- Hofmann A, Paul M. Resection of colorectal liver metastases. *World J Surg* 1995; 19: 59-71.

[21] Gayowski TJ, Iwatsuki S, Madariaga JR, et al. Experience in hepatic resection for metastatic colorectal cancer: analysis of clinical and pathological risk factors. *Surgery* 1994; 116: 703-711.

[22] Rosen CB, Nagorney DM, Taswell HF et al. Perioperative blood transfusion and determinants of survival after liver resection for metastatic colorectal carcinoma. *Ann Surg* 1992; 216: 492-505.

[23] Nordlinger B, Park R, Delva E, Quilichini M, Hannoun L, Huguet C. Hepatic resection for colorectal liver metastases. *Ann Surg* 1987; 205: 256-263.

[24] Hughes KS, Simons R, Songhorabodi , et al. resection of the liver for colorectal carcinoma metastases: a multi-institutional study of indications for resection. *Surgery* 1988; 103: 278-288.

[25] Fong Y, Cohen AM Fortner JG, et al. Liver resection for colorectal metastase. *J Clin Onc* 1997; 15: 938-946.

[26] Cobourn CS, Makowka L, Langer B, Taylor B, Falk R. Examination of patient selection and outcome for hepatic resection for metastatic disease. *Surg Gynecol Obstet* 1987; 165: 239-246.

[27] Schlag P, Hohenberger P, Herfarth C. Resection of liver metastases in colorectal cancer: Competitive analysis of treatment results in synchronous vs metachronous metastases. *Eur J Surg Oncol* 1990; 16: 360-365.

[28] Doci R, Gennari L, Bignami P, Montalto F, Morabito A, Bozzetti F. One hundred patients with hepatic metastases from colorectal cancer treated by resection: analysis of prognostic determinants.

[29] Younes RN, Rogatko A, Brennan MF.The influence of intraoperative hypotention and perioperative blood transfusion on disease free survival in patients with complete resection of colorectal liver metastases. *Ann Surg* 1991; 214:107-113.

[30] Scheele J, Stanl R, Altendorf-Hofmann A, Gall FP. Indicators of prognosis after hepatic resection for colorectal secondaries. *Surgery* 1991; 110: 13-29.

[31] Cady B, Stone MD, McDermott WV Jr, et al. Technical and biological factors in disease free survival after hepatic resection for colorectal cancer metastases. *Arch Surg* 1992; 127: 561-569.

[32] Adson MA 1987 Resection of liver metastases – when it is worthwhile? *World Journal of surgery* 11: 511-520

[33] Nordingler B, Jack D, Guiget M et al 1992 Surgical resection of hepatic metastases. Multicentric retrospective study by the French Ass of Surgery.In Nordlinger B, Jaeck D. Treatment of hepatic metastases of colorectal cancer. *Springer Paris*: pag 129-146

[34] Scheele J, Stangl R, Altendorf Hofmann A. Hepatic metastases from colorectal carcinoma: impact of surgical resection on the natural history. *British Journal of Surgery* 77: 1241-1246.

[35] Scheele J, Altendorf-Hofmann A, Stangl R, Schmidt K 1996 Chirurgische Resektion kolorektalerLebermetastaten: Goldstandard fur solitare und resektable Herde. *Swiss surgery, Supplement* 4:4-17.

[36] Butler J, Attiyet F F, Daly J M 1986 Hepatic resection for metastases of the colon and rectum. *Surg Gynecol Obster* 162:109-113.

[37] Scheele, A Altendorf-Hofman. "Surgical treatment of liver metastase" Ch. 75 pag. 1475-1502 In. *Surgery of the liver and biliary tract Third Edit Vol II W:B*:

[38] Chai NG, Chi Ming Lam, Ronnie Tung Ping Poon, Victor AI, Wai Kuen Tso and Sheung Tat Fan. Thermal ablative therapy for malignant liver tumors: A critical appraisal. *J Gastroent and Hepat* 2003 18, 616-629.

[39] Nordlinger B, Vaillant JC, Guiget M, et al. Survival benefit of repeat repeat liver resection for current colorectal liver metastases: 143 cases. Associatione Francaise de Chirurgie . *Journal of Clinical Oncology* 1994. 12: 1491-1496.

[40] Bradley AL, chapman Wc, Wright JK, et al. Surgical experience with hepatic colorectal metastasis. *American surgeon* 1999; 65: 560-566.

[41] Martin JK, O'Connell MJ, Wieand HS et al. Intra-arterial floxuridine vs systemic fluoruracil for hepatic metastases from colorectal cancer. A randomized trial. *Arch Surg*. 1990; 125: 1022-7.

[42] Harmantas A, Rotstein LE, Langer B. regional vs systemic chemoterapy in the treatment of colorectal carcinoma metastatic to the liver. Is there a survival difference? Meta-analysis of the published literature. *Cancer* 1996; 78: 1639-45.

[43] Gruttadauria S, Lauro A, Marino I, et al : Intraoperative radiofrequency thermal ablation combined with liver resection for extensive colorectal metastases disease. *Hepatology* 32 (4,Pt 2 of 2): 622 A, 2000.

[44] Choti MA, Bulkley GB, Management of hepatic metastases. *Liver TX Surg* 1999; 5: 65-80

[45] Cromheecke M, de Jong KP, Hoekstra HJ, Current treatment for colorectal cancer metastatic to the liver. *Eur J Surg Onc* 1999; 25:451-463.

[46] Hugh TJ, Kinsella AR, Poston GJ. Management strategies for colorectal liver metastases. *Part II Surg Oncol* 1997; 6:31-48.

[47] Kemeny NE, Atiq OT. Non surgical treatment for liver metastases. *Baillieres Best Pract Res Clin Gastroenterol* 1999; 13: 593-610.

[48] Dodd GD, Lees WR, Lee FT, Minimally invasive treatment of malignant hepatic tumors. *Radiology* 213 P: 58,1999.

[49] Solbiati L., Livraghi T., Goldberg S.N., Ierace T., Meloni F., Dellanoce M., Cova L., Halpern E.H., Gazelle G.S. Percutaneous radio-frequency ablation of hepatic metastases from colorectal cancer: long-term results in 117 patients. *Radiology* October 2001.

[50] Strasberg I, Linheman. Radiofrequency ablation of liver tumors. *Curr Probl Surg* 2003; 40: 449-498.

[51] Hyunchul Rhim, Gerald Dodd III, Radiofrequency thermal ablation of liver tumors. *Review* 1998 September.

[52] Lu DS, Raman ss, Vodopich dj, wang m, sayre j, lassman c: Effect of vessel size on creation of hepatic radiofrequency lesions in pigs: assessment of the 'heat sink' effect. *AJR Am J Roentgenol* 2002;178: 47-51.

[53] Patterson EJ, Scudamore CH, Owen DA, Nagy AG, Buczkoski AK, Radiofrequency ablation of porcine liver in vivo: effect of blood flow and treatment time on lesion size. *Ann Surg.* 1998; 227: 559-65.

[54] Goldberg SN, Hahn PF, Tanabe KK, et al. Percutaneous radiofrequency tissue ablation: does perfusion mediated tissue cooling limit coagulation necrosis? *J Vasc. Inter Radiol.* 1998; 9: 101-11.

[55] Rossi S Garbagnati F, De Francesco I, et al Relationship between the shape and size of radiofrequency induced thermal lesions and heoatic vascularization. *Tumori* 1999; 85: 128-32.

[56] Rossi S, Garbagnati F, Lencioni R, et al. Percutaneous radiofrequency thermal ablation of nonresectable hepatocellular carcinoma after occlusion of tumor blood supply. *Radiology* 2000; 217: 119-26.

[57] Francica G, Marone G., Solbiati L, et al. Hemobilia, intrahepatic hematoma and acute thrombosis with cavernomatous transformation of the portal vein after percutaneous thermoablation of a liver metastasis.*Eropean radiology*. 10,926-929 (2000).

[58] Dominique E, El Otmany, Goharin A, Attalah D, de Baere T, Intraductal cooling of the main bile ducts during intraoperative radiofrequency ablation. *J Surg. Oncol Suppl* 2001; 76: 297-300.

[59] Elias D, Ouellet F,Bellon N, Pignon JP, Pocard M, Lasser P Extrahepatic disease does not contraindicate hepatectomy for colorectal liver metastases. *British J of Surg* 2003; 90: 567-574.

[60] Curley SA, Izzo F, Delrio P et al Radiofrequency ablation of unresectable primary and metastatic hepatic malignancies: results in 123 pts. *Ann Surg*. 230: 1-8, 1999.

[61] Cuschieri A., Bracken J., Boni L.: Initial experience with laparoscopic ultrasound-guided radiofrequency thermal ablation of hepatic tumors. *Endoscopy* 31:318-321, 1999.

[62] Wallace JR, Christians KK, Quiroz F et al. Ablation of liver metastsis: Is preoperative imaging sufficiently accurate? *J Gastrointestinal Surgery* 2001;5: 98-107.

[63] Mazziotti A., Grazi GL. Intraoperative ultrasound –diagnostic aspects in liver surgery In surgery of the liver and biliary tract, TRHIRD EDITION *L.H. Blumgart, Y Fong*. Volume 1: 499-507.

[64] Luck AJ, Maddern GJ. Intraoperative abdominal ultrasonography. *British Journal of Surgery Volume 86 (1)*. 1999: 5-16.

[65] Conlon R, Jacobs M, Dasgupta D, et al. The value of intraoperative ultrasound during hepatic resection compared with improved magnetic resonance imaging. *European Journal of Ultrasound* 16; 3: 2003, 211-216.

[66] Gozzetti G, Mazziotti A, Bolondi L, et al. Intraoperative ultrasonography in surgery for liver tumors. *Surgery* 1986;99:523-530.

[67] Castaing D, Emond J, Kunstlinger F et al. Utility of operative ultrasound in the surgical management of liver tumors. *ANN SURG* 1986;204: 600-605.

[68] Parker Ga, Lawrence W Jr, Horsley JS III, et al. Intraoperative ultrasound of the liver affects operative decision making. *Ann Surg*. 1989; 209:569-577.

[69] Staren ED, Gambla M, Deziel DJ, et al. Intraoperative ultrasound in the management of liver neoplasm. *Am Surg* 1997; 63; 591-597.

[70] Elias D., Debaere T., Muttillo I., Cavalcanti A., Coyle C., Roche A.: Intraoperative use of readiofrequency treatment allows an increase in the rate of curatice liver resection. *J. Surg. Oncol*. 67:190-191, 1998.

[71] McGahan J.P., Dodd G.D.: Radiofrequency ablation of the liver: current status. *A.J.R.* 176:3-16, 2001.

[72] Patterson EJ, Scudamore CH, Owen DA, Nagy AG, Buczkowski AK. Radiofrequency ablation of porcine liver in vivo: effects of blood flow and treatment time on lesion size. *Ann Surg*. 1998; 227: 559-65.

[73] Scott DJ, Young WN, Watumull Lm et al. Accuracy and effectiveness of laparoscopic versus open hepatic radiofrequency ablation. *Surg Endosc*. 2001; 15: 135-140.

[74] Goldberg SN, Solbiati L, Gazelle GS, Tanabe K, Compton CC, Mueller PR. Treatment of intrahepatic malignancy with radiofrequency ablation: radiologic-pathologic correlation in 16 patients. *AJR Am J Roentgenol* 1997; 166 (Suppl): 121-122 (Abstract).

[75] Rossi S. Buscarini E, Garbagnati F, Di Stasi M, Quaretti P, Rago M *et al.* Percutaneous treatment of small hepatic tumors by an expandable radiofrequency needle electrode. *AJR Am J Roentgenol* 1998; 170: 1015-1022.

[76] Siperstein A., Garland A., Engle K., et al. Local recurrence after laparoscopic radiofrequency thermal ablation of hepatic tumors [see comments]. Ann Surg Oncol 2000; 7:106-13.

[77] Dick EA, Taylor-Robinson Sd, Thomas HC et al. ablative therapy for liver tumors ( Review) 54refs *Gut* 2002; 50: 733-739.

[78] Izzo F. Other Thermal Ablation Techniques: Microwave and Interstitial Laser Ablation of Liver Tumors. *Annals of Surgical oncology* 2003;10 (5): 491-497.

[79] Iannitti DA, Dupuy DE, Mayo-Smith WW, Murphy B. Hepatic radiofrequency ablation. *Arch Surg* 2002; 137:422-6; discussion 427.

[80] Wood TF, Rose DM, Chung M, Allegra DP, Foshag LJ, Bilchik AJ. Radiofrequency ablation of 231 unresectable hepatic tumors: indications, limitations, and complications. *Ann Surg Oncol* 2000;7:593-600.
[81] Buchalter S., Crain M., Kreisberg R.: Regulation of lactate metabolism *in vivo*. D*iabetes Metab. Rev*. 5:379-391, 1989.
[82] Kreisberg R.: Lactate homeostasis and lactic acidosis. *Ann Intern. Med.* 92:227-237, 1980
[83] Fath, J.J., Ascher N.L., Konstantinided F.N., et al: Metabolism during hepatic transplantation: indicators of allograft function. *Surgery* 96:664-674, 1984.
[84] De Gasperi A., Mazza E., Corti A., et al: Lactate blood levels in the perioperative period of orthotopic liver transplantation. *Int. J. Clin. Lab. Res*. 27:123-128, 1997.
[85] Orii R., Sugawara Y., Hayashida M., et al: Peri-operative blood lactate levels in recipients of living-related liver transplantation. *Transplantation* 69:2124-2127, 2000.
[86] Gruttadauria S., Lauro A., Doria C. et al. Resezioni (Ro) Per Il Trattamento Di Metastasi Epatiche Da Tumore ColoRettale. *Tumori Volume 1, Number 3*, May-June 2002 S 107.
[87] Siperstein A., Garland A., Engle K., et al. Laparoscopic radiofrequency ablation of primary and metastatic liver tumors. *Tech Considerations Surg Endosc* 2000; 14:400-5.
[88] Liu JB, Goldberg BB, Merton DA, Rawool NM, Neddleman L, Forsberg F. The role of contrast-enhanced sonography for radiofrequency ablation of liver tumors. *J Ultrasound Med* 2001; 20:517-23.
[89] Vogl TJ, Muller PK, Hammerstingl R. et al. Malignant liver tumors treated with MR imaging-guided laser-induced thermotherapy: technique and prospective results. *Radiology* 1995; 196:257-65.
[90] Huppert PE, Trubenbach J, Schick F, Pereira P, Konig C, Claussen CD. MRI-guided percutanetos radiofrequency ablation of hepatic neoplasms-first technical and clinical experiences. [German] *ROFO-Fortschritte auf dem Gebeit der Rontgenstrahlen und der Bildgebenden V* 2000; 172:692-700.
[91] Anderson GSBA, Brinkmann F, Soulen MC et al. FDG Positron Emission Tomography in the Surveillance of Hepatic Tumors Treated with Radiofrequency ablation *Clinical Nuclear Medicne* 2003. 28 (3);192-197.
[92] De Baere T, Elias D, Dromain C, et al. Radiofrequency ablation of 100 hepatic metastases with a mean follow-up of more than 1 year. AJR. *AJR Am J Roentgenol* 2000; 175:619-25.
[93] Rossi S, Di Stasi M, Buscarini E, et al. Percutaneous RF interstitial thermal ablation in the treatment of hepatic cancer,. *AJR Am J Roentgenol* 1996; 167:759-68.
[94] Seidenfeld J., Kron A., Aronson N.: Radiofrequency ablation of unresectable liver metastases. *J Am Coll Surg* Vol 195, No. 3, September 2002.
[95] De Baere T, Elias D, Dromain C, et al. Radiofrequency ablation of 100 hepatic metastases with a mean follow-up of more than 1 year. AJR. *AJR Am J Roentgenol* 2000; 175:619-25.
[96] Machi J. Radiofrequency ablation for multiple hepatic metastases. *Ann Surg Oncol* 2001; 8:379-80.

[97] American Cancer Society. Cancer facts and figures. Washington , DC: *American Cancer Society*, 1999; 23: 198-202.

[98] Garre C. Contribution to surgery of the liver. *BurnsBeitr Klin Chir* 1888; 4: 181.

[99] Elias D. Goharin A., El Otmany A., Taieb J., Duvillard P., Lasser P., De Baere T. Usefulness of intraoperative radiofrequency thermoablation of liver tumors associated or not with hepatectomy. *European Journal of Surgical Oncology* 2000; 26:763-769.

[100] Nordlinger B, Guiguet M, Vaillant JC, Balladur P, Boudjema K, Bachellier P, Jaeck D. Surgical resection of colorectal carcinoma metastases to the liver. A prognostic scoring system to improve case selection, based on 1568 patients. Association Francaise de Chirurgie. *Cancer* 1996; 77:1254-62.

[101] Cady B, Jenkins RL, Steele GD Jr, Lewis WD, Stone MD, McDermott WV, Jessup JM, Bothe A, Lalor P, Lovett EJ, Lavin P, Linehan DC. Surgical margin in hepatic resection for colorectal metastasis: a critical and improvable determinant of outcome. *Ann Surg* 1998; 227: 566-71.

[102] Yamamoto J, Shimada K, Kosuge T, Yamasaki S, Sakamoto M, Fukuda H. Factors influencing survival of patients undergoing hepatectomy for colorectal metastases. *Br J Surg* 1999; 86: 332-7.

[103] Ueno H, Mochizuki H, Hatsuse K, Yamamoto T. Indicators for treatment strategies of colorectal liver metastases. *Ann Surg* 2000; 231: 59-66.

[104] Seifert JK, Bottger TC, Weigel TF, Gonner U, Junginger T. Prognostic factors following liver resection for hepatic metastases from colorectal cancer. *Hepatogastroenterology* 2000; 47: 239-46.

[105] Minagawa M, Makuuchi M, Torzilli G, Takayama T, Kawasaki S, Kosuge T, Yamamoto J, Imamura H. Extension of the frontiers of surgical indications in the treatment of liver metastases from colorectal cancer: long-term results. *Ann Surg* 2000; 231: 487-99.

[106] Lise M, Bacchetti S, Da Pian P., Nitti D, Pilati P. Patterns of recurrence after resection of colorectal liver metastases: prediction by models of outcome analysis. *World J Surg* 2001; 25: 638-44.

[107] Yamada H, Kondo S, Okushiba S, Morikawa T, Katoh H. Analysis of predictive factors for recurrence after hepatectomy for colorectal liver metastases. *World J Surg* 2001; 25: 1129-33.

[108] Scheele J, Stangl R, Alterndorf-Hofmann A. Hepatic metastases from colorectal carcinoma: impact of surgical resection on the natural history. *Br J Surg* 1990; 77: 1241-6.

[109] Topal B, Flamen P, Aerts R, D'Hoore A, Filez L, Van Cutsem E, Mortelmans L, Penninckx F. Clinical value of whole-body positron emission tomography in potentially curable colorectal liver metastases. *Eur J Surg Oncol* 2001; 27: 175-9.

[110] Solbiati L, Ierace T, Goldberg SN, Sironi S, Livraghi T, Fiocca R *et al.* Percutaneous US-guided radio-frequency tissue ablation of liver metastases: treatment and follow-up in 16 patients. *Radiology* 1997; 202: 195-203.

[111] Livraghi T, Goldberg SN, Monti F, Bizzini A, Lazzaroni S, Meloni F *et al.* Saline-enhanced radio-frequency tissue ablation in the treatment of liver metastases. *Radiology* 1997; 202: 205-210.

[112] Solbiati L, Goldberg SN, Ierace T, Livraghi T, Meloni f, Dellanoce M *et al.* Hepatic metastases: percutaneous radio-frequency ablation with cooled-tip electrodes. *Radiology* 1997; 205: 367-373.

[113] Jiao LR, Hansen PD, Havlik R, Mitry R, Mitry RR, Pignatelli M, Habib N. Clinical short-term results of radiofrequency ablation in primary and secondary liver tumors. *Am J Surg* 1999; 177: 303-306.

[114] Goldberg SN, Kamel IR, Kruskal, et al. AJR Am J Roentgenol. 2002Jul;179 (1): 93-101.

[115] Bismuth H, Adam R, Levi F, et al. Resection of nonresectable liver metastases from colorectal cancer after neoadyuvant chemotherapy. *Ann Surg* 1996; 224: 509-520.

[116] Yasuno M, Tori T, TakahashiK, et al. Results of the hepatic resection of liver metastases from colorectal carcinoma after continuos hepatic arterial infusion of chemotherapy. New strategy for unresectable liver metastases. Anti Cancer Treatment sixth International Congress Paris France February 6-9, 1996, meeting abstrcat N. 383: 137.

[117] Clavien PA., Selzner N., Morse M et al. Down staging of hepatocellular carcinoma and liver metastases from colorectal cancer by selective intra-arterial chemotherapy. *Surgery* 2002Apr; 13 (4): 433-442.

[118] Kadry Z, Clavien PA. New treatments with curative intent for metastatic colorectal liver cancer. *Expert Opin Pharmacother*. 2002 Aug; 3 (8): 1191-1197.

[119] Lencioni R, Goletti O, Armilotta, et al. Radiofrequency thermal ablation of liver metastases with cooled tip electrode needle: results and pilot clinical trial. *Eur radiol* 1998: 8: 1205-1211.

In: Liver Cancer: New Research
Editor: Felix Lee, pp. 79-99
ISBN 1-59454-182-5


*Chapter IV*

# Strategies for Inferior Phrenic Arteriography and Transcatheter Arterial Chemoembolization in Patients with Hepatocellular Carcinoma

***Kwang-Hun Lee***[3]
Department of Radiology and Research Institute of Radiological Science,
Yonsei University College of Medicine, Seoul, Republic of Korea

## Abstract

### Purpose

To establish the strategies for inferior phrenic arteriography and transcatheter arterial chemoembolization (TACE) in patients with hepatocellular carcinoma (HCC) including when to perform, how to perform, and hemodynamic changes of the inferior phrenic artery (IPA).

### Materials and Methods

One hundred eight patients with HCC underwent a total of 310 sessions (mean, 2.87 sessions) of TACE of the IPA. Chemoembolization was performed with an emulsion of iodized oil (lipiodol) and doxorubicin hydrochloride (adriamycin), and gelatin sponge particles. The criteria for inferior phrenic arteriography were: 1) location of HCC in the bare area (S1, S2, S7), and adrenal metastasis on CT scan even in the first session of

[3] Department of Radiology, YongDong Severance Hospital, 146-92 Dokok-Dong, Kangnam-Ku, Seoul 135-270, Republic of Korea, Telephone: 82-2-3497-3510, FAX: 82-2-3462-5472, E-mail: doctorlkh@yumc.yonsei.ac.kr

TACE, 2) presence of non-staining area on hepatic arteriography, 3) mismatch of the size of the HCC mass between CT scan and hepatic arteriography, 4) presence of non-enhancing portion of the mass on CT hepatic arteriography, 5) absence or wash-out of lipiodol in the IPA territory on CT scan after the first session of TACE, 6) deprivation of the hepatic arteries due to repeated chemoembolization or occlusion of the hepatic arteries as a complication of a percutaneously implanted port-a-cath system.

## Results

In the first session, 40 patients (37%) underwent chemoembolization of the IPA. The remaining 68 patients (63%) underwent after the first session. Right IPA supply was in 105 patients (97.2%). Left IPA supply was in five patients (4.6%). The most of tumor (78.3%, 94 of 120 nodules) is located at S7 and S8. But, other segments (S4, S6, S1, and S2) and inferior vena cava also involved by IPA parasitization. As much as 26.6% (32 of 120 nodules) is located at deeper liver parenchyma away from the capsule. Seventy five small HCC less than 2cm sized which have IPA parasitization are found reaching 62.5% (75 of 120 nodules). Independent parasitic supply of IPA was in 79 nodules (65.8%), dependent parasitic supply was in 8 nodules (6.7%), and exclusive parasitic supply was in 33 nodules (27.5%). There was no procedure-related mortality and major morbidity.

## Conclusion

It is important to suspect the possibility of blood supply of the IPA into the HCC. TACE through the IPA can be performed safely and effectively. Interventionists should know various situation of the parasitization of the IPA into the HCC for the treatment of the patients with HCC.

## Index Terms:

Interventional procedures; Liver neoplasms, angiography; Liver neoplasms, blood supply; Liver neoplasms, chemotherapeutic infusion

# INTRODUCTION

Since transcatheter arterial chemoembolization (TACE) into the hepatic artery was performed as to the unresectable hepatocellular carcinoma (HCC) in early 1980, the TACE has been acknowledged as the effective treatment modality to improve the prognosis of unresectable or inoperable HCC patient and performed all over the world up to the present [1, 2]. As experiences are accumulated, favorable results regarding the resectable HCC have been reported by performing either selective segmental or subsegmental chemoembolization [3-9], and some authors assert it is good to primarily perform the subsegmental TACE as its efficiency is equivalent to the one of surgical resection if superselective subsegmental chemoembolization is available [8, 9]. If injecting the mixture of emulsion of iodized oil (lipiodol) and anticancer drug through the superselected feeding artery into the tumor, the tumor portion is filled with the mixture of lipiodol and anticancer drug and then the portal branches around the tumor is filled through the arterioportal shunt, so we may acquire the effect to interrupt the portal blood flow around the tumor, and then if embolizing the feeding artery with the gelatin sponge particle, arterial blood flow is also interrupted. Surrounding normal liver parenchyma including the tumor may be interrupted the arterial blood flow and portal blood flow as well, so the tumor and surrounding liver parenchyma are infracted and we may technically acquire the complete necrosis without any recurrence.

However, if the size of HCC is originally large or hepatic artery is injured by previous chemoembolization, the extrahepatic collateral is formed with easy, so ensure to perform the chemoembolization only after checking if it is supplied by the hepatic artery and extrahepatic collateral arteries as well [10-12]. Many extrahepatic collateral routes could be found during the TACE and included: periportal collateral arising from the gastroduodenal artery or pancreaticoduodenal arcade, right and left inferior phrenic artery (IPA), right and left gastric artery, pancreaticoduodenal arcade supplying the gastroduodenal and proper hepatic arteries, right and left internal mammary artery and superior epigastric artery, intercostal artery, lumbar artery, adrenal arteries, capsular branches of the right renal artery, branches of the middle or right colic artery and omental branches. Of those collaterals, the most commonly encountered collateral route during the TACE may be the IPA. Therefore, recognition of the HCC feeding from the IPA and performance of TACE into IPA are important. The purpose of this study was to introduce the general performance of the TACE in our institution and to establish the strategies for inferior phrenic arteriography and chemoembolization in patients with HCC including when to perform, how to perform, and the hemodynamic changes of the IPA.

## Materials and Methods

### Patients

From January 1996 to December 2003, a total of 1203 sessions of TACE were performed in 561 consecutive patients with HCC. Our institutional review board approved the procedure, and informed consent was obtained from each patient or from their legal guardian.

One hundred eight of the 561 (19%) patients with HCC who required TACE of the IPA were included in this study, retrospectively. There were 75 men and 33 women with ages ranging from 33 to 72 years (mean, 54 years). Thirty seven patients were in Child-Pugh class A, 60 patients in B, and 11 patients in C. Underlying diseases are follow as: B viral cirrhosis in 96 patients, C viral cirrhosis in 5 patients, alcoholic cirrhosis in 5 patients, and non-cirrhosis in 2 patients.

Generally, TACE was contraindicated when the main portal vein was occluded by tumor thrombus invasion, massive transtumoral shunt into the portal or hepatic vein. In these cases, catheter-directed chemoinfusion or port-a-catheter chemoinfusion could be performed. If there is no functional hepatopetal portal flow by severe portal vein hypertension without portal vein thrombosis or total bilirubin > 3mg/dl, it may be construed to be relative contraindication. However, TACE may be performed carefully according to the tumor size, number, and multi-segmental distribution. Thus, for the patients without functional hepatopetal portal flow or Child-Pugh class C with high total bilirubin, indication of TACE is available only when the subsegmental TACE may be performed through the superselection of only feeding artery. If segmental TACE is required for the large size of tumor or showing multi-segmental distribution, the TACE may not be performed at once, and it must be performed several times by following up the liver function. If main portal vein is not tumor thrombus but benign thrombotic occlusion and collateral hepatopetal portal flow is formed, the TACE may be performed. When the HCC is presented as the icteric HCC by invading the bile duct, we perform the TACE if superselection of HCC feeder invading the bile duct is available after the jaundice or biliary infection control through the performance of percutaneous transhepatic biliary drainage, and if it is not available, we performed the catheter-directed chemoinfusion or port-a-catheter chemoinfusion.

### Pre-procedure Imaging

Pre-procedural imagings of three-phasic abdominal dynamic CT scan or MR imaging have been performed within one month. Ensure to check the segmental location and number of HCC, and the presence or absence of the thrombus in the portal vein through pre-procedural imaging. The selective TACE may become easy by finding the feeder with easy by means of prefiguring the segmental location of HCC. However, make sure to remember that all segment 7, 8, and 4 branch of the hepatic artery may be functioned as the feeding artery by severe hepatic arterial anatomic variation in the liver dome area. For the HCC of subcapsular or exophytic location, engage in the procedure by prejudging the angiographic evaluation by means of selecting another artery other than hepatic artery in consideration of parasitic supply from non-hepatic artery.

### Monitoring During the Procedure

Ensure to perform the monitoring of EKG, pulse rate, blood pressure and O2 saturation for all patients all the times, from entering the angioroom to leaving the angioroom after the treatment.

## Chemoembolization into Hepatic Arteries

One of the both common femoral artery access was punctured by modified Seldinger's technique with 18-gauge disposable Angiocath. And then, 0.035 inch hydrophilic guide wire (Terumo, Tokyo, Japan) was inserted. A 5-F angiographic sheath was inserted routinely over the guide wire. A 1,000mL of normal saline mixed with 5,000 IU of heparin was used for catheter flushing and instruments washing. Angiography should be obtained by digital subtraction method, so called digital subtraction angiography (DSA). As an angiographic catheter, 5-F Rosch Hepatic (Cook, Bloomington, IN, U.S.A) or Yashiro (Terumo, Tokyo, Japan) catheter was used. First, indirect portography via superior mesenteric artery and/or celiac-splenic artery with a 5-F angiographic catheter was obtained. Even if the portal vein is not obstructed by the thrombus, there may be no hepatopetal flow by the intrahepatic portal hypertension, so safe TACE procedure is promised by performing the hepatic arteriography and chemoembolization after checking the level of functional hepatopetal portal flow through the performance of indirect portography. And then, hepatic arteriographies were obtained with regard to the anatomic variations of the hepatic artery. It is recommendable to get only the hepatic artery visualized by selecting the common hepatic artery in normal hepatic artery anatomy.

When the arteriography was performed at celiac axis, the angiographic evaluation for liver nodule may become suboptimal by the reduced contrast media flowed in the hepatic artery, and also the HCC of left lobe of the liver may become masking by the staining of stomach and spleen resulted from the contrast media flowed in the left gastric artery and splenic artery. Most of HCC patients are the case of liver cirrhosis-related, so splenic artery is under the condition of hypertrophy. Accordingly, more contrast media flow in the splenic artery rather than the hepatic artery, and it shows the problem that lateral segment of left lobe of the liver is masked by the enlarged spleen staining.

For the case that right hepatic artery shows an arising variation in the superior mesenteric artery (so called replaced right hepatic artery), catheter tip is selected to the replaced right hepatic artery if slowly taking out the catheter under the hand injection of contrast media after inserting 5-F Rosch Hepatic catheter into the portion which is deeper than the portion where the replaced right hepatic artery arises in the superior mesenteric artery proximal. For the case showing anatomic variation of hepaticomesenteric trunk or celiacomesenteric trunk, perform the arteriography by selecting 0.035 inch hydrophilic guide wire. For the case that left hepatic artery shows an arising variation from left gastric artery, you may perform the arteriography by selecting the left gastric artery only with catheter work. However, make a selection using 0.035 inch hydrophilic guide wire for the most cases. When angulation of left gastric artery is severe, insertion of 5-F angiographic catheter may become hard, or it may come off during breathing or injecting the contrast media even if insertion is available. In this case, to avoid the catheterization-related complications such as dissection by the excessive insertion, it is recommendable to perform the arteriography using the 3-F coaxial microcatheter after accessing to left hepatic artery.

After the completion of the diagnostic angiography, segmental or subsegmental chemoembolization procedures were performed with use of a 3-F coaxial microcatheters (Renegade; Boston Scientific, Natick, NA or Micro-ferret; Cook, Bloomington, IN or SP; Terumo, Tokyo, Japan). In principle, the chemoembolization was performed by super-selecting only the feeding artery in order to prevent the hepatic function impairment caused by chemoembolization. For the superselection of feeding artery, the ability to classify the feeding artery and non-feeding artery is required. Normal feeding artery shows the aspect of hypertrophy and tortuous. However, it is not easy to classify the feeding artery for the case of small HCC, or when vascularity is sufficiently developed as overall hepatic arteries are hypertrophy and tortuous under the condition of severe liver cirrhosis. It will be helpful to perform the segmental arteriography using 3-F coaxial microcatheter with the segmental location of tumor inferred to some degree in the pre-procedural imaging. Also, for the case showing the nodule in right lobe of the liver which is overlapped by several segmental arteries in the hepatic arteriography using 5-F catheter in the anterior-posterior projection DSA, it will be helpful to repeat the arteriography by performing the right anterior oblique projection DSA of about 15 degree.

When numbers of feeders were existed, we performed the chemoembolization into the minor feeder at first, and then performed the chemoembolization into the major feeder. If performing the chemoembolization of major feeder first, the tumor staining may become masked by the minor feeder resulted from the up-taken artifact of iodized oil in the tumor and result incomplete chemoembolization.

Make sure to comply with following three principles when performing the arteriography after selecting the peripheral branch of hepatic artery using the microcatheter. First, when taking out the microguide wire, it is important to slowly take out the microguide wire not to get the air bubble produced by the friction and negative pressure between the microcatheter and the microguide wire. Second, even if you are very careful, a small amount of air bubble may remain in the microcatheter, so ensure to perform the arteriography after removing the air bubble through the aspiration of blood with the syringe. If performing the arteriography with the air remained in the microcatheter, air embolism is induced in the feeding artery and an effective chemoembolization is not guaranteed. Third, upon performing the aspiration with the syringe, ensure not to perform the arteriography if the blood is not freely aspired, and perform the arteriography using the power injector only after checking if the blood is freely aspired and test injection of the contrast media with hand injection as when the blood is not freely aspired, which means the microcatheter's being wedged on the arterial wall; if injecting the contrast media with the power injector, TACE procedure may be fail by the produced dissection. When superselected to the small feeding artery, it is safe to perform the arteriography with hand injection.

Chemoembolic agent which composed of the mixture of lipiodol and doxorubicin hydrochloride (adriamycin) was injected into the feeder with a selective manner through the 3-F coaxial microcatheter. For the small nodular HCC showing the subsegmental location, where superselection was available, we performed the chemoembolization up to the portal vein side including hepatic artery by performing the subsegmental chemoembolization to enable the lipiodol to backflow up to the surrounding portal branch after filling up the tumor in order to reduce the marginal recurrence by enabling the chemoembolization up to the portal vein side as HCC is supplied with blood from the hepatic artery and portal vein as well when it shows extracapsular invasion. When feeding artery was involved into numbers of subsegmental branches and there were numbers of nodular HCCs in a segment, we performed the segmental chemoembolization. And then, about $1^3$ mm sized gelatin sponge particles which mixed by heparinized normal saline and non-ionic contrast media with 1:2 ratio were injected into the feeder for transient embolization of the feeding artery. When the hepatic artery is injured by the repeated TACE, if using the gelatin sponge particle, it only becomes the proximal embolization, and next session of TACE becomes hard by the aggravated hepatic artery injury and post-TACE liver failure is caused, so gelatin sponge particle is not used when the hepatic arteries are injured.

## Chemoembolization into the IPA

Even in the first session of chemoembolization, inferior phrenic arteriography was performed when tumor supply from IPA was suspected. When the lipiodol was uptake by previous hepatic artery TACE, we performed the inferior phrenic angiography before performing the hepatic angiography and chemoembolization if it is available because if performing the hepatic artery TACE first, the lipiodol is uptake in the HCC and surrounding liver parenchyma, so it may be hard to precisely evaluate the parasitization of the IPA for the lipiodol artifact when performing the IPA angiography next. Specially, even if the newly developed HCC nodule is not abutted to the surface of the bare area but is away from the surface in the patient who received repeated TACE, the nodule may receive parasitic supply from IPA, so we confirmed IPA arteriography necessarily.

The criteria for inferior phrenic arteriography were: 1) location of HCC in the bare area (S1, S2, S7), and adrenal metastasis on CT scan even in the first session of TACE, 2) presence of non-staining area on hepatic arteriography, 3) mismatch of the size of the HCC mass between CT scan and hepatic arteriography, 4) presence of non-enhancing portion of the mass on CT hepatic arteriography, 5) absence or wash-out of lipiodol in the IPA territory on CT scan after the first session of TACE, 6) deprivation of the hepatic arteries due to repeated chemoembolization or occlusion of the hepatic arteries as a complication of a percutaneously implanted port-a-cath system.

We may find the IPA by searching with the contrast media injected with hand using 5-F Rosch Hepatic catheter or Yashiro catheter at the celiac axis just above, proximal portion of the celiac axis, between the celiac axis and right renal artery, and right renal artery. Once the orifice of the IPA was selected to 5-F catheter, we performed the arteriography with the hand injection of 10ml syringe.

It is the most difficult to select the IPA when it is arising in the proximal portion of the celiac axis. Attempt the selection with 3-F coaxial microcatheter and 0.018 inch guide wire after partially hanging 5-F catheter on the orifice of the celiac axis. If it is not successful, direct insertion of 5-F catheter into the IPA may be possible with 0.035 inch hydrophilic guide wire.

If the orifice of the IPA is securely selected with 5-F catheter, insertion of 3-F coaxial microcatheter is easy. When the IPA is searched using 5-F Rosch Hepatic or Yashiro catheter, but it is not securely selected to the orifice of the IPA, inserting 3-F coaxial microcatheter may be fail. At this time, you may insert 3-F coaxial microcatheter by securely selecting the orifice of the IPA after changing to 5-F Cobra (C1) catheter.

When 5-F catheter arteriography was insufficient, we performed the arteriography through 3-F coaxial microcatheter. When performing the arteriography by selecting superior adrenal artery arising in the proximal of right IPA, contrast media must be injected with hand instead of power injector as the rupture may occur if injecting in fine adrenal branch with the power injector. Chemoembolic agent and chemoembolization method of the IPA was the same performed in the hepatic artery. When both anterior branch and posterior branch supplied the parasitic to the HCC, we performed the chemoembolization at once, and when supply was available in only one branch out of two, we performed the chemoembolization by selecting only feeding branch. When super-selection was hard for the thin branch of the IPA supplying the parasitization or when chemoembolic agent was passing to innocent larger distal branch if performing the chemoinfusion in the proximal, or when there was benign transpleural IPA to pulmonary artery shunt in the distal branch of the IPA, we performed the proximal chemoembolization after performing the microcoil embolization in the distal branch in advance because if chemoembolic agent is delivered to innocent branch, whole IPA territory is emboloized, so the complications such as severe ischemic shoulder pain, paralysis of the diaphragm, transpleural lung shunt and pulmonary embolization may be induced and effective drug delivery to the tumor is not available.

Rarely, HCC is extended up to suprahepatic segment of inferior vena cava or right atrium by invading the hepatic vein and right IPA performs the duty of supply, and for this case, if performing the chemoembolization with the mixture of lipiodol and adriamycin, it is immediately shunt through the tumor thrombus and only the pulmonary embolization is induced, so cisplatin [cis-diamminedichloroplatinum (CDDP)] chemoinfusion becomes available.

When there was stenosis or occlusion in the orifice of the IPA, we attempt the entry into 3-F coaxial microcatheter after wedging in the orifice using 5-F catheter, and if it was not still available, we performed the chemoembolization by selecting the collateral route to 3-F coaxial microcatheter.

## Dosage Limit of Chemotherapeutic Agent and Iodized Oil

Commonly, mixture of adriamycin 50mg and lipiodol 10ml was used. Adriamycin was well mixed with the lipiodol for its lipophilic property. Dosage of adriamycin did not exceed 50mg. Dosage of lipiodol was specified not to exceed 10ml. However, the dosage of up to 20ml was used when there was no disease in the lung parenchyma with large tumor size and good liver function, ensure to inject the lipiodol by carefully checking if the shunt to the hepatic vein is well performed in the fluoroscopy at this time.

When thrombus of HCC was accompanied in the portal vein, hepatic vein, inferior vena cava, or right atrium, we infused the mixture of adriamycin and lipiodol for the nodular component after performing the cisplatin chemoinfusion - dosage 2 mg/Kg; infusion time 15~20 minutes.

## Contrast Media

In general, angiography and chemoembolization procedures were performed with non-ionic iodine contrast media (Visipaque; Amersham). If the patient showed the allergic reactions to the iodine contrast media, however, MR contrast media (Omniscan; Amersham) was used for arteriography and chemoembolization procedures. When the indirect portography was performed via superior mesenteric artery, the usual amount of injected non-ionic iodine contrast media was 30ml (3ml per sec x 10sec). When the indirect portography was performed via celiac-splenic artery, the usual amount of injected non-ionic iodine contrast media was 30—35ml (6—7ml per sec x 5sec). Common hepatic arteriography was performed in cases without anatomic variation of the hepatic artery, injected amount of non-ionic iodine contrast media was 20—25ml (4—5ml per sec x 5sec). When either left hepatic artery was arising from left gastric artery, or there was anatomic variation that the hepatic artery is arising from superior mesenteric artery (replaced right hepatic artery), we performed the arteriography by selecting the left gastric artery and replaced right hepatic artery to 5-F angiographic catheter in principle. The injected non-ionic iodine contrast media was set to 15-20ml (3—4ml per sec x 5sec). When the arteriography performed at segmental hepatic artery via 3-F coaxial microcatheter, the amount of non-ionic iodine contrast media was 5ml (1ml per sec x 5sec). When the arteriography performed at subsegmental hepatic artery via 3-F coaxial microcatheter, the amount of non-ionic iodine contrast media was 1.5—3ml (0.5—1ml per sec x 3sec). When the tumor feeding artery was super-selected, we made the verification through the hand injection using 1ml syringe.

When performing the TACE using the MR contrast media, it must be used under the condition of less than 60ml, so we performed the segmental and subsegmental arteriography by selecting only segment, where tumor is located, in the CT or MR imaging without performing the indirect portography.

## Drugs Used During the TACE

The most commonly and always used drug during the TACE is the analgesics because the ischemic pain is inevitable during the chemoembolization. Because the cooperation with the patient is very important during the procedure of TACE, avoidance of the sedative drugs is better. For pain control, usually non-sedative intravenous analgesics, Pethidine (Demerol) is used. This drug has some side effects such as nausea, vomiting, and dizziness, so it is administered to 25mg in the first, and if the pain persists, it is recommendable to additionally administer by 25mg and dosage of more than 75mg is not used. At the time of intravenous administration, analgesic effect of Demerol appear within 5 minutes, so it is good to administer 25mg of Demerol before performing the chemoembolization after the superselection of feeding artery. This drug has the effect to reduce the blood pressure to some degree for the pain-induced hypertension including pain control function. When non-selectively performing the chemoembolization for the IPA, shoulder pain may become severe. At this time, if performing the chemoembolization after injecting about 2% lidocaine hydrochloride 5ml, it will be helpful to reduce the pain.

Pain and tension induced hypertension is also frequent problem during the TACE. For the mild blood pressure elevation, if administering the Demerol to intravenous, pain control becomes available and blood pressure may be reduced, so ensure to recheck if blood pressure is reduced after 5 minutes. If hypertension is severe in the beginning, or blood pressure is not reduced after 5 minutes of intravenous administration of the Demerol, administer the Nifedipine (Adalat) 10—20mg to the sublingual, and if it is not controlled after administering the Adalat, perform continuous drop infusion to the intravenous route in the rate of 2—7 mg/hour by diluting the Isosorbide dinitrate (Isoket) in normal saline.

Sufficient lipiodol uptake may not be achieved in the HCC nodule by causing arterial spasm in the middle of intra-arterial injection of the mixture of adriamycin and lipiodol for its high viscosity and chemotoxicity. At this time, if slowly injecting Papaverin (Papaverin) 0.5ml mixed with normal saline 2ml, vasospasm is immediately resolved and successful chemoembolization may be achieved. However, patients feel severe pain when going through papavein injection and chemoembolization process. This process involves dilatation of the artery supplying non-tumorous parenchyma as well as tumor feeding artery. That leads to chemoembolizaton of non-tumorous liver parenchyma, and therefore, severe ischemic pain.

Rarely, the sinus bradycardia may be developed during the selective chemoembolization. As previously stated, for the most chemoembolization, hypertension is often developed for the pain and tension in the middle of procedure. However, hypotension is rarely developed may be from pain shock. If hypotension is measured on the monitor, quickly check the ECG waveform and pulse rate, and confirm if heart motion becomes slow in the fluoroscopy. At this circumstance, intravenous administration of the Atropin (Atropin sulfate) 1ample (0.5mg) is very effective, and the blood pressure and heart rate are recovered immediately.

## DEFINITIONS

Parasitization or parasitic supply means that the HCC is supplied by the non-hepatic systemic artery. The patterns of the parasitic supply of the IPA to the HCC were classified into the three types: independent parasitic supply, dependent parasitic supply, and exclusive parasitic supply pattern. Independent parasitic supply of the IPA means that some portions of HCC, where IPA supplies the parasitic, are not supplied in the hepatic artery. In other words, as to a HCC mass, the portion where hepatic artery supplies and the portion where IPA supplies are different. Dependent parasitic supply of the IPA means that some portions of HCC, where IPA supplies the parasitic, accord to the portion supplied in the hepatic artery or included in the portion supplied in the hepatic artery. The exclusive parasitic supply of the IPA means that whole HCC is supplied only in the IPA without any hepatic arterial supply.

## FOLLOW-UP PROTOCOLS

As long as there was no allergic reaction in non-ionic iodine contrast media, we followed up with three-phasic abdomen dynamic CT scan, and if the patient showed an allergic reaction against the iodine contrast media, we followed up with three-phasic liver dynamic MR imaging. We performed the follow-up imaging 3 weeks, 3 months, 6 months, 9 months and 12 months after the TACE for the first year, and then we performed it every 6 months. If recurring in the middle of follow-up, we repeated the follow-up in the previously stated interval.

## RESULTS

One hundred eight patients with HCC underwent a total of 310 sessions (mean, 2.87 sessions) of TACE of the IPA. Forty patients (37%) required chemoembolization of the IPA even in the first session. The remaining 68 patients (63%) required chemoembolization of the IPA after the first session.

Right IPA supply was in 105 patients (97.2%). Left IPA supply was in five patients (4.6%) (Fig 1). Of the five patients who received a parasitic supply from the left IPA, both right and left IPA parasitization of the HCC was existing in two patients. In the remaining three patients, only the left IPA parasitization was noted.

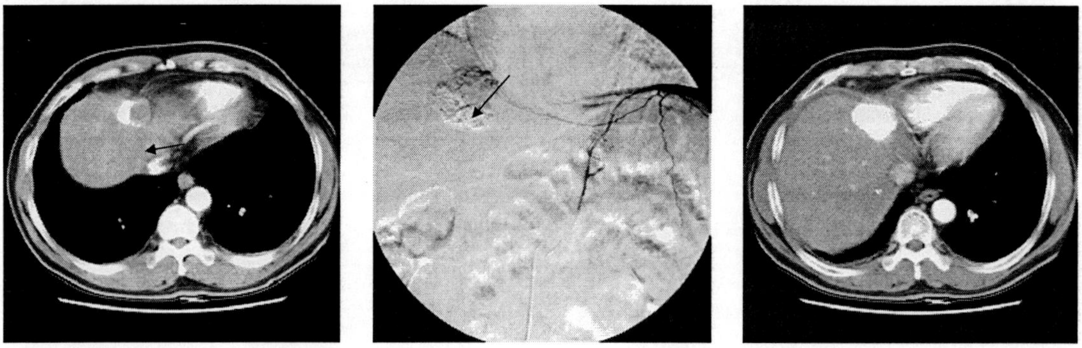

Fig 1. HCC supplied from left IPA
A. Arterial phase of abdomen dynamic CT scan shows lipiodol defect area (arrow) at previous lipiodol uptake lesion in liver dome S4 which means marginal recurrence.
B. Left IPA arteriography shows parasitic supply of tumor staining (arrow). And TACE was successfully performed through this left IPA. Hepatic arteriography did not demonstrated tumor staining (not shown).
C. One month follow-up CT scan shows compact lipiodol uptake at the previous defect area. This lesion did not recurred for three years follow-up period.

**Table 1. Relationship Between the HCC Supplied from IPA and the Segment, Capsule of the Liver, and the Size.**

| Tumor Location | Distance from Capsule | Tumor Size |
|---|---|---|
| Segment 7 (n=56) | Exophytic (n=16) | < 1cm (n=28) |
| Segment 8 (n=38) | Capsule Abutting (n=72) | 1—2cm (n=47) |
| Segment 4 (n=10) | Apart from Capsule (n=32) | 2.1—3cm (n=28) |
| Segment 6 (n=6) | 5mm—2cm deeper from capsule | 3.1—5cm (n=3) |
| Segment 1 (n=4) | | > 5cm (n=14) |
| Segment 2 (n=4) | | |
| Right atrium (n=2) | | |

Note—a total of 120 HCC nodules in 108 patients.

Relationship between the HCC supplied from the IPA and the segment of the location, distance from the capsule of the liver, and the size of the HCC were presented at Table 1. The most of tumor (78.3%, 94 of 120 nodules) is located at S7 and S8. The remainders are located at S4, S6, S1, and S2. Furthermore, right IPA supply is found at thrombus of HCC extended into the suprahepatic segment of the inferior vena cava (Fig 2). With regard to the nodular HCC supplied by IPA and the liver capsule, 73.3% (88 of 120 nodules) is abutted to the liver capsule or is exophytic. But as much as 26.6% (32 of 120 nodules) is located at deeper liver parenchyma away from the capsule (Fig 3). Regarding the size of tumor, 75 small HCC less than 2cm out of 120 nodules which have IPA parasitization are found reaching 62.5% (75 of 120 nodules).

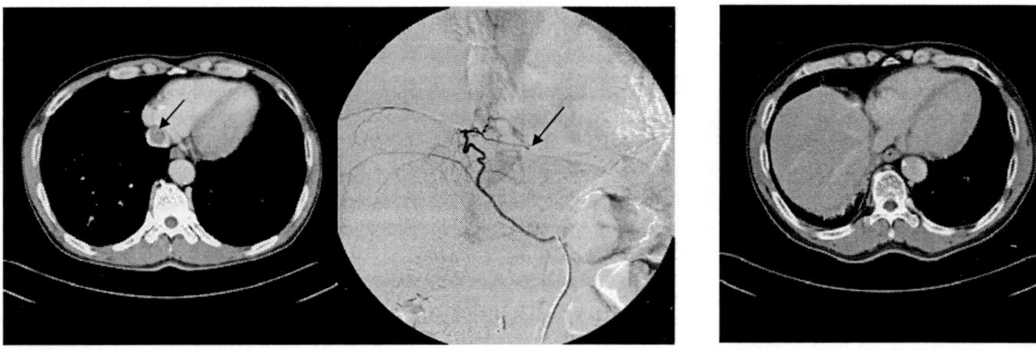

Fig 2. HCC tumor thrombus extending into the suprahepatic segment of the inferior vena cava that is supplied from right IPA.
A. Portal phase of abdomen dynamic CT scan shows HCC tumor thrombus (arrow) in the suprahepatic segment of the inferior vena cava which is extended through the left hepatic vein.
B. Right IPA arteriography shows the hypervascular tumor thrombus staining (arrow). CDDP chemoinfusion therapy was performed repeatedly three times for one month interval.
C. Follow-up CT scan shows absence of the previously noted tumor thrombus. Liver parenchymal HCC and tumor thrombus in left hepatic vein were also completely resolved.

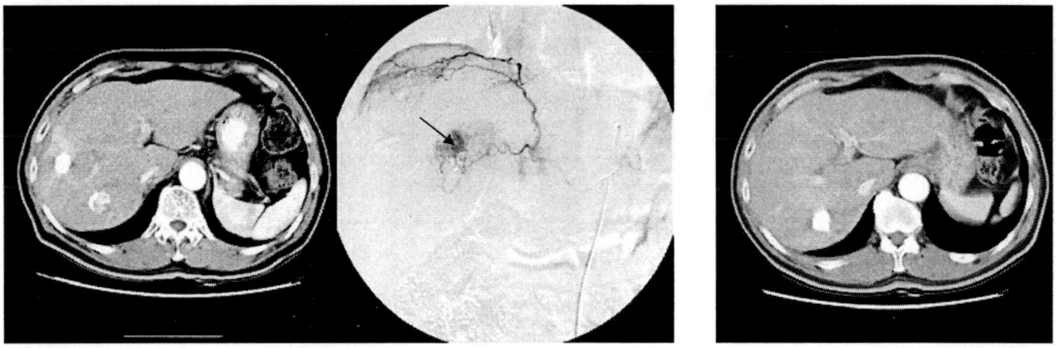

Fig 3. Right IPA parasitization into the HCC located in deeper liver parenchyma apart from the liver capsule.
A. Arterial phase of abdomen dynamic CT scan shows recurred nodular HCC (arrow) in S7 about 2cm apart from the liver capsule.
B. Right IPA arteriography shows exclusive parasitic supply pattern of hypervascular nodular tumor staining (arrow) from posterior branch of the right IPA. Selective TACE into the posterior branch of the IPA was performed successfully.
C. Follow-up CT scan shows compact lipiodol uptake. This lesion did not recurred for three years follow-up period.

**Table 2. Characters of 33 Nodular HCC Which Received Exclusive Pattern of IPA Parasitization in 28 Patients.**

| Previous No. of TACE | Tumor Size | Segment | Relationship between HCC and Liver Capsule |
|---|---|---|---|
| 1—8 session(s) | 4mm—3cm | S7 (n=17) | exophytic (n=3) |
| (mean, 2.8) | (mean, 1.3cm) | S8 (n=12) | abut (n=12) |
| | | S4 (n=2) | apart from capsule (n=18) |
| | | S1 (N=2) | |

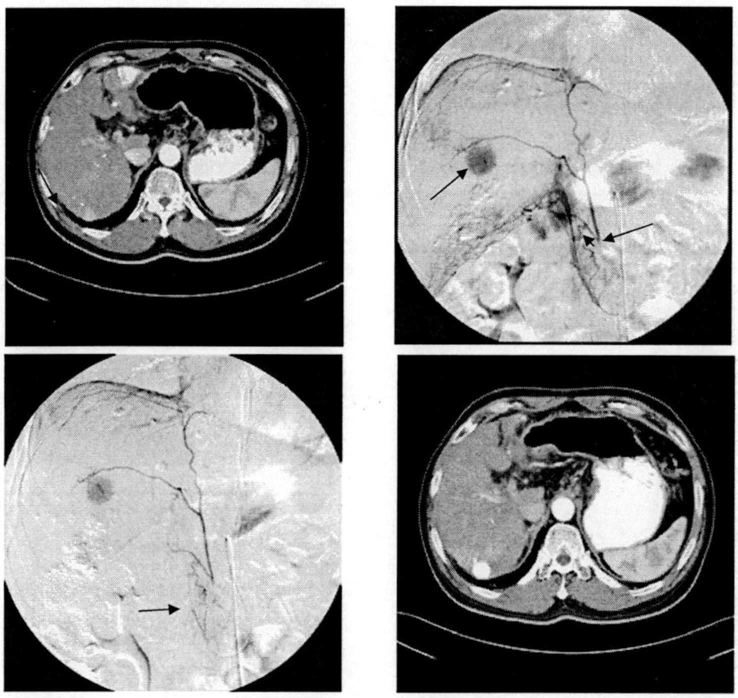

Fig 4. TACE into the IPA through the collateral route.
A. Arterial phase of abdomen dynamic CT shows small nodular HCC (arrow) in S7 subcapsular location.
B. Arteriography of the right renal capsular artery shows right IPA opacification through the collateral route (arrowheads) with hypervascular nodular tumor staining (thin arrow) exclusively fed by posterior branch of the right IPA. Note the occluded orifice of the right IPA (thick arrow).
C. The collateral route was selected with 3-F coaxial microcatheter, and TACE was performed successfully via this collateral route. Arrow indicates the tip of the microcatheter.
D. Follow-up CT scan shows compact lipiodol uptake. This lesion did not recurred for one year follow-up period.

Independent parasitic supply of IPA was in 79 nodules (65.8%), dependent parasitic supply was in 8 nodules (6.7%), and exclusive parasitic supply (Fig 1, Fig 3) was in 33 nodules (27.5%). Characters of nodular HCC which had exclusive parasitic supply pattern of IPA are presented in Table 2. All patients with exclusive parasitic supply pattern have had injury of the hepatic arteries from previous repeated hepatic arterial TACE. In case 18 out of

33 nodular HCC (54.5%) which have exclusive parasitic supply pattern by IPA, the location of those nodules was in deeper liver parenchyma apart from the liver capsule.

Arteriography and chemoembolization of IPA before hepatic artery chemoembolization was performed in 68 patients (62.9%) who have had large iodized oil uptake mass from previous TACE.

Five patients have had occlusion of the right IPA orifice: two patients had collateral connection with the right renal capsular artery, one with the proximal superior mesenteric artery, one with the hepatic parenchymal artery, and one with the left IPA. TACE could be possible in all patients via the collateral route (Fig 4).

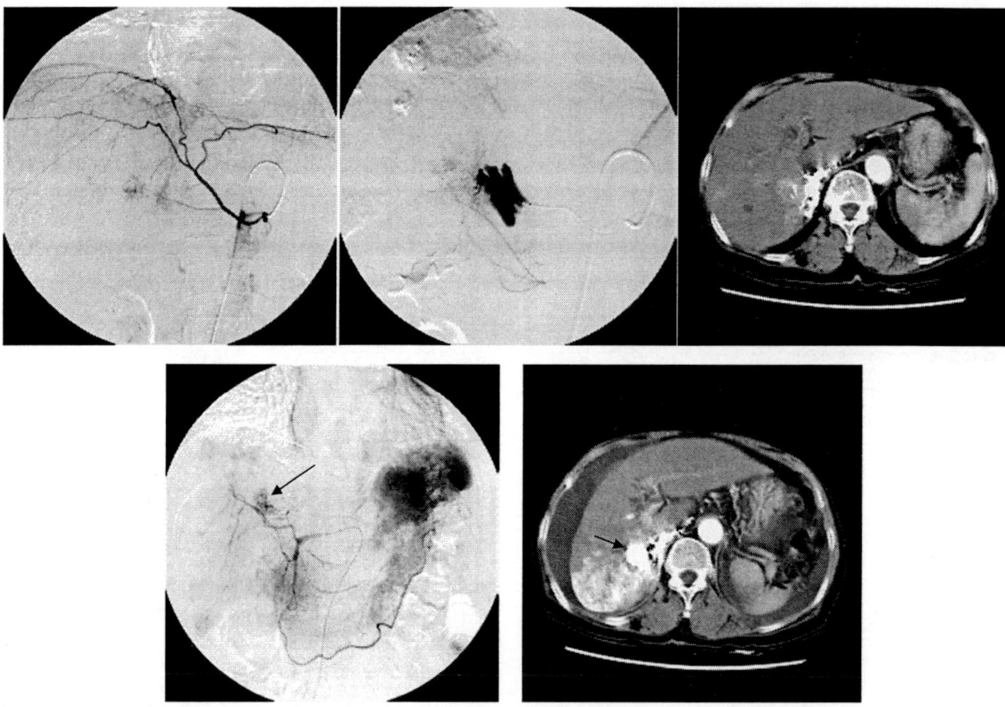

Fig 5. Rupture of the tumor feeding superior adrenal artery during the arteriography. Remodeling of the hepatic artery.
A. S7 nodular HCC staining (arrowhead) was exclusively fed by superior adrenal artery (arrow).
B. Rupture of the superior adrenal artery occurred during the selective arteriography using the power injector. Note the extravasated contrast media (arrows). TACE was incomplete, and embolization was performed with gelatin sponge particle and microcoil to prevent bleeding. Although the patient complained severe pain, vital signs were stable.
C. Follow-up CT scan shows nodular HCC (arrow) in S7 deeper liver parenchyma apart from the liver capsule without lipiodol uptake. Note the extravasated lipiodol in the retroperitoneal space (arrowheads).
D. Follow-up hepatic arteriography shows hypervascular nodular tumor staining (arrow) which was supplied from superior adrenal artery. This phenomenon was the redistribution of the tumor feeding artery due to the occlusion of the previously supplying feeder. So, successful TACE was possible through the hepatic artery.
E. Follow-up CT shows compact uptake of the lipiodol (arrow). This lesion did not recurred for two years follow-up period.

In one case with exclusive parasitic supply pattern of IPA is fed by the superior adrenal artery off right IPA. Superior adrenal artery is ruptured in this patient when the angiography is performed by the method of contrast media with 1 ml/sec x 3 sec with power injector 800 psi via superselected 3-F coaxial microcatherter. At that time, TACE was incomplete. Fortunately, however, TACE was successful to redistribute feeder two months later by way of supplying hepatic arterial branch (Fig 5).

Other parasitic supply arteries were associated in 24 patients (22.2%) with renal capsular artery, adrenal artery, omental branch, right intercostal artery, right subcostal artery, right and left internal mammary artery (Fig 6).

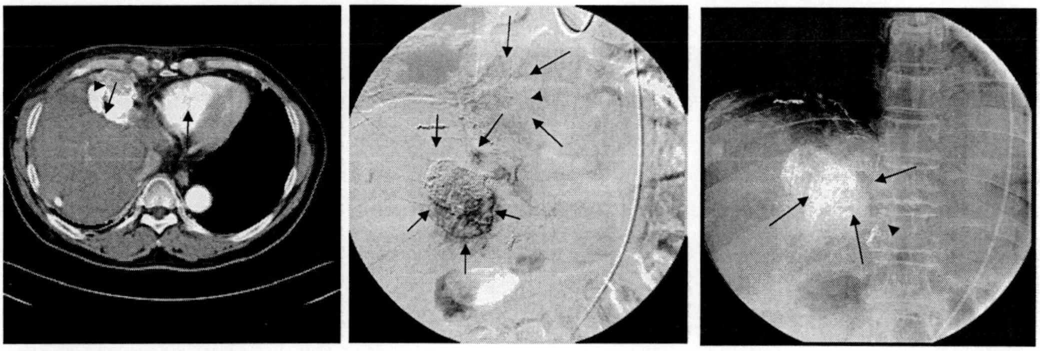

Fig 6. Other parasitic artery.
A. Arterial phase of abdomen dynamic CT scan shows marginal recurred HCC (arrow) in S4 ventral aspect. The patient received previous one session of hepatic artery and right IPA TACE.
B. Right internal mammary arteriography shows hypervascular tumor staining (thick arrows) corresponding to the CT scan. Note the course of the 3-F coaxial microcatheter (arrowheads) suggest that the right internal mammary artery was selected. Microcoils (thin arrows) along the diaphragm area were in the right IPA that was used at previous TACE into the right IPA for protective and effective TACE.
C. Successful TACE was performed into the musculophrenic branches of the right internal mammary artery. Note the large nodular lipiodol uptake area (arrows) and protective microcoils (arrowhead) in superior epigastric branch of the right internal mammary artery.

Two patients with ruptured HCC had right IPA parasitization. In one case, right IPA parasitization was responsible for marginal recurrence without hepatic artery supply. In the other case, omental branch and right IPA parasatization were responsible for marginal recurrence without suppling hepatic artery.

Affected shoulder pain was tolerable in all except one patient. Two patients complained intolerable severe back pain persisted for a week due to retroperitoneal fat necrosis from chemoembolization of the superior adrenal artery off right IPA. One patient was ruptured at superior adrenal artery during the course of chemoembolization with mixture of adriamycin and lipiodol through 3-F coaxial microcatheter. And the other one was ruptured at superior adrenal artery during the arteriography through 3-F coaxial microcatheter after the superior adrenal artery was superselected. Their vital was stable and they were underwent transcatheter arterial embolization with gelatin sponge particle and microcoil. No bleeding was found. Two patients were complicated with lipiodol lung embolization through the transpleural IPA to pulmonary artery shunt. Cough and sputum were persisted for two months, but recovered with conservative management. Two patients had passive lung atelectasis in right lower lobe basal segments. This phenomenon might be due to the paralysis of the diaphragm probably from the TACE-induced ischemic complication. However, they were asymptomatic.

# Discussion

## Arteries of the Diaphragm [13, 14]

The arteries of the diaphragm ramify on both its superior and inferior surfaces. The arteries supplying the superior surface of the diaphragm are pericardiacophrenic and musculophrenic branches of the internal mammary artery, and superior phrenic arteries arising from the thoracic aorta. The arteries supplying the inferior surface of the diaphragm are the IPAs. The most common extrahepatic collateral artery which has parasitic supply to the HCC is the IPA. The IPAs may arise from the front of the abdominal aorta just below the aortic hiatus and immediately above the origin of the celiac trunk as a first branch of the abdominal aorta. Also, they may arise from the celiac trunk either separately or by a single stem common to both sides. Furthermore, the IPA may also arise from the renal arteries, and other aberrancies occur. It is important to be aware of where the IPA is arising so that selective arteriography can be conducted right away, skipping unnecessary aortography step.

The IPA branches several superior adrenal arteries. And then, the IPA divides into an anterior and a posterior branch. The posterior branch is usually branched more early and runs posteriorly and lateralward toward the ribs and anastomoses with the terminals of the intercostals and superior phrenic arteries. The anterior branch is usually located more cranially than the posterior one and ramifies anteriorly and medialward on the under side of the diaphragm, anastomosing with the same branch of the other side and with the terminals of the musculophrenic and pericardiacophrenic arteries. Successful selective TACE in correlation of cross-sectional imaging and angiographic finding can be guaranteed only when you are fully aware of the anatomy of IPA branching pattern and superior adrenal arteries.

## Nerves of the Diaphragm: Referred Pain from the Diaphragm and Paralysis of the Diaphragm [13, 14]

The phrenic nerves supply the entire motor fibers to the diaphragm and also the sensory fibers of the pain and proprioception to most of the central portion of the diaphragm. The phrenic nerve arises from the ventral rami of C3—C5 of the cervical plexus of the spinal cord. Small peripheral parts of the diaphragm receive their sensory nerve supply from the lower intercostals nerves and the subcostal nerves.

Pain from the diaphragm radiates to two different areas because of the difference in the sensory nerve supply of the diaphragm. Pain resulting from irritation of the diaphragmatic pleura or the diaphragmatic peritoneum is referred to the shoulder region, the area of skin supplied by the C3 through C5 segments of the spinal cord. These segments also contribute ventral rami to the phrenic nerves. Irritation of the peripheral regions of the diaphragm, innervated by the inferior intercostals nerves, is referred to the skin over the costal margins of the anterolateral abdominal wall. Intra-venous analgesics and intra-arterial lidocaine injection may be helpful for pain reduction.

Paralysis of the diaphragm may occur from the severe pain or ischemia of the motor nerve fibers, resulting passive lung atelectasis. Most patients with passive lung atelectasis were asymptomatic.

## Other Collaterals to Find

In one study [15], of the 30 patients with HCC located in ventral hepatic area directly beneath the diaphragm, 10 patients had internal mammary artery feeding, and of those who had internal mammary arterial feeding, seven patients also had IPA feeding. This result proved potential communication and overlapping arterial supplying area between the IPA and internal mammary artery.

The IPA has many anastomotic connections, including the musculophrenic artery and pericardiacophrenic artery off internal mammary artery, the intercostals artery, and subcapsular branches of hepatic arterial branch in the diaphragm [16, 17]. Therefore, in case residual viable portion of HCC or recurrence is seen after TACE of IPA, selective arteriography of the aforementioned branches that could potentially form anastomosis with IPA should be performed.

## Understanding about IPA Territory

The right and left IPAs run along the inferior surface of the diaphragm, and their branches are in direct contact with the liver in the region in which no parietal peritoneum covers the diaphragm, the "bare area" of the liver. Portions of liver S1, S2, and S7 form this bare area. Certainly, the IPA frequently supplies lesions located in these segments [15].

However, in our study, parasitic supply of the IPA to the HCC was noted not only the lesions in the bare area (S1, S2, and S7) but also the lesions in the S4, S6, S8, and right atrium. Tanabe et al. [18] also reported that parasitic supply of the IPA to the HCC located in S4 and S8. Basically, IPA parasitization of HCC at S1, S2, and S7 area is considered as the right thing to do because IPA supplies liver through bare area. More importantly, nodules in non-bare area such as S4, S6, and S8 can also have parasitization of the IPA when hepatic artery is damaged.

## When to Perform IPA Chemoembolization

Classically, IPA arteriography and chemoembolization in patients with HCC is essential when the hepatic arteries are injured from previous TACE and other procedures. Tanabe et al. [18] observed that HCC that have not had previous treatment may also have their blood supply from an IPA in one of the 14 patients. In this study, the chemoembolization of the IPA even in the first session without previous chemoembolization is required in forty patients

(37%) of 108 patients. In case of large HCC, patients not previously chemoembolized has a possibility of IPA parasitization, and therefore, need IPA chemoembolization in the first session. In reality however, first session of TACE is limited to hepatic artery due to the safe dosage of chemotherapeutic agent and iodized oil, and IPA chemoembolization can be performed in the next session. In this case, being aware of where IPA is arising and in what degree it is supplying parasitic tumor through arteriography will help with the next session of TACE.

When HCC location is at bare area, IPA arteriography is a must even in the first session of TACE. From the second session of TACE, IPA arteriography should always be conducted regardless of HCC location when HCC seen in CT or MRI are not all seen in hepatic arteriography.

## Non-tumorous Pleural and Pulmonary Staining by IPA

Because of the IPA is one of the systemic arteries that contribute to the transpleural systemic-pulmonary artery anastomosis, non-tumorous staining at the pleura and lung parenchyma may be visualized by IPA arteriography when the pulmonary abnormalities involve the lung base [19].

It should be differentiated from the true tumor staining to avoid useless TACE and to prevent unwarranted lipiodol embolization of the pulmonary artery. Lee et al. [20] described the detailed angiographic findings of the pleural and pulmonary staining which mimicking a tumor staining of HCC during the IPA arteriography. They asserted that the clue of these findings is the sequential visualization of the IPA, pulmonary arteries, and pulmonary veins. At first, the tortuous peripheral branches of the IPA are visualized, and then the peripheral fine branches of the pulmonary arteries are appeared with staining of the lung parenchyma at the lung base. Finally, the draining pulmonary veins can be seen (Fig 7). Oblique view of the DSA also may be helpful for distinguishing the inflammatory staining and the nodular tumor staining. Interventionists should know this non-tumorous angiographic finding of the IPA to avoid the useless TACE which can result unhappy embolization of the pulmonary arteries and veins.

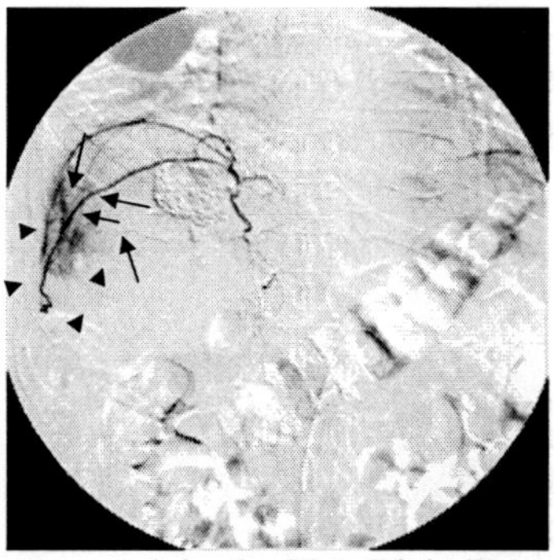

Fig 7. Non-tumorous pleural and pulmonary staining by IPA. Right IPA arteriography shows wedge-shaped lung parenchymal staining (arrowheads) from anterior branches (thin arrows) of the right IPA at right costophrenic angle area. Draining pulmonary vein is visualized (thick arrows).

## SUMMARY

According to the our results of the TACE of the IPA, we recommend the strategies of the arteriography and chemoembolization of the IPA as bellows:

1. It is necessary to check IPA arteriography even though TACE is being performed for the first time when HCC is exophytic or capsular abutting in liver dome area (S7, S8, S4, and S2) or caudate lobe of the liver (S1).

2. It is mandatory to conduct IPA arteriography especially when hepatic artery is injured by repeated hepatic artery TACE since IPA can still supply HCC, regardless of tumor location segment, capsule abutment, and tumor size. It is important to remember that when hepatic artery is injured, IPA is capable of supplying other liver segments and HCC in deeper liver parenchyma area apart from the capsule regardless of bare area. Small HCC less than 2cm can be supplied from parasitization of IPA. In case of newly developed HCC after repeated TACE, the staining of HCC may not be seen in hepatic artery arteriography due to the injury of hepatic artery and may be parasitized exclusively from IPA.

3. Right IPA arteriography should also be performed as well as hepatic artery arteriography if large lipiodol uptake mass is at bare area and there is a possibility of recurrence. Our protocol in such a case is do not proceed with TACE right after hepatic artery arteriography even though there is a HCC supplied by hepatic artery but also check IPA arteriography following hepatic artery angiography. That is because tumor staining by IPA might not be clearly seen if IPA arteriography is followed by TACE of hepatic artery due to digital subtraction artifact caused by lipiodol injected into hepatic artery.

4. It is important to always consider the possibility of parasitic supply by left IPA although the occurrence is very rare. In this case, right lobe of the liver dome area (S7 and S8) as well as left lobe of the liver S2 and S4 can also happen. If the mass is large, parasitization by left IPA is possible when parasitic supply by right IPA is not sufficient. Even thought the mass is small, parasitic supply by left IPA is also possible if hepatic artery and right IPA are damaged by previous multi-session of TACE. Though there is no injury of right IPA, parasitization from left IPA may be possible when right IPA is hypoplastic and left IPA is dominant.

5. It is highly recommended that benign transpleural shunt and true tumor parasitic supply should be differentiated in order to avoid unnecessary procedure of chemoembolization and procedure-related complications.

6. Protective and effective TACE is possible if TACE is performed following microcoil embolization of distal portion of IPA in case IPA distal is not involved in tumor supply or there is benign transpleural shunt at the distal of IPA with parasitic tumor supply at the proximal of IPA.

7. If the tumor size seen in CT and the staining of tumor size and configuration checked in hapatic arteriography and right IPA arteriography do not match, other collaterals such as renal capsular artery, adrenal artery, omental branch, contralateral left IPA, right intercostal artery, right and left internal mammary artery should also be examined.

8. When there is a transtumoral connection between hepatic artery and IPA, sufficient lipiodol uptake might not be achieved with proximal IPA chemoembolization. That is because the mixture of chemotherapeutic agent and lipiodol that is hand injected from

proximal IPA is not fully delivered into tumor due to the flow from hapatic artery into the tumor. A solution to such a case is to select tumor feeding artery and wedge the microcatheter in the feeding artery wall and hand inject. By doing so, drug delivery can be achieved. In other words, superselective TACE in every IPA TACE ensures effective and safe TACE.

9. Arteriography using power injector is prohibited when unhypertrophied superior adrenal artery is superselcted. The reason is that rupture can result from pressure injection and incomplete TACE is resulted. When arteriography is necessary in order to check feeding, it should be done with hand injection.

10. If there is a patient with ruptured HCC with IPA parasitization, IPA arteriography as well as hepatic arteriography should be done because HCC rupture from IPA feeding could happen, very rare though.

## Conclusion

Reported results about the effect of TACE through collaterals were comparable to the rates for usual TACE through the hepatic artery [12, 21, 22]. For effective TACE of the HCC, therefore, recognition of the presence of extrahepatic tumor feeders is crucial because adequate embolization of the collateral tumor feeders as well as the hepatic arteries is equally important. The IPA is one of the most common extrahepatic tumor feeders, therefore, it is too important to evaluate the presence of tumor blood supply from the IPA and to perform chemoembolization.

## References

[1] Yamada R, Sato M, Kawabata M, Nakatsuka H, Nakamura K, Takashima S. Hepatic artery embolization in 120 patients with unresectable hepatoma. *Radiology* 1983; 148:397-401.

[2] Nakamura H, Mitani T, Murakami T, et al. Five-year survival after transcatheter chemoembolization for hepatocellular carcinoma. *Cancer Chemother Pharmacol* 1994; 33 Suppl:S89-92.

[3] Nakamura H, Oi H, Hori S, et al. Outcome of localized hepatocellular carcinoma treated with segmental arterioportal chemoembolization. *Cancer Chemother Pharmacol* 1992; 31 Suppl:S69-71.

[4] Matsui O, Kadoya M, Yoshikawa J, et al. Small hepatocellular carcinoma: treatment with subsegmental transcatheter arterial embolization. *Radiology* 1993; 188:79-83.

[5] Matsuo N, Uchida H, Nishimine K, et al. Segmental transcatheter hepatic artery chemoembolization with iodized oil for hepatocellular carcinoma: antitumor effect and influence on normal tissue. *J Vasc Interv Radiol* 1993; 4:543-549.

[6] Nishimine K, Uchida H, Matsuo N, et al. Segmental transarterial chemoembolization with Lipiodol mixed with anticancer drugs for nonresectable hepatocellular carcinoma: follow-up CT and therapeutic results. *Cancer Chemother Pharmacol* 1994; 33 Suppl:S60-68.

[7] Matsui O, Kadoya M, Yoshikawa J, Gabata T, Takashima T, Demachi H. Subsegmental transcatheter arterial embolization for small hepatocellular carcinomas: local therapeutic effect and 5-year survival rate. *Cancer Chemother Pharmacol* 1994; 33 Suppl:S84-88.

[8] Itsubo M, Koike K, Tsuno S, et al. Subsegmental transcatheter arterial embolization for small hepatocellular carcinoma. *Hepatogastroenterology* 2002; 49:735-739.

[9] Iwamoto S, Sanefuji H, Okuda K. Angiographic subsegmentectomy for the treatment of patients with small hepatocellular carcinoma. *Cancer* 2003; 97:1051-1056.

[10] Charnsangavej C, Chuang VP, Wallace S, Soo CS, Bowers T. Angiographic classification of hepatic arterial collaterals. *Radiology* 1982; 144:485-494.

[11] Soo CS, Chuang VP, Wallace S, Charnsangavej C, Carrasco H. Treatment of hepatic neoplasm through extrahepatic collaterals. *Radiology* 1983; 147:45-49.

[12] Shibata T, Kojima N, Tabuchi T, Itoh K, Konishi J. Transcatheter arterial chemoembolization through collateral arteries for hepatocellular carcinoma after arterial occlusion. *Radiat Med* 1998; 16:251-256.

[13] Moore KL, Dalley AF. Abdomen. In: Kelly PJ, ed. Clinically oriented anatomy. 4th ed. Philadelphia, Lippincott Williams & Wilkins, 1999; 174-330.

[14] Woodburne RT, Burkel WE. The abdomen. In: Woodburne RT, Burkel WE, eds. Essentials of human anatomy. 8th ed. New York, *Oxford University Press, Inc.*, 1988; 407-508.

[15] Nakai M, Sato M, Kawai N, et al. Hepatocellular carcinoma: involvement of the internal mammary artery. *Radiology* 2001; 219:147-152.

[16] Michels NA. Collateral arterial pathways to the liver after ligation of the hepatic artery and removal of the celiac axis. *Cancer* 1953; 6:708-724.

[17] Reimann B, Lierse W, Schreiber HW. Anastomoses between the segmental arteries of the liver and phrenicohepatic arterio-arterial anastomoses. *Langenbecks Arch Chir* 1983; 359:81-92.

[18] Tanabe N, Iwasaki T, Chida N, et al. Hepatocellular carcinomas supplied by inferior phrenic arteries. *Acta Radiol* 1998; 39:443-446.

[19] Webb WR, Jacobs RP. Transpleural abdominal systemic artery-pulmonary artery anastomosis in patients with chronic pulmonary infection. *AJR* 1977; 129:233-236.

[20] Lee DH, Hwang JC, Lim SM, Yoon HK, Sung KB, Song HY. Pleural and pulmonary staining at inferior phrenic arteriography mimicking a tumor staining of hepatocellular carcinoma. *Cardiovasc Intervent Radiol* 2000; 23:109-113.

[21] Ikeda K, Kumada H, Saitoh S, Arase Y, Chayama K. Effect of repeated transcatheter arterial embolization on the survival time in patients with hepatocellular carcinoma. An analysis by the Cox proportional hazard model. *Cancer* 1991; 68:2150-2154.

[22] Taniguchi K, Nakata K, Kato Y, et al. Treatment of hepatocellular carcinoma with transcatheter arterial embolization. Analysis of prognostic factors. *Cancer* 1994; 73:1341-1345.

In: Liver Cancer: New Research
Editor: Felix Lee, pp. 101-117

ISBN 1-59454-182-5


*Chapter V*

# Mdm-2 Over-Expression in Hepatitis B x Antigen Positive Hepatocellular Carcinoma

***Jie Liu,*** [1,*] ***Helena M. G. P. V. Reis,*** [1,*] ***Zhaorui Lian,*** [1,*]
***Jingbo Pan,*** [1,*] ***Li Li,*** [1,*] ***Mark A. Feitelson,*** [1,†,*,4] ***Minghua Zhu,*** [2,‡]
***Meng-Chao Wu*** [2]***, Hong-Yang Wang*** [2]***, Patrick Arbuthno*** [3,§]
***and Michael C. Kew*** [3,§]

[1]Thomas Jefferson University, [2]Second Military Medical University, [3]University of the Witwatersrand

[*]Dept of Pathology, Anatomy and Cell Biology, Thomas Jefferson University, Philadelphia, PA, USA 19107

[†]Department of Microbiology and Immunology, Kimmel Cancer Center, Thomas Jefferson University, Philadelphia, PA, USA 19107

[‡]Department of Pathology, Second Military Medical University, Shanghai, 200433 People's Republic of China.

[§]Department of Medical Biochemistry, University of the Witwatersrand, 7 York Road, Parktown, Johannesburg 2193, South Africa.

[¶]Shanghai Eastern Hospital & Institute of Hepatobiliary Surgery, Second Military Medical University, Shanghai, 200436, People's Republic of China.

[4]Corresponding author name and address: Mark A. Feitelson, Ph.D., Room 222 Alumni Hall, Department of Pathology, Anatomy and Cell Biology, Thomas Jefferson University, 1020 Locust Street, Philadelphia, PA 19107. Phone: 215-503-1036; Fax: 215-503-9982; email: Mark.Feitelson@jefferson.edu

## ABSTRACT

The oncogene, *mdm-2*, is over-expressed in a fraction of hepatocellular carcinomas (HCC), suggesting that it is important in tumor pathogenesis. HBV encoded x antigen (HBxAg) is also closely associated with the development of HCC. To determine whether mdm-2 over-expression in HCC correlates with HBxAg, expression, HCC tissues from HBV carriers were stained for HBxAg and mdm-2 by immunohistochemistry. Mdm-2 was over-expressed in the nuclei of tumor cells in 25 of 37 HCC tissues examined (67%), and its over-expression correlated with that of HBxAg in the cytoplasm of the same cells. Using different HBxAg mutants, it was shown that HBxAg *trans*-activation function correlated with elevated endogenous *mdm-2* mRNA levels. HBxAg also *trans*-activated the *mdm-2* promoter in an exogenously added reporter gene construct in p53 null Hep3B cells. These results suggest that mdm-2 is frequently over-expressed in HBV associated HCC, and that it appears to be a transcriptional target for HBxAg. Hence, HBxAg mediated *trans*-activation may contribute importantly to the up-regulated expression of mdm-2 in HCC.

**Key words:** hepatitis B virus, HBxAg, Hepatocellular carcinoma, Mdm-2

## INTRODUCTION

Chronic hepatitis B virus (HBV) infection is associated with a high risk for the development of hepatitis, cirrhosis, and hepatocellular carcinoma (HCC) in an estimated 350 million people worldwide (Feitelson, 1992; Tiollais, Pourcel & Dejean, 1985). The pathogenesis of chronic infection and development of HCC is considered to be, in part, immune mediated (Chisari, 1997), although the persistent expression of the HBV encoded x antigen (HBxAg) also contributes to tumor formation (Feitelson & Duan, 1997; Henkler & Koshy, 1996). HBxAg mRNA and protein are over-expressed in the livers of patients with chronic liver disease (Diamantis et al, 1992; Paterlini et al, 1995; Wang, London & Feitelson, 1991; Wang et al, 1991). In addition, HBxAg stimulates the cell cycle (Benn & Schneider, 1995; Koike et al, 1994a), transforms cell lines (Hohne et al, 1990; Shirakata et al, 1989), and is strongly associated with the development of HCC in transgenic mice (Kim et al, 1991; Koike et al, 1994). HBxAg may promote hepatocellular growth and survival by activating several signal transduction pathways (Benn & Schneider, 1994; Klein & Schneider, 1997; Lee & Yun, 1998; Su & Schneider, 1996), and by directly binding to and stimulating the activities of cellular transcription factors (Autunovic, Lemieux and Cromlish, 1993; Barnabas, Hai & Andrisani, 1997; Henkler & Koshy, 1996; Lauer et al, 1994; Maguire, Hoeffler & Siddiqui, 1991; Qadri, Maguire & Siddiqui, 1995), suggesting possible mechanism(s) whereby HBxAg contributes to the development of HCC.

HBxAg also binds to and inactivates the tumor suppressor, p53 (Feitelson, et al, 1993; Truant et al, 1995; Wang et al, 1994). Loss of p53 by point mutations (Ng et al, 1994; Nishida et al, 1993; Volkmann et al, 1994), deletions of the p53 locus (Murakami et al, 1991; Nishida et al, 1993), or by integration of viral DNA in or near the p53 gene (Slagle, Zhou &

Butel, 1991), suggest that the integrity of the *p53* gene is important in preventing HCC. This is supported by the finding that wild type p53 suppresses the tumorigenic phenotype of human hepatoma cells (Puisieux, Ponchel & Ozturk, 1993; Xu et al, 1996). In HCC, inactivating p53 mutations appear to be associated with late stage tumor progression (Murakami et al, 1991; Teramoto et al, 1994). The finding that many human HCCs have normal p53 (Bourdon et al, 1995; Buetow et al, 1992; Hosono et al, 1993), that X transgenic mice that develop HCC have normal p53 (Ueda et al, 1995), and that there is an inverse relationship between HBxAg expression and p53 mutation (Greenblatt et al, 1997), suggest that HBxAg acts directly upon wild type p53. In fact, in recent studies, most of the p53 detected by staining in HCC tissue was wild type (Bourdon et al, 1995; Greenblatt et al, 1997; Ueda et al, 1995), suggesting a mechanism other than mutation was responsible for the stabilization and accumulation of p53 in HCC tissues.

In a variety of human tumors, elevated levels of wild type p53 correlate with elevated levels of the p53 effector, mdm-2 (Blaydes et al, 1997; Keleti et al, 1996; Pruneri et al, 1997). Up-regulated wild type p53 and mdm-2 have also been reported in a subset of HCCs (Endo et al. 2000; Qiu et al, 1998; Zhu et al, 2003). Given that mdm-2 binds to and triggers the ubiquitin-mediated degradation of p53, and that p53 stimulates *mdm-2* gene expression, documents the presence of an auto-regulatory feedback loop which helps to regulate growth and survival (Wu et al, 1993). The findings that HBxAg binds to and functionally inactivates wild type p53 *in vitro* (Feitelson et al, 1993; Truant et al, 1995; Wang et al, 1994) and *in vivo* (Ueda et al, 1995), brings up the question as to how *mdm-2* gene expression remains up-regulated in the absence of functional wild type p53. Hence, experiments were designed to verify whether mdm-2 was overexpressed in HCC, and if so, whether its over-expression was linked to the presence and function of HBxAg.

# Materials and Methods

## Patients and Tissues

The HCC and surrounding nontumor liver tissues used for analysis were obtained from two different sets of patients. Twenty-three paired tumor/nontumor samples came from as many Chinese patients who had undergone surgery for the removal of their tumors. Most patients lived in and around Xi'an, and were treated at the Fourth Military Medical University. Blocks of fresh frozen tumor (HCC) and corresponding nontumor (liver) tissues were available for each patient. In a few patients where enough surgical material was available, tumor and surrounding nontumor tissue were dissected, separately snap frozen, and stored at –80°C for further analysis. In 13 of these patients, sequence analysis of the p53 exons 4-9 had been previously determined (Greenblatt *et al*, 1997). Fourteen additional paired tumor/nontumor samples were obtained from South African patients. Additional characteristics of the South African and Chinese patients have been published (Greenblatt et al, 1997; Lian et al, 1999). In all cases, tissues were procured for diagnostic purposes and then made available for these studies. Uninfected human liver from 10 individuals who lived in Xijing, China were available as controls.

## Immunohistochemical Staining

Several different primary antibodies were used in this study. The anti-mdm-2 was a purified mouse monoclonal antibody (clone IF2) (Oncogene Research Products, Cambridge, MA) which was used at a dilution of 1:80 on tissue sections. The anti-p53 was also a purified mouse monoclonal antibody raised against a conformational epitope of wild-type p53 (Ab-5) (Oncogene Research Products) and was also used at a dilution of 1:80 for staining. The anti-HBx was a previously characterized peptide antibody (Feitelson & Clayton, 1990; Feitelson, Clayton and Blumberg, 1990) used for immunohistochemical detection of HBxAg (Wang, London & Feitelson, 1991; Wang et al, 1991) at a dilution of 1:5000.

Staining was carried out with each antibody on consecutive fresh frozen sections using the DAKO EnVision$^+$ System (peroxidase labeled polymer kit) to detect the binding of mouse or rabbit primary antibodies (DAKO, Carpenteria, CA). Detection was carried out using DAKO Liquid DAB$^+$, which is based on a horseradish peroxidase (HRP)-labeled polymer conjugated to a secondary antibody. For staining, slides were deparaffinized, rehydrated, and then antigen retrieval was performed by using the DAKO Antigen Retrieval Solution at 95°C for 20 min. Slides were then predigested with 0.1% trypsin in 0.1% $CaCl_2$ (pH 7.8) at room temperature (RT) for 10 min. Endogenous peroxidase was blocked with 1% $H_2O_2$ (30% $H_2O_2$, Fisher Scientific, Pittsburgh, PA) on the slides for 15 min at RT. The slides were air dried and then treated with 1% BSA for 20 min. at RT. Primary antibodies made up in Antibody Diluent (DAKO) were incubated at 4°C overnight. The slides were then washed 3X with Tris-buffered saline (pH 7.5). Staining was then conducted using the DAKO EnVision$^+$ System, followed by liquid DAB$^+$ Substrate chromogen solution, and finally counterstained with Hematoxylin (Sigma Chemical Co., St. Louis, MO). For negative controls, an equivalent dilution of normal mouse IgG (Vector Labs, Burlingame, CA) or rabbit preimmune serum were used in place of primary antibody. The specificity of HBxAg staining was also assessed by preabsorption of the primary antibody with an excess of immunizing antigen (X peptide) prior to staining, and by staining uninfected liver (Wang, London & Feitelson, 1991; Wang et al, 1991). For mdm-2 and p53, uninfected liver sections were also stained with anti-mdm-2, anti-p53 or normal mouse IgG.

Grading for HBxAg immunostaining was evaluated as previously described (Schindl et al, 2001) using a combination of staining intensity and the percent of positive cells. Staining intensity was scored as 1 (weak), 2 (moderate) or 3 (strong), while the percent positive cells was scored as 1 (< 10% positive), 2 (11-50% positive), 3 (51-80% positive) or 4 (>81% positive). The combined scores identified tissues that were negative (0 points), weakly stained (3 points), moderately stained (4-5 points), or strongly stained (6-7 points).

Immunostaining for p53 and mdm-2 was also evaluated as previously described (Endo et al, 2000; Lu et al, 2002). Expression of both antigens were considered to be up-regulated when the percent of positive cells was between 10 and 25% (+), between 25 and 50% (++), or was > 50% (+++) (Pacinda et al, 1996). For HBxAg, p53, and mdm-2, a total of 1000 hepatocytes were counted over 3-5 random fields at a magnification of 400x.

## Plasmids

The HBxAg expression plasmid, pcDNA3-HBx, was constructed using a 621 bp fragment of HBV DNA (Valenzuela et al, 1980) containing the X promoter, the full length X open reading frame, and the HBV polyadenylation site. This fragment was cloned downstream from the early cytomegalovirus promoter at the *Hind* III/*Kpn* I sites within pTTW-1 (a kind gift from Dr. William Mason).

The plasmid pGL2-HIV-LTR was constructed as described (Lian et al, 1999), in which the firefly luciferase gene was placed under the transcriptional control of the human immunodeficiency virus long terminal repeat. This recombinant was used to test the *trans*-activation properties of wild type and mutant HBxAg constructs, since the HIV-LTR is responsive to *trans*-activation by wild type HBxAg (Twu et al, 1989).

pNA(mdm2)-CAT, in which the bacterial chloramphenicol acetyltransferase (CAT) gene is under control of the *mdm-2* promoter, was a kind gift from Dr. Moshe Oren.

## CAT Assay

pNA(mdm2)-CAT was transiently cotransfected into Hep3B (human hepatoma) (Aden et al, 1979) cells, as described (Lian et al, 1999). At 48 hrs post-transfection, CAT activity was measured in cell lysates in a CAT specific ELISA according to manufacturer's instructions (Roche, Indianapolis, IN).

## Cell Lines

HepG2 cells, a differentiated cell line derived from a human hepatoblastoma (Aden et al, 1979), and Hep3B cells, a human hepatocellular carcinoma cell line (Aden et al, 1979), were cultured on type-1 rat tail collagen coated tissue culture dishes or plates, exactly as described (Lian et al, 1999).

## Construction of HBxAg Mutants and Their Expression in HepG2 Cells

pcDNA3-HBx was used as starting material for generating mutations within the X gene. Deletions corresponding to a loss of 10, 20, 30 or 40 amino acids from either end of HBxAg were generated by PCR. An internal deletion spanning HBxAg residues 78-115, inclusive (XMR), was also made by PCR amplifying the 5' and 3' regions of the X gene exclusive of the deleted residues with two pairs of specific primers. Additional details about the construction of these mutants have been previously published (Lian et al, 1999). Verification that the correct mutants were made and cloned properly was carried out by DNA sequence analysis. Maxipreps were then prepared from transformed DH5$\alpha$ cells grown overnight in ampicillin. Validation that the mutant clones encode stable products of only the expected size was assessed by *in vitro* translation, immunoprecipitation with anti-x, and sodium dodecyl sulfate/polyacrylamide gel electrophorsis (SDS/PAGE) (Sun et al, 1998). Once the stability of the HBxAg mutants were established, they were used to stably transfect HepG2 cells using Superfect (QIAGEN, Chatsworth, CA), followed by selection in G418.

### *Northern and Western Blot Analysis*

Total cellular RNA was isolated from $2x10^6$ tissue culture cells according to the enclosed instructions (QIAGEN). Two and a half micrograms of total cellular RNA were separated on 2% formaldehyde, 1% agarose gels, and transfered to Nytran nylon filters using the Turboblotter rapid downward transfer system (both from Schleicher & Schuell, Keene, NH). The filters were hybridized with an appropriate DNA probe labeled with $\alpha$-$^{32}$P-dCTP (3000Ci/mmol; Amersham, Piscataway, NJ) using a random-priming kit (Amersham Life Science, Arlington Heights, IL). The probes consisted of a 500-bp PCR product spanning the HBV X ORF (nts 1366-1847), a 1.8kb *Bam*H1 fragment from the human wild type *p53* pcDNA3 clone (a kind gift from Dr. Ed Mercer), and a 400 bp *Nsi*1/*Apa*1 mdm-2 gene fragment from the 5' region of the gene (kindly provided by Dr. Moshe Oren). The relative levels of transcripts were obtained by densitometric analysis of autoradiograms with an Imaging Densitometer (Model GS-670, BioRad, Hercules, CA) and normalized to the levels of the housekeeping gene transcript encoding glyceraldehyde 3-phosphate dehydrogenase (G3PDH).

Lysates prepared from 5 x $10^6$ HepG2X cells were assayed for HBxAg by western blotting using a mixture of rabbit anti-x peptide antibodies, as described (Feitelson & Clayton, 1990; Feitelson, Clayton and Blumberg, 1990). Horseradish peroxidase conjugated goat anti-rabbit Ig (Accurate, Westbury, NY) and ECL substrate (Amersham, Arlington Heights, Ill) were used for detection. For western blotting of mdm-2, 0.5 grams of tumor or nontumor was homogenized, analyzed by SDS/PAGE, and then transferred onto immobilon membranes, as described (Feitelson et al, 1993). The primary antibody, anti-mdm-2 was the same as that used for immunohistochemistry, except that the dilution used was 1:200. Other details of western blotting have been previously published.

### *Statistical Analysis*

The relationship between HBxAg, p53 and mdm-2 by immunohistochemistry was determined by calculating the significance, p, using the Chi-square ($x^2$) test in 2 x 2 comparisons. Values were significant when $p < 0.05$.

## Results

### Detection of HBxAg, p53 and mdm-2 in Tumor and Nontumor Tissue

Tumor and surrounding nontumor tissue from each of 23 Chinese patients and 14 South African patients were stained for mdm-2, p53, and for HBxAg. Overall, HBxAg was a common marker in tumors from both sets of patients, with 20 of 23 Chinese (87%) and 11 of 14 South African (85%) patients staining positive (Table 1). These observations were similar to those reported earlier (Wang, London & Feitelson, 1991; Wang et al, 1991). HBxAg was detectable in tumors from 14 or 15 HBsAg carriers of Chinese origin (93%) and in 7 of 7 carriers from South Africa (100%), but was also detected in 6 of 8 HBsAg negative Chinese patients (75%) and in 4 of 7 South African patients (57%). These results suggest that HBxAg is prevalent in both HBsAg positive and negative HCC patients, as reported earlier (Zhu et al, 1993). Interestingly, most of the HBsAg negative cases from both groups of patients had detectable levels of one or more viral antibodies (Greenblatt et al, 1997; Lian et al, 1999), implying underlying HBV infection. Importantly, 19 Chinese (83%) and 6 South Africans (46%) had detectable mdm-2 in tumor and, to a much more limited extent, in surrounding nontumor cells, suggesting that mdm-2 expression is commonly elevated in HCC. These are also similar with earlier observations (Luo, Cheng & Feng, 2001; Qiu et al, 1998; Schlott et al, 1999). However, statistical analysis showed a highly significant correlation between mdm-2 and HBxAg expression in both Chinese and African populations ($x^2$ = 14.9, $p < 0.001$), suggesting higher levels of mdm-2 in the presence of HBxAg. This was further supported by the finding of no mdm-2 staining in 6 of 6 HBxAg negative HCCs (Table 1) and of little mdm-2 (and no HBxAg) staining in fresh frozen sections from all 10 uninfected livers. Hence, HBxAg expression appeared to be linked in some way to enhanced mdm-2 expression in HCC.

**Table 1. Immunohistochemistry of HBxAg, p53, and mdm-2 in HCC**

| Number of positive patients | | | | Markers | | | Total (%) |
|---|---|---|---|---|---|---|---|
| Chinese | | African | | HBxAg | p53 | mdm-2 | |
| $HBs^+$ | $HBs^-$ | $HBs^+$ | $HBs^-$ | | | | |
| 7 | 3 | 2 | 0 | + | + | + | 12 (32) |
| 7 | 2 | 2 | 2 | + | - | + | 13 (35) |
| 0 | 0 | 2 | 1 | + | + | - | 3 (8) |
| 0 | 1 | 1 | 1 | + | - | - | 3 (8) |
| 1 | 2 | 0 | 3 | - | - | - | 6 (16) |
| 15 | 8[a] | 7 | 7[b] | 31 | 15 | 25 | 37 |

[a]Seven of these eight patients had detectable anti-HBc, anti-HBs and/or anti-HBe (Greenblatt et al, 1997; Lian et al, 1999). The single patient without detectable antibodies was also negative for HBxAg, p53 and mdm-2 in the liver.
[b]Five of these seven patients had detectable anti-HBc, anti-HBs and/or anti-HBe. One patient positive for HBxAg but negative for p53 and mdm-2, and one patient negative for all three markers were also negative for HBV antibodies.

The situation with p53 was a little different. Although p53 staining in the nuclei of tumor cells was observed in 15 of 37 patients (41%), and was present in 12 tumors from as many patients who were also positive for mdm-2, there was little overlap in the cells that were positive for both proteins within a single tumor, and statistical analysis failed to show a correlation between these markers as well ($x^2$ = 1.78, $p > 0.1$), as noted earlier (Luo, Cheng & Feng, 2001). However, the statistical relationship between HBxAg and p53 was just within significance ($x^2$ = 4.88, $p < 0.05$), which is consistent with the binding of HBxAg to wild type p53 in hepatocarcinogenesis (Ueda et al, 1995).

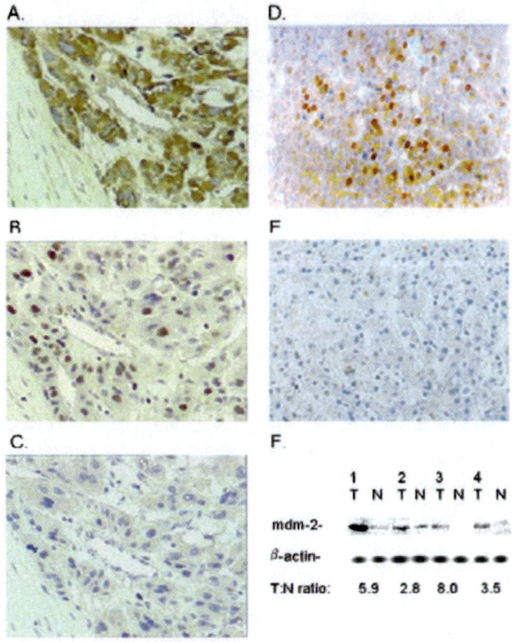


Fig. 1. Immunohistochemical staining for **(A)** HBxAg or **(B)** mdm-2 on consecutive fresh frozen tumor sections from an HCC patient. In **(C)**, a consecutive section of tissue is stained with preimmune rabbit serum. In each panel, the tumor margin is delineated by a fibrous capsule in the lower left. Positive signals are indicated by a brown color. **D.** Double staining for mdm-2 (red staining, mostly nuclear) and HBxAg (tan staining, mostly cytoplasmic) in HCC cells **(D)** and in an uninfected liver **(E)**. **(F)** Western blot analysis of mdm-2 in tumor (T) and nontumor (N) from each of four patients. The relative amounts of □-actin in each lane are also presented. Finally, the ratio of mdm-2 in each T/N pair were calculated from the scanned images of the mdm-2 western blot.

## Relationship Between mdm-2 Over-Expression and p53 Gene Status

Previous work had shown that p53 over-expression in HBxAg positive hepatocytes and HCC cells was associated with the stabilization of wild type p53 (Greenblatt et al, 1997; Ueda et al, 1995). The use of antibodies that detect an epitope on wild type p53 suggest that the latter is observed in most of the HCCs studied herein. To prove this, fresh frozen sections from 13 Chinese patients with known p53 gene status (either wild type or mutant) were stained for mdm-2. The results show up-regulated mdm-2 expression in 9 out of 10 patients (90%) with a wild type p53 gene, and in 2 out of 3 patients (67%) with mutant p53 gene (Table 2). Again, there was no correlation between p53 and mdm-2 staining in these patients ($p > 0.25$), suggesting that elevated mdm-2 does not seem to be associated with elevated wild type p53 in these tumors. This implies that there must be other mechanism(s) responsible for the elevated mdm-2 expression observed in the majority of HCC.

**Table 2. Immunohistochemistry of HBxAg and mdm-2 Among Chinese Patients with a Wild Type or Mutant p53 Gene.**

| | HBsAg | Markers in Tumor | | |
|---|---|---|---|---|
| | (serum) | HBxAg | p53[a] | mdm-2 |
| 1 | + | + | - | + |
| 2 | + | + | + | + |
| 3 | + | + | + | + |
| 4 | + | + | - | + |
| 5 | + | + | - | + |
| 6 | - | + | + | + |
| 7 | + | + | - | + |
| 8 | - | + | + | + |
| 9 | - | + | + | + |
| 10 | - | + | + | + |
| 11 | - | + | - | - |
| 12 | - | - | - | - |
| 13 | - | + | - | + |

[a]A point mutation at p53 codon 236 (patient 7), 249 (patient 9), or 298 (patient 11) was detected by PCR amplication and sequencing of p53 exons 4-9, inclusive (Greenblatt et al., 1997). For codons 236 and 298, the point mutations result in a translation STOP codon, while the 249 mutation is associated with aflatoxin exposure (Bressac et al, 1991; Hsu et al, 1991), which converts an arginine to a serine. All other patients had wild type p53 by the same criteria.

## Relationship Between HBxAg trans-Activation and mdm-2 Expression

The statistically significant relationship between HBxAg and mdm-2 expression (Table 1) is consistent with the possibility that elevated mdm-2 expression may result from the trans-activation activity of HBxAg. To test this hypothesis, a series of HBxAg mutants were made and shown to make the appropriate in vitro translation products (data not shown). Plasmids encoding each of these polypeptides were then individually transfected into HepG2 cells. Initial characterization of these cell lines by northern blot analysis showed that each line expressed the expected mRNA from the recombinant gene (Figure 2A). The corresponding HBxAg associated polypeptides were then identified by western blot analysis of lysates from the same cell lines (Figure 2B). These combined results demonstrate that wild type and mutant HBxAg mRNAs and polypeptides were made by each of the stably transfected cultures. The levels of endogenous p53 and mdm-2 mRNAs in each of these clones were then assessed by northern blot analysis. Corresponding northern blots of mdm-2 mRNA from which the gel scans in Figure 2C were based, are presented in Figure 2D. Figure 2E shows the corresponding western blots of endogenous mdm-2 protein from each of the cell lines. Separate cultures of each of these HepG2 derived clones were transiently transfected with pGL-HIV-LTR to assess the trans-activation activity of each HBxAg polypeptide (Figure 2F). The results show a direct correlation between HBxAg trans-activation activity and the levels of mdm-2 mRNA and protein, but no correlation between HBxAg trans-activation and the levels of p53 mRNA (Figure 2C). These results are consistent with the hypothesis that HBxAg trans-activation function may stimulate the expression of mdm-2 in HCC cells.

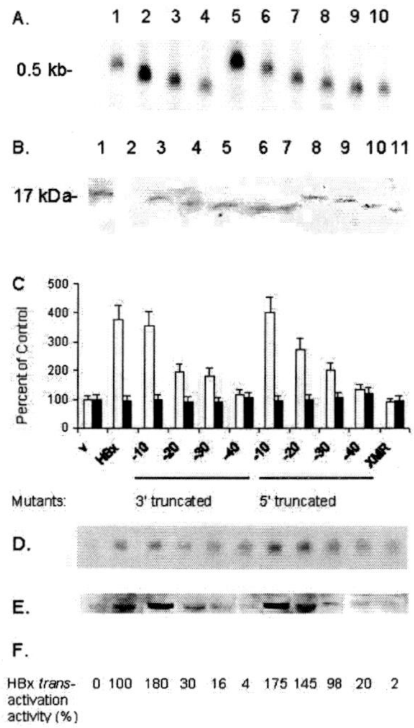


Fig. 2. Characterization of HepG2 clones stably transfected with pcDNA3, pcDNA3-HBx, or with pcDNA expression plasmids encoding different mutants of HBxAg. **(A)** Northern blot analysis of ten individual HepG2 clones, each stably transfected with a different pcDNA3 expression plasmid, making an X mRNA 3' truncated by 30 (lane 1), 60 (lane 2), 90 (lane 3) and 120 (lane 4) base pairs. Lane 5 is the mRNA encoding full length HBxAg. Lanes 6-9 consist of X mRNAs 5' truncated by 30 (lane 6), 60 (lane 7), 90 (lane 8) and 120 (lane 9) base pairs. Lane 10 is the mRNA that encodes XMR. **(B)**. Western blot analysis of the HBxAg related polypeptides encoded by the transcripts in panel **A**. HepG2 cells stably transfected with pcDNA3-HBx, which encodes full length HBxAg (lane 1), or with vector (pcDNA3) alone (lane 2). Different HepG2 cultures were transfected with pcDNA3 plasmids encoding HBxAg polypeptides lacking the carboxy-terminal 10 (lane 3), 20 (lane 4), 30 (lane 5) or 40 (lane 6) amino acids, or with XMR (lane 7). Other cultures were stably transfected with plasmids encoding HBxAg polypeptides lacking the amino-terminal 10 (lane 8), 20 (lane 9), 30 (lane 10) or 40 (lane 11) amino acids. **(C)** Gel scans from the northern blot analyses of endogenous mdm-2 or p53 mRNAs in HepG2 cells stably expressing various HBxAg encoding constructs. HepG2 cells were stably transfected with pcDNA3 vector (v), with pcDNA3 encoding wild type HBxAg (HBx), with HBx mutants progressively truncated at their 3' or 5' ends by the indicated numbers of amino acid residues, or with the internally deleted XMR mutant. Mdm-2 mRNA levels are indicated by white bars while p53 mRNA levels are indicated by black bars, and the results plotted relative to the G3PDH control. The results reflect the average of three independent experiments. **(D)** Northern blot analysis of mdm2 mRNAs from HepG2 cells expressing the various HBx deletion mutants in panel **(C)**. **(E)** Western blot analysis of mdm-2 proteins from HepG2 cells expressing the various HBx deletion mutants. **(F)** The corresponding *trans*-activation activities of the individual HBx plasmids in transiently transfected HepG2 cells, in which pGL2-HIV-1-LTR was used as the reporter, were determined for comparison.

### The mdm-2 Promoter as a Target for HBxAg trans-activation

The correlation between endogenous mdm-2 mRNA levels with HBxAg *trans*-activation activity (Figure 2) suggests that mdm-2 may be a target for HBxAg. To test this hypothesis more thoroughly, a reporter plasmid in which the CAT gene was expressed from the mdm-2 promoter, was transiently cotransfected into Hep3B cells (which are p53 null) along with increasing amounts of pcDNA3-HBx. The results show that HBxAg stimulates the *mdm-2* promoter up to 4.4 ± 0.4 fold in a dose dependent manner (Figure 3). Parallel experiments using pcDNA3 plasmids expressing each of the HBxAg mutants again showed a correlation between HBxAg *trans*-activation activity and mdm-2 promoter activity (data not shown). This data suggests that HBxAg stimulates the *mdm-2* promoter in liver cells.

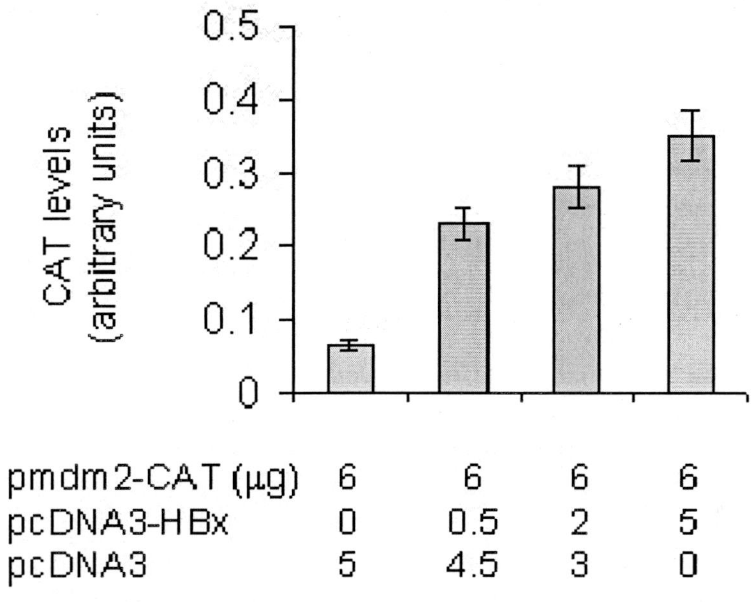


Fig. 3. *Trans*-activation of the mdm-2 promoter by HBxAg. Hep3B cells were transiently transfected with the indicated amounts of each plasmd, and CAT activity was determined by ELISA in cell lysates 48 hours post transfection. The results are based upon 3 independent experiments, each done in duplicate.

## DISCUSSION

There have now been several reports suggesting an elevated expression of apparently wild type p53 in HCC (Bourdon et al, 1995; Buetow et al, 1992; Hosono et al, 1993). Wild type *p53* gene status has been verified in HBxAg positive tumors from patients by p53 exon sequencing (Greenblatt et al, 1997) and from X transgenic mice that develop HCC by PCR/single stranded conformational polymorphism analysis (Ueda et al, 1995). In HCC, as in other tumor types, elevated wild type p53 expression is often accompanied by an increase in the levels of mdm-2 (Blaydes et al, 1997; Keleti et al, 1996; Momand & Zambetti 1997; Pruneri et al, 1997; Qiu et al, 1998). During chronic HBV infection, HBx mRNA and protein accumulate in infected hepatocytes (Diamantis et al, 1992; Paterlini et al, 1995; Wang, London & Feitelson, 1991; Wang et al, 1991), eventually binding to and inactivating virtually all of the endogenous wild type p53 (Ueda et al, 1995). This may disrupt the p53/mdm-2 autoregulatory loop (Wu et al, 1993), by inactivating wild type p53 (Feitelson et al, 1993; Truant et al, 1995; Wang et al, 1994), and triggering an increase in mdm-2. In several reports, up-regulated expression of mdm-2 is associated with HCC progression and invasiveness (Qiu et al, 1998; Zhu et al, 2003), suggesting that HBxAg may promote later stages of tumorigenesis, in part, by this mechanism.

These observations, however, raise the question as to how mdm-2 expression is stimulated in HCC. A common mechanism whereby mdm-2 is over-expressed involves genomic amplification of the *mdm-2* gene (Momand & Zambetti, 1997), and there is some evidence for this in a small fraction of HCCs (Zondervan et al, 2000). Elevated mdm-2 activity has also been found associated with promoter methylation of the $p14^{ARF}$ gene, whose product acts as a tumor suppressor by binding to and sequestering mdm-2 in the nucleoli of liver cells (Edamoto et al, 2003). Selected mutations with the mdm-2 protein, which increase mdm-2 activity, have also been found in a modest number of HCCs (Schlott et al, 2002). However, the observations that HBxAg up-regulates mdm-2 mRNA in liver cells (Figure 2) by stimulating the mdm-2 promoter in a p53 independent manner (Figure 3), suggests that HBxAg targets mdm-2 in place of wild type p53 in hepatocarcinogenesis. This conclusion is further supported by the statistically significant correlation between HBxAg and mdm-2 staining in HCC tissues, and the lack of correlation between elevated mdm-2 and p53 (Table 1). In addition, the observation that HBxAg inhibits the proteasome *in vitro* (Hu et al, 1999), which is responsible for the degradation of both mdm-2 and p53 (Chang et al, 1998; Maki, Huibregtse & Howley, 1996), provides another mechanism whereby HBxAg may up-regulate the expression of mdm-2 in the presence of elevated levels of wild type, but inactive, p53.

The mechanisms whereby wild type p53 expression is either up-regulated or stabilized in HBxAg positive tumors (Figure 1) remains to be fully understood. In this context, there is recent evidence that the phosphorylation of p53 at selected sites alter its binding to mdm-2 (Sakaguchi et al, 2000) and the ability of p53 to stimulate the transcription of *mdm-2* (Nakamura et al, 2000) or other effector genes (Appella & Anderson, 2000). Given that HBxAg stimulates several signal transduction pathways involving protein kinases in a series of phosphorylation cascades (Benn & Schneider, 1994; Klein & Schneider, 1997; Lee & Yun, 1998; Su & Schneider, 1996), it is possible that one or more of these pathways alters the phosphorylation state of p53 and the normal functioning of the p53/mdm-2 autoregulatory loop. These mechanisms may complement the apparent transcriptional targeting of mdm-2 by HBxAg outlined in this work, resulting in an excess of mdm-2 in the presence of stabilized, but functionally inactivated p53. Additional studies are now underway to explore the contributions of these possible mechanisms to HBxAg associated hepatocellular transformation.

**Acknowledgements.** This work was funded by National Institutes of Health grants CA48656 and CA66971 to MF. JL and ZL were partially supported by the Oncology Research Faculty Development Program from NCI.

## REFERENCES


Aden, D. P., Fogel, A., Plotkin, S., Damjanov, I., & Knowles, B. B. (1979). Controlled synthesis of HBsAg in a differentiated human liver carcinoma-derived cell line. *Nature, 282,* 615-617.

Appella, E., & Anderson, C. W. (2000). Signaling to p53: breaking the posttranslational modification code. *Pathologie et Biologie, 48,* 227-245.

Autunovic, J., Lemieux, N., & Cromlish, J. A. (1993). The 17kDa HBx protein encoded by hepatitis B virus interacts with the activation domains of Oct-1, and functions as a co-activator in the activation and repression of a human U6 promoter. *Cellular and Molecular Biology Research, 39,* 463-482.

Barnabas, S., Hai, T., & Andrisani, O. M. (1997). The hepatitis B virus X protein enhances the DNA binding potential and transcription efficacy of bZip transcription factors. *Journal of Biological Chemistry, 272,* 20684-20690.

Benn, J., & Schneider, R. J. (1994). Hepatitis B virus HBx protein activates ras-GTP complex formation and establishes a ras, raf, MAP kinase signaling cascade. *Proceedings of the National Acadamy of Sciences of the United States of America, 91,* 10350-10354.

Benn, J., & Schneider, R. J. (1995). Hepatitis B virus HBx protein deregulates cell cycle checkpoint controls. *Proceedings of the National Academy of Sciences of the United States of America, 92,* 11215-11219.

Blaydes, J. P., Gire, V., Rowson, J. M., & Wynford-Thomas, D. (1997). Tolerance of high levels of wild type p53 in transformed epithelial cells dependent on autoregulation by mdm-2. *Oncogene, 14,* 1859-1868.

Bourdon, J. C., D'Errico, A., Paterlini, P., Grigioni, W., May, E., & Bebuire, B. (1995). p53 protein accumulation in European hepatocellular carcinoma is not always dependent on *p53* gene mutation. *Gastroenterology, 108,* 1176-1182.

Bressac, B., Kew, M., Wands, J., & Ozturk, M. (1991). Selective G to T mutations of p53 gene in hepatocellular carcinoma from southern Africa. *Nature. 350:429-431.*

Buetow, E. H., Sheffield, V. C., Zhu, M., Zhou, T., Shen, F. M, Hino, O., Smith, M., McMahon, B. J., Lanier, A. P., London, W. T., Redeker, A. G., & Govindarajan, S. (1992). Low frequency of p53 mutations observed in a diverse collection of primary hepatocellular carcinomas. *Proceedings of the National Academy of Sciences of the United States of America, 89,* 622-626.

Chang, Y. C., Lee, Y. S., Tejima, T., Tanaka, K., Omura, S., Heintz, N. H., Mitsui, Y,. & Magae, J. (1998). mdm2 and bax, downstream mediators of the p53 response, are degraded by the ubiquitin-proteasome pathway. *Cell Growth & Differentiation, 9,* 79-84.

Chisari, F. V. (1997). Cytotoxic T cells and viral hepatitis. *Journal of Clinical Investigation, 99,* 1472-1477.

Diamantis, I. D., McGandy, C. E., Chen, T. J., Liaw, Y. F., Gudat, F., & Bianchi, L. (1992). Hepatitis B X gene expression in hepatocellular carcinoma. *Journal of Hepatology, 15,* 400-403.

Edamoto, Y., Hara, A., Biernat, W., Terracciano, L., Cathomas, G., Riehle, H. M., Matsuda, M., Fujii, H., Scoazec, J. Y., & Ohgaki, H. (2003). Alterations in RB1, p53 and Wnt pathways in hepatocellular carcinomas associated with hepatitis C, hepatitis B and alcoholic cirrhosis. *International Journal of Cancer, 106,* 334-341.

Endo, K., Ueda, T., Ohta, T., & Terada, T. (2000). Protein expression of MDM2 and its clinicopathological relationships in human hepatocellular carcinoma. *Liver, 20,* 209-215.

Feitelson, M. A. (1992). Hepatitis B virus infection and primary hepatocellular carcinoma. *Clinical Microbiology Reviews, 5,* 275-301.

Feitelson, M. A., & Clayton, M. M. (1990). X antigen polypeptides in the sera of hepatitis B virus infected patients. *Virology, 177,* 367-371.

Feitelson, M. A., Clayton, M. M., & Blumberg, B. S. (1990). The X antigen/antibody markers in hepadnavirus infections. I. Presence and significance of the hepadnavirus X gene product(s) in serum. *Gastroenterology, 98,* 1071-1078.

Feitelson, M. A., & Duan, L. X. (1997). Hepatitis B virus X antigen in the pathogenesis of chronic infections and the development of hepatocellular carcinoma. *American Journal of Pathology, 150,* 1141-1157.

Feitelson, M. A., Zhu, M., Duan, L. X., & London, W. T. (1993). HBxAg and p53 are associated *in vitro* and in liver tissues from patients with primary hepatocellular carcinoma. *Oncogene, 8,* 1109-1117.

Greenblatt, M. S., Feitelson, M. A., Zhu, M., Bennett, W. P., Welsh, J. A., Jones, R. A., Borkowski, A., & Harris, C. C. (1997). Integrity of p53 in hepatitis B x antigen positive and negative hepatocellular carcinomas. *Cancer Research, 57,* 426-432.

Henkler, F., & Koshy, R. (1996). Hepatitis B virus transcriptional activators: mechanisms and possible role in oncogenesis. *Journal of Viral Hepatitis, 3,* 109-121.

Hohne, M., Schaefer, S., Seifer, M., Feitelson, M. A., Paul, D., & Gerlich, W. H. (1990). Malignant transformation of immortalized transgenic hepatocytes after transfection with hepatitis B virus DNA. *EMBO Journal, 9,* 1137-1145.

Hosono, S., Chou, M. J., Lee, C. S., & Shih, C. (1993). Infrequent mutation of *p53* gene in hepatitis B virus primary hepatocellular carcinomas. *Oncogene, 8,* 491-496.

Hsu IC. Metcalf RA. Sun T. Welsh JA. Wang NJ. Harris CC. (1991). Mutational hotspot in the p53 gene in human hepatocellular carcinomas. *Nature. 350,* 427-428.

Hu, Z., Zhang, Z., Doo, E., Coux, O., Goldberg, A. L., & Liang, T. J. (1999). Hepatitis B virus X protein is both a substrate and a potential inhibitor of the proteasome complex. *Journal of Virology, 73,* 7231-7340.

Keleti, J., Quezado, M. M., Abaza, M. M., Reffeld, M., & Tsolos, M. (1996). The mdm-2 oncoprotein is over-expressed in rhabdomyosarcoma cell lines and stabilizes wild type p53 protein. *American Journal of Pathology, 149,* 143-151.

Kim, C. M., Koike, K., Saito, I., Miyamura, T., & Jay, G. (1991). HBx gene of hepatitis B virus induces liver cancer in transgenic mice. *Nature, 351,* 317-320.

Klein, N. P., & Schneider, R. J. (1997). Activation of src family kinases by hepatitis B virus HBx protein and coupled signaling to ras. *Molecular and Cellular Biology, 17,* 6427-6436.

Koike, K., Moriya, K., Iino, S., Yotsuyanagi, H., Endo, Y., Miyamura, T., & Kurokawa, K. (1994). High-level expression of hepatitis B virus HBx gene and hepatocarcinogenesis in transgenic mice. *Hepatology, 19,* 810-819.

Koike, K., Moriya, K., Yotsuyanagi, H., Iino, S., & Kurokawa, K. (1994a). Induction of cell cycle progression by hepatitis B virus HBx gene expression in quiescent mouse fibroblasts. *Journal of Clinical Investigation, 94,* 44-49.

Lauer, U., Weiss, L., Lip, M., Hofschneider, P. H., & Kekule, A. S. (1994). The hepatitis B virus presS2/St transactivator utilizes AP-1 and other transcription factors for trans-activation. *Hepatology, 19,* 23-31.

Lee, Y. H. & Yun, Y. (1998). HBx protein of hepatitis B virus activates Jak1-STAT signaling. *Journal of Biological Chemistry, 273,* 25510-25515.

Lian, Z., Pan, J., Liu, J., Zhu, M., Arbuthnot, P., Kew, M. C., & Feitelson, M. A. (1999). The translation initiation factor, SUI1, may be a target of hepatitis B x antigen in hepatocarcinogenesis. *Oncogene, 18,* 1677-1687.

Lu, M. L., Wikman, F., Orntoft, T. F., Charytonowicz, E., Rabbani, F., Zhang, Z., Dalbagni, G., Pohar, K. S., Yu, G.. Cordon-Cardo, C. (2002). Impact of alterations affecting the p53 pathway in bladder cancer on clinical outcome, assessed by conventional and array-based methods. *Clinical Cancer Research, 8,* 171-9.

Luo, Y. L., Cheng, R. X., & Feng, D. Y. (2001). Role of functional inactivation of p53 from mdm2 over-expression in hepatocarcinogenesis. *Bulletin of Hunan Medical University, 26,* 13-16.

Maguire, H. F., Hoeffler, J. P., & Siddiqui, A. (1991). HBV X protein alters the DNA binding specificity of CREB and ATF-2 by protein-protein interactions. *Science, 52,* 842-844.

Maki, C. G., Huibregtse, J. M., & Howley, P. M. (1996). *In vivo* ubiquitination and proteasome-mediated degradation of p53. *Cancer Research, 56,* 2649-2654.

Momand, J., & Zambetti, G. P. (1997). Mdm-2: "Big Brother" of p53. *Journal of Cellular Biochemistry, 64,* 343-352.

Murakami, Y., Hayashi, K., Hirohashi, S., & Sekiya, T. (1991). Aberrations of the tumor suppressor *p53* and retinoblastoma genes in human hepatocellular carcinomas. *Cancer Research, 51,* 5520-5525.

Nakamura, K., Sun, Y., Yokoyama, Y., Ferris, D., Singh, N., Ichikawa, T., Shinozjuka, K., Kunitoma, M., & Colburn, N. (2000). Phosphorylation status and function of p53 are inversely related to protein kinase C activation. *Anticancer Research, 20,* 1-6.

Ng, I. O. L., Chung, L. P., Tsang, S. W. Y., Lam, C. L., Lai, E. C. S., Fan, S. T., & Fan, M. (1994). *p53* gene mutation spectrum I hepatocellular carcinomas in Hong Kong Chinese. *Oncogene, 9,* 985-990.

Nishida, N., Fukuda, Y., Kokuryu, H., Toguchida, J., Yandell, D. W., Ikenega, M., Imura, H., & Ishizaki, K. (1993). Role and mutational heterogeneity of the *p53* gene in hepatocellular carcinoma. *Cancer Research, 53,* 368-372.

Pacinda, S. J., Ledet, S. C., Gondo, M. M., Langston, C., Brown, R. W., Carmona, P. A., Franklin, R. B., Roggli, V. L., Cagle, P. T. (1996). p53 and MDM2 immunostaining in pulmonary blastomas and bronchogenic carcinomas. *Human Pathology, 27,* 542-546.

Paterlini, P., Poussin, K., Kew, M., Franco, D., & Brechot C. (1995). Selective accumulation of the X transcript of hepatitis B virus in patients negative for hepatitis B surface antigen with hepatocellular carcinoma. *Hepatology, 21,* 313-321.

Pruneri, G., Pignataro, L., Carboni, N., Luminari, S., Capaccio, P., Neri, A., & Buffa, R. (1997). Mdm-2 oncoprotein overexpression in laryngeal squamous cell carcinoma: Association with wild type p53 accumulation. *Modern Pathology, 10,* 785-792.

Puisieux, A., Ponchel, F., & Ozturk, M. (1993). p53 as a growth suppressor gene in HBV related hepatocellular carcinoma cells. *Oncogene, 8,* 487-490.

Qadri, I., Maguire, H. F., & Siddiqui, A. (1995). Hepatitis B virus *trans*-activator protein X interacts with the TATA-binding protein. *Proceedings of the National Academy of Sciences of the United States of America, 92,* 1003-1007.

Qiu, S. J., Ye, S. L., Wu, Z. Q., Tang, Z. Y., & Liu, Y. K. (1998). The expression of the *mdm2* gene may be related to the aberration of the *p53* gene in human hepatocellular carcinoma. *Journal of Cancer Research & Clinical Oncology, 124,* 253-258.

Sakaguchi, K., Saito, S., Higashimoto, Y., Roy, S., Anderson, C. W., & Appella, E. (2000). Damage-mediated phosphorylaton of human p53 threonine 18 through a cascade mediated by a casein 1-like kinase. *Journal of Biological Chemistry, 275,* 9278-9283.

Schindl, M., Oberhuber, G., Obermair, A., Schoppmann, S. F., Karner, B., Birner, P. (2001). Overexpression of Id-1 protein is a marker for unfavorable prognosis in early-stage cervical cancer. *Cancer Research, 61,* 5703-6.

Schlott, T., Ahrens, K., Ruschenburg, I., Reimer, S., Hartmann, H., & Droese, M. (1999). Different gene expression of MDM2, GAGE-1, -2 and FHIT in hepatocellular carcinoma and focal nodular hyperplasia. *British Journal of Cancer 80,* 73-78.

Schlott, T., Scharf, J. G., Gorzel, C., Middel, P., & Spring, H. (2002). Cirrhotic livers reveal genetic changes in the MDM2-p14ARF system of cell cycle regulators. *British Journal of Cancer, 86,* 1290-1296.

Shirakata, Y., Kawada, M., Fujiki, Y., Sano, H., Oda, M., Yaginuma, K., Kobayashi, M., & Koike, K. (1989). The X gene of hepatitis B virus induced growth stimulation and tumorigenic transformation of mouse NIH3T3 cells. *Japanese Journal of Cancer Research, 80,* 617-621.

Slagle, B. L., Zhou, Y. Z., & Butel, J. S. (1991). Hepatitis B virus integration event in human chromosome 17p near the *p53* gene identifies the region of the chromosome commonly deleted in virus-positive hepatocellular carcinomas. *Cancer Research, 51,* 49-54.

Su, F., & Schneider, R. J. (1996). Hepatitis B virus HBx protein activates transcription factor NF-□B by acting on multiple cytoplasmic inhibitors of *rel*-related proteins. *Journal of Virology, 70,* 4558-4566.

Sun, B. S., Zhu, X., Clayton, M. M., & Feitelson, M. A. (1998). Identification of a protein isolated from senescent human cells that binds to hepatitis B virus X antigen. *Hepatology, 27,* 228-239.

Teramoto, T., Satonaka, K., Kitazawa, S., Fujimori, T., Hayashi, K., & Maeda, S. (1994). *p53* gene abnormalities are closely related to hepatoviral infections and occur at a late stage of hepatocarcinogenesis. *Cancer Research, 54,* 231-235.

Tiollais, P., Pourcel, C., & Dejean A. (1985). The hepatitis B virus. *Nature, 317,* 489-495.

Truant, R., Antunovic, J., Greenblatt, J., Prives, C., & Cromlish, J. A. (1995). Direct interaction of the hepatitis B virus HBx protein with p53 response element-directed transactivation. *Journal of Virology, 69,* 1851-1859

Twu, J. S., Rosen, C. A., Haseltine, W. A., & Robinson, W. S. (1989). Identification of a region within the human immunodeficiency virus type 1 long terminal repeat that is essential for trans-activation by the hepatitis B virus gene X. *Journal of Virology, 63,* 2857-2860.

Ueda, H., Ullrich, S. J., Ngo, L., Gangemi, D., Kappel, C. A., Feitelson, M. A., & Jay, G. (1995). Functional inactivation but not structural mutation of p53 causes liver cancer. *Nature Genetics, 9,* 41-47.

Valenzuela, P., Quiroga, M., Zaldivar, J., Gray, P., & Rutter, W. J. (1980). The nucleotide sequence of the hepatitis B viral genome and the identification of the major viral genes. In: *Animal Virus Genetics.* Fields BN, Jaenisch R and Fox CF (eds.). Academic Press, San Diego, 57-70.

Volkmann, M., Hofmann, W. J., Muller, M., Rath, U., Otto, G., Zentgraf, H., & Galle, P. R. (1994). p53 overexpression is frequent in European hepatocellular carcinoma and largely independent of the codon 249 hot spot mutation. *Oncogene, 9,* 195-204.

Wang, W., London, W. T., & Feitelson, M. A. (1991). Hepatitis B x antigen in hepatitis B virus carrier patients with liver cancer. *Cancer Research, 51,* 4971-4977.

Wang, W., London, W. T., Lega, L., & Feitelson, M. A. (1991). Hepatitis B x antigen in liver from carrier patients with chronic hepatitis and cirrhosis. *Hepatology, 14,* 29-37.

Wang, X. W., Forrester, K., Yeh, H., Feitelson, M. A., Gu, J.-r., & Harris, C. C. (1994). Hepatitis B virus X protein inhibits p53 sequence-specific DNA binding, transcriptional activity, and association with transcription factor ERCC3. *Proceedings of the National Academy of Sciences of the United States of America, 91,* 2230-2234

Wu, X., Bayle, H., Olson, D., & Levine, A. J. (1993). The p53-mdm-2 autoregulatory feedback loop. *Genes & Development, 7,* 1126-1132.

Xu, G. W., Sun, Z. T., Forrester, K., Wang, X. W., Coursen, J., & Harris, C. C. (1996). Tissue-specific growth suppression and chemosensitivity promotion in human hepatocellular carcinoma cells by retroviral-mediated transfer of the wild type *p53* gene. *Hepatology, 24,* 1264-1268.

Zhu, M., London, W. T., Duan, L. X., & Feitelson, M. A. (1993). The value of hepatitis B x antigen as a prognostic marker in the development of hepatocellular carcinoma. *International Journal of Cancer, 55,* 571-576.

Zhu, M. H., Ni, C. R., Zhu, Z., Li, F. M., & Zhang, S. M. (2003). Determination of expression of eight p53-related genes in hepatocellular carcinoma with tissue microarrays. *Aizheng, 22,* 680-685.

Zondervan, P. E., Wink, J., Alers, J. C., Jzermans, J. N., Schalm, S. W., de Man, R. A., & van Dekken, H. (2000). Molecular cytogenetic evaluation of virus-associated and non-viral hepatocellular carcinoma: analysis of 26 carcinomas and 12 concurrent dysplasias. *Journal of Pathology, 192,* 207-215.

In: Liver Cancer: New Research
Editor: Felix Lee, pp. 119-159

ISBN 1-59454-182-5


*Chapter VI*

# Understanding Mechanisms of Hepatocarcinogenicity of the Breast Cancer Drug Tamoxifen at the Molecular Level: Relative Risks to Women Versus Rodents.

***Ian N. H. White[1,5] and Karen Brown[2]***

[1]MRC Molecular Endocrinology Group, Dept of Cancer Studies and Molecular Medicine, University of Leicester, Leicester, LE2 7LX UK.

[2]Cancer Biomarkers and Prevention Group, The Biocentre, University of Leicester, Leicester, LE1 7RH, UK.

## ABSTRACT

Tamoxifen has been used successfully as adjuvant therapy in the treatment of breast cancer since the 1970's. Epidemiological investigations showed this drug might increase the incidence of new primary malignancies, such as liver, endometrial or colorectal cancers. Life-time dosing of rats with tamoxifen showed there was a dose dependent increase in the incidence of hepatocellular carcinomas in the treated animals. Since human liver tumors often take decades to develop, it was hoped that by understanding the mechanisms of carcinogenicity in rodents, it might be possible to assess the risks to women taking this class of drug. In rats, tamoxifen dosing leads to hepatic DNA damage, detected by techniques such as $^{32}$P-postlabeling. Little or no such damage could be detected in non-target organs such as kidney, lung or spleen. Tamoxifen is converted by CYP's, to the putative active metabolite, α-hydroxytamoxifen that, following conjugation

[5] Address for correspondence: Ian N.H. White, MRC Molecular Endocrinology Group, Dept of Cancer Studies and Molecular Medicine, University of Leicester, Leicester, LE2 7LX UK. Telephone 44-116-223-1851Email: iw6@le.ac.uk

with sulfate, gives an electrophile that is highly reactive towards DNA. Using insect baculovirus expressed human CYPs, in combination with liquid chromatography-mass spectrometry, it was shown that only CYP3A4 was able to carry out α-hydroxylation. With [$^{14}$C] tamoxifen as substrate and employing the highly sensitive technique of accelerator mass spectrometry, only CYP3A4 was able to catalyze the covalent binding of this drug to DNA. However, Phase 2 glucuronidation conjugates α-hydroxytamoxifen to a stable non-toxic glucuronide. This glucuronidation reaction in human liver is over 50 fold higher than in rats and protects against the toxicity. The present evidence suggests that in women, tamoxifen hepatocarcinogenicity will not be a problem.

## INTRODUCTION

Tamoxifen, first introduced in the 1970s, is now first line therapy for estrogen receptor positive breast cancers. Chemically, tamoxifen is a triphenylethylene (Fig. 1) and competes with estradiol by binding to the same ligand binding domain of the estrogen receptor [1]. Concerns were raised when it was found that in the rat, long-term administration leads to the development of hepatocellular carcinomas [2]. Until recently, it was not clear if tamoxifen was exerting its hepatocarcinogenic effects through an epigenetic mechanism, promoting endogenous DNA lesions via estrogen receptor mediated actions or was genotoxic, either directly or through some electrophilic metabolite. With millions of women taking this drug therapeutically or potentially as a chemopreventive agent against breast cancer, it became important to assess the human epidemiological evidence and understand the mechanisms of hepatocarcinogenesis in rats.

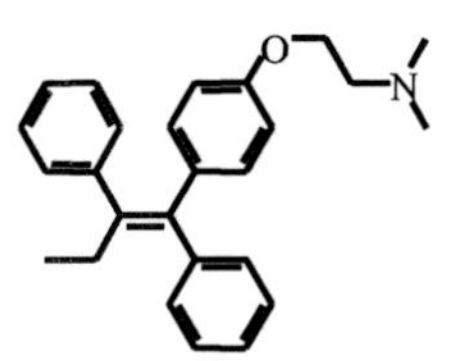

Tamoxifen, I

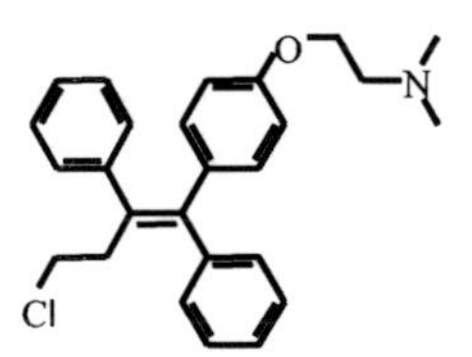

Toremifene, II

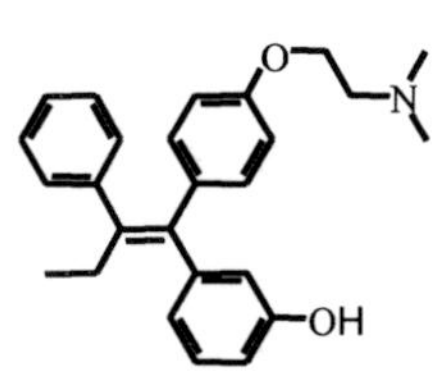

Droloxifene,3210

Figure 1. Chemical structures of tamoxifen (I), toremifene (II) and droloxifene (III).

## THE USE OF TAMOXIFEN IN THE TREATMENT OF BREAST CANCER

At the present time, more than 3 million women have been treated with tamoxifen [3]. It is undoubtedly effective. Meta-analysis of clinical trials involving 37,000 individuals showed therapy is associated with about a 47% reduction in tumor recurrence for estrogen receptor positive tumors during ~10 years of follow-up [4]. However, in those women with low or zero estrogen-receptor levels in their primary tumor, the benefits of tamoxifen appear to be small. Analysis of the most effective duration of treatment through 7 years of follow-up suggests 5 years is optimum [5]. In the year 2000 there was a 25% reduction of mortality rates due to breast cancer in the UK and USA, in women between the ages of 20-69 years, which has been attributed in part to the efficacy of tamoxifen treatment [6]. Furthermore, the potential use of this drug as a chemopreventive agent is being established [7, 8]. A number of clinical trials have shown that giving tamoxifen to healthy women can reduce the early incidence of breast cancer by about 40% [9] and tamoxifen treated patients have a significantly lower incidence of contralateral breast cancers. Tamoxifen is most beneficial for younger women with an elevated risk of breast cancer [10], although it was estimated that in the US, in the year 2000, over 65 million women aged 35-79 years without breast cancer might benefit from tamoxifen chemoprevention [11].

## TAMOXIFEN TREATMENT FOR HEPATOCELLULAR CARCINOMA IN HUMANS

Somewhat bizarrely, in the light of our current understanding of the genotoxic action of tamoxifen in rat liver, this drug has been used to treat hepatocellular carcinomas in men and women. A high proportion of patients present with hepatocellular carcinoma inoperable at diagnosis and have a dismal prognosis. In the past, some believed that tamoxifen might inhibit proliferation in estrogen receptor positive hepatocellular carcinomas in a similar way to that seen in breast, even though most tumors are estrogen receptor negative. A possible rationale for this treatment may have been based on the finding that increased estrogen exposure in the form of oral contraceptives leads to an increased incidence of liver adenomas, nodular hyperplasia and hepatocellular carcinomas in women [12]. It might seem logical, therefore, to treat liver tumors with an estrogen antagonist such as tamoxifen. Against this, there is now evidence that certain oral contraceptives themselves are liver genotoxins. In rats, after daily oral administration of ethynylestradiol (0.075 mg), hyperplastic nodules are seen in the liver within 4 months and hepatocellular carcinoma in about 8% of treated rats at 12 months. DNA adducts, determined by $^{32}$P-postlabeling were detected after 4 months dosing at levels of 73 adducts/$10^8$ nucleotides [13].

The doses of tamoxifen used for the treatment of hepatocellular carcinoma are 60 or 120mg/day. Clinical trials have shown convincingly that tamoxifen is not effective as therapy for hepatocellular carcinoma. In fact, a multi-centre study suggested that there may be a significantly higher risk of death in the tamoxifen treated (120 mg/day) compared with the placebo groups [14]. Meta-analysis of 7 trials, involving 898 patients showed tamoxifen to have no anti-tumor effects and no survival benefits [15].

## Adverse Effects of Tamoxifen Treatment in Women

While there is a clear therapeutic advantage to women with breast cancer taking antiestrogens such as tamoxifen, its use in healthy women needs to be assessed more stringently, especially if the drugs are to be taken on a daily basis over a number of years. The most commonly reported short-term side effects of tamoxifen include hot flushes, tachycardia and nausea. Tamoxifen and estradiol exert their effects through many different cellular targets in human tissue (Fig. 2). Five or more years of tamoxifen use results in a small increase in the incidence of cataracts [16]. More life threatening are thromboembolic events which are significantly increased with tamoxifen, although these occur in less than 1% of treated women [17]. Perhaps the most serious concerns come from epidemiological investigations, initially based on data of Rutqvist *et al.* [18], that suggested this drug might increase the incidence of new primary malignancies, such as liver, endometrial and colorectal cancers (Table 1). A number of other studies since that time have confirmed the increased incidence for endometrial cancers. Reviewing all of the data available in 1996, the International Agency for Research on Cancer (IARC) concluded that in humans there is sufficient evidence for the carcinogenicity of tamoxifen in increasing the risk for endometrial cancer but there is inadequate evidence in humans for the carcinogenicity of tamoxifen in other organs [2]. The absolute risks from tamoxifen of endometrial cancer, stroke, pulmonary embolism or deep vein thrombosis increase with age [10].

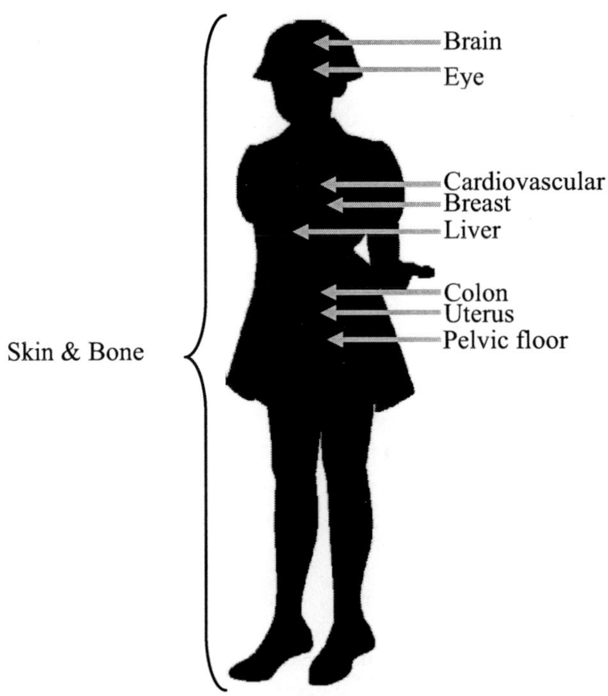


Figure 2. Potential target organs in women for the action of estradiol and estrogen receptor modulators.

In the liver, unlike uterine endometrium, rates of cell proliferation are very low. Uterine tumors associated with tamoxifen treatment appear relatively rapidly over a 5 year follow up period, although with longer follow up times, the incidence does continue to increase [18]. Based on the evidence from radiation exposure, such as thorotrast, hepatocellular carcinomas in humans may take decades to develop [19].

**Table 1. Liver, colon and uterine primary malignancies in women treated with tamoxifen[6]**

| Study | | Tamoxifen treated | Control group | Risk ratio (95% CI) |
|---|---|---|---|---|
| Rutqvist *et al.* [18] | Number: | 1372 | 1357 | |
| Median follow up 9 yrs | Dose: | 40 mg/kg/day | | |
| | Liver/ biliary tract | 3 | 1 | 2.9 (0.3 - 28.2) |
| | Colon | 13 | 6 | 2.1 (0.8-5.6) |
| | Endometrium | 23 | 4 | 5.6 (1.9-16.2) |
| Curtis *et al.* [138] | Number: | 14,358 | 72,965 | |
| SEER | Dose: | ? | | |
| | Liver | 3, O/E=1.10 | 8, O/E= 0.35 | |
| | Colon | 80 O/E=1.04 | 613 O/E=0.94 | |
| | Endometrium | 73 O/E=2.03 | 384 O/E=1.23 | 2.03 (1.59-2.55) |
| Fisher *et al.* [17] | Number: | 1419 | 1424 | |
| NSABP B-14. | Dose: | 20 mg/kg/day | | |
| ~5 years follow up | | | | |
| | Liver | None observed | | |
| | Colon | 10 | 11 | P= 0.98 |
| | Endometrium | 0 | 15 | 7.5 |
| Fisher *et al.* [139] | Number: | 6681 | 6707 | |
| NSABP P-1. Median | Dose: | 20 mg/kg/day | | |
| follow up 4.55 years | | | | |
| | Liver | 0 | 0 | |
| | Colon | 11 | 9 | |
| | Endometrium | 36 | 15 | 2.53 (1.35- 4.97) |

## Liver Tumors in Rats Treated With Tamoxifen

Treatment of rats with tamoxifen (20 mg/kg body wt/day) for 52 weeks results in the formation of liver hyperplastic nodules. Such nodules are not seen in rats treated for 1 day, 2 or 12 weeks [20]. In a study carried out in the UK to GLP standards, male and female rats were given 5, 20, and 35 mg/kg of tamoxifen/day. After 2 years, there was a dose dependent

[6] Results show some of the major investigations and are not a comprehensive survey.

increase in the incidence of liver tumors in the treated animals (Table 2). The majority of the neoplasms were hepatocellular carcinomas showing a well differentiated trabecular pattern while some tumors were glandular in type (Fig. 3A, B) [21]. There was no evidence for an increase in tumor incidence at any other site including the uterus. Interestingly, these results showed there to be no real difference in the incidence of liver tumors between male and female rats.

**Table 2. Liver tumors in Wistar-derived rats given oral tamoxifen[7]**

| Dose (mg/kg) | 0 | 5 | 25 | 35 |
|---|---|---|---|---|
| **Males** | | | | |
| Number of animals | 102 | 51 | 51 | 51 |
| Hepatocellular adenoma | 1 | 8 | 11 | 8 |
| Hepatocellular carcinoma | 1 | 8 | 34 | 34 |
| Hepato/cholangiocellular carcinoma | 0 | 0 | 2 | 5 |
| **Females** | | | | |
| Number of animals | 104 | 52 | 52 | 52 |
| Hepatocellular adenoma | 1 | 2 | 6 | 9 |
| Hepatocellular carcinoma | 0 | 6 | 37 | 37 |
| Hepato/cholangiocellular carcinoma | 0 | 0 | 4 | 5 |

The hepatocarcinogenic effects of tamoxifen were confirmed by various other groups in a number of different strains. Williams *et al.* [22] gave tamoxifen by daily gavage to groups of 55 to 57 female Sprague-Dawley rats at doses of 2.8, 11.3 or 45.2 mg/kg. Dosing started when the animals were 6 weeks of age and continued for up to 1 year with two recovery segments, 4 weeks of recovery after 6 months of exposure and 3 months of recovery after 12 months of exposure. At 6 months dosing with 45.2 mg/kg tamoxifen, hepatocellular adenomas and carcinomas were observed in 71 and 29% of rats respectively and at 12 months, the adenomas were present in 50% and carcinomas in 75% of high dose rats. In the 11.3 mg/kg dose group, liver lesions were not found until 12 months when 50% of animals had adenomas and 10%, carcinomas. At 2.8 mg/kg, no hepatoproliferative changes were found.

In order to establish if there were any strain differences in the response of rats to tamoxifen, 10 female Fischer F344, Wistar and Lewis rats were fed either normal diet or one containing 420 ppm tamoxifen [23]. Although the food intake was not uniform throughout the dosing period, the level of tamoxifen corresponded to a dose of about 40 mg/kg/day. Altered hepatic foci were evident in haematoxylin and eosin stained sections from all 3 strains of rat after 3 months exposure to tamoxifen and there was a treatment related increase in the number of glutathione S-transferase P positive foci (Fig. 3C). Such foci were 10 and 20 fold higher in Wistar and Lewis rats respectively than in F344 animals. There was a marked strain difference in the time to development of tumors. After 11 months, all of the Wistar and

[7]Data taken from Greaves *et al* [21].

Lewis rats had developed liver carcinoma, while the Fischer rats developed liver carcinoma by 20 months. Depression in cell proliferation, relative to age-matched controls, was seen in the livers of Fischer rats after six months of exposure to tamoxifen, in contrast to an increase in the Wistar and Lewis rats. This observation is consistent with the promotion of foci to tumors and the subsequent progression of tumors to carcinomas in the latter two strains.

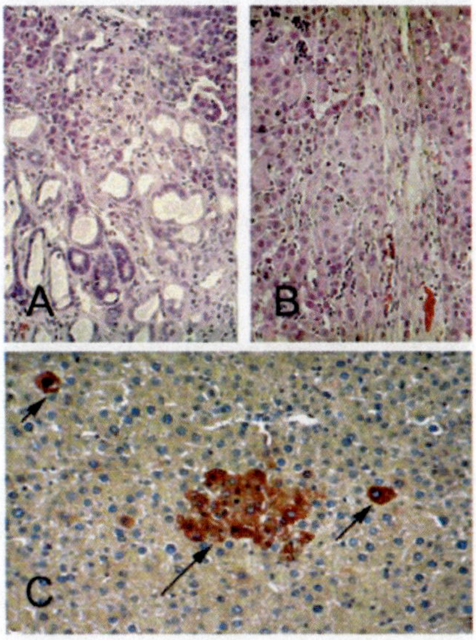


Figure 3. Hepatocellular tumors from high dose rat liver at 2 years: A, showing glandular pattern; B, an infiltrating solid carcinoma. Hematoxylin and eosin. Original magnification x 170. Figure provided by Dr Peter Greaves, MRC Toxicology Unit.

Phenobarbital treatment is able to promote liver tumor development. Wistar rats were given 3 months dietary tamoxifen (420 ppm) and then treatment was discontinued. In one group, phenobarbital was included in their drinking water and in this group, liver carcinomas were seen after 9 months (3 out of 6 animals) whereas no tumors were seen in groups given tamoxifen alone or phenobarbital alone [24]. Developing this theme, Carthew *et al* [25] examined what length of exposure to dietary tamoxifen (420 ppm) was needed in order to induce liver tumors in female Wistar rats. With a group size of 36, animals were fed for zero, 1, 4, 8 or 12 weeks and then left for lifetime for tumor assessment. No tumors were seen after treatment for 1 week but 2, 3 and 11 tumors were detected after the initial 4, 8 and 12 weeks exposure, clearly showing a dose-response relationship with respect to duration of tamoxifen exposure and lifetime risk of liver cancer. It is interesting that the putative active metabolite, α-hydroxytamoxifen when given to Wistar/Han rats for 10 days at a dose level of 40 mg/kg, results in levels of hepatic DNA damage (~3000 adducts/$10^8$ nucleotides), equivalent to those seen after long-term tamoxifen dosing. However, no liver tumors were seen after 13 months even with phenobarbital promotion [26]. This suggests that tamoxifen induced DNA damage alone is insufficient to result in tumor formation and additional promotion/progression steps are required.

Tamoxifen is a selective liver carcinogen in the rat and although the time to tumor formation may vary, all strains of rats investigated are susceptible. The study of Greaves *et al* [21] showed that lung metastases were found at the higher dose levels but there have been no reports of primary tumors in organs other than the liver. It perhaps should be emphasised that the doses of tamoxifen used in these studies in rats that resulted in liver tumor formation (11.3 to 45.2 mg/kg day) are far beyond that used in women for therapeutic purposes. As mentioned above, the present 20 mg daily dose for a 60 kg women is equivalent to ~0.3 mg/kg.

In understanding mechanisms of action, structure activity studies have been carried out examining the effects of long-term dosing of rats with analogues of tamoxifen. Toremifene (Fig. 1, II) has a chloroethyl side chain instead of the ethyl side chain of tamoxifen. Astonishingly at the time, toremifene, when given by daily gavage at 0, 12 or 24 mg/kg and in a pilot study, 48 mg/kg, to female Sprague-Dawley rats, resulted in no hepatocarcinogenic activity and actually reduced the incidence of altered liver cell foci and glutathione S-transferase P immunoreactivity [27, 28]. In a 2 year dietary study with toremifene at doses of 0, 0.12, 1.2, 5.0 and 12 mg/kg/day, using both male and female rats and a group size of 50, no preneoplastic or neoplastic lesions and no obvious toxicity could be observed [29]. Similarly, with droloxifene, (3-hydroxytamoxifen Fig. 1, III), a two-year oral dosing study with Sprague-Dawley rats at 4, 12, 36 or 90 mg/kg, failed to result in hepatocellular carcinomas [30]. Both toremifene and droloxifene bind to estrogen receptors in a similar manner to tamoxifen so it was difficult to understand if tamoxifen was exerting its hepatocarcinogenic effects via interaction with these receptors why toremifene and droloxifene were without effect.

## Clastogenic Effects of Tamoxifen in Isolated Rat Hepatocytes

Although tamoxifen is negative in standard tests for unscheduled DNA synthesis, exposure of rat hepatocytes to tamoxifen *in vitro*, did result in the induction of unscheduled DNA synthesis, when preparations from rats which had been pre-treated with tamoxifen were used [31]. This suggested tamoxifen might induce enzymes responsible for its own activation. Studies of Sargent *et al.*, [32, 33] showed tamoxifen induces both structural and numerical changes in chromosomes of rat hepatocytes. Female Sprague-Dawley rats were given a single dose of 35 mg/kg of tamoxifen, toremifene or idoxifene and one day following treatment, the hepatocytes were isolated and cultured for 47 h. Colcemid was added for 3 h prior to harvest of the hepatocytes for karyotypic evaluation. Tamoxifen and toremifene resulted in aneuploidy in 85 and 50 % of the cells respectively while idoxifene resulted in a 57 % aneuploidy incidence. The level of aneuploidy in solvent-treated rats was around 3%. A similar incidence of aneuploidy was seen following treatment of Wistar rats with either tamoxifen or toremifene while droloxifene gave a weak ~10% increase [34]. It is interesting that dosing of rats with droloxifene, idoxifene or toremifene results in little or no hepatic DNA damage when determined by other methods such as $^{32}$P-postlabeling or accelerator mass spectrometry *(see below).* This makes is difficult to conclude if such findings are relevant in predicting possible human risk.

## Long-Term Effects in Mice Treated With Tamoxifen

Currently in the US, major programs are underway supported by the NIH and AACR using mouse models to simulate human cancers [35]. However, no study using mice of any strain, treated with tamoxifen, has shown the development of hepatocellular carcinomas. In the original long-term investigations, Alderley Park mice were given 5 or 50 mg/kg orally for 3 months then kept for up to 12 months on a diet containing tamoxifen to give similar doses. Only skeletal abnormalities were seen in the older dosed mice and no liver tumors. It is known that the susceptibility of different strains of mice to hepatocarcinogens can differ markedly. In one study, tamoxifen was administered in the diet at a dose corresponding initially to about 120 mg/kg/day to three stains of female mice (B6C3F1, C57BL/6 and DBA/2) with 15-mice/treatment group. After 8 weeks, the concentration in the diet was reduced by one third to give a daily dose of around 40 mg/kg, done in order to reduce the development of skeletal abnormalities (kyphosis). Up to two years, there was no treatment related increase in liver tumors in any of the mouse strains with or without phenobarbital promotion [36]. Tamoxifen was detected in the mouse livers, but at levels 50 times lower than those reported in a comparable rat study. Results suggest that the pharmacokinetics of tamoxifen in the mouse differ significantly from the rat. Much higher rates of hepatic Phase 1 metabolism convert tamoxifen to less hepatotoxic 4-hydroxytamoxifen and tamoxifen *N*-oxide (see below). Thus AUCs for tamoxifen and *N*-desmethyltamoxifen are approximately 4 times greater in the rat than the mouse after equivalent doses of tamoxifen (200 mg/kg) [37].

## Effects on Hamster Livers

Far fewer studies have been carried out in hamsters than in rats but there is no evidence to suggest that tamoxifen is a hepatocarcinogen in this species. For example, Liehr *et al* [38] implanted groups of 7 to 12 male Syrian hamsters with pellets of either tamoxifen or estradiol (25mg) or both together. After 7 months, kidney tumors were seen in the estradiol treated animals but the tumor incidence was reduced by joint exposure to estradiol and tamoxifen. There were no reports of liver tumors. In the light of our current knowledge on metabolic activation, it seems probable that the doses of tamoxifen used in this study would not be high enough to result in sufficient hepatic DNA damage to give liver tumors. In another study, between 5 and 20 Armenian hamsters, a rodent that is especially sensitive to hepatotoxic effects of exogenous estrogens, were given subcutaneous implants of phytoestrogen zeranol on day 0 and 94. One group was then given subcutaneous tamoxifen (5 mg/animal) twice a week up to day 32 and then once weekly until day 202, when they were killed. The incidence of hepatocellular carcinomas in hamsters receiving zeranol alone was about 60 % and this was reduced to about 1 to 2% with tamoxifen treatment [39]. Zeranol induces acute hepatotoxicity and is the primary initiator of subsequent hepatic carcinogenesis. It was concluded that the blocking action of both effects by tamoxifen, suggested in this particular instance acute hepatotoxicity and promotion of hepatic carcinogenesis were mediated through estrogen receptor pathways, although follow up studies were not carried out to confirm this.

## TAMOXIFEN ABSORPTION, DISTRIBUTION AND METABOLISM

Tamoxifen is well absorbed after its oral administration but there are wide variations between individuals, which at least in part may reflect differences in hepatic metabolism. The steady state plasma concentrations in humans receiving a therapeutic dose of 20mg/kg/day are 150-300 ng/ml [40-42]. Tamoxifen is highly lipophilic. The great majority of the drug is bound to proteins in plasma but levels of tamoxifen and its Phase I metabolites are 10 to 100 fold higher in tissues than in serum [37, 43]. It is extensively metabolized after oral administration in rats and in women. Fig. 4 shows the major Phase I metabolites identified in plasma of treated women by LC-electrospray ionization – mass spectrometry [44, 45]. These include *N*-desmethyltamoxifen and 4-hydroxytamoxifen. In the liver of breast cancer patients, the concentrations of tamoxifen and *N*-desmethyltamoxifen were broadly similar between ~1000 to 15,000 ng/g. In human liver (but not rodents), appreciable concentrations of *N,N*-didesmethyltamoxifen (1000 to 3000 ng/g) accumulate. Only trace amounts (27-89 ng/g) of 4-hydroxytamoxifen are detected. In a study involving 6 breast cancer patients who had received the drug for between 2 and 45 months, tamoxifen levels between 159 and 5572 ng/g were reported [46]. In this study, no quantitation of tamoxifen metabolites was carried out.

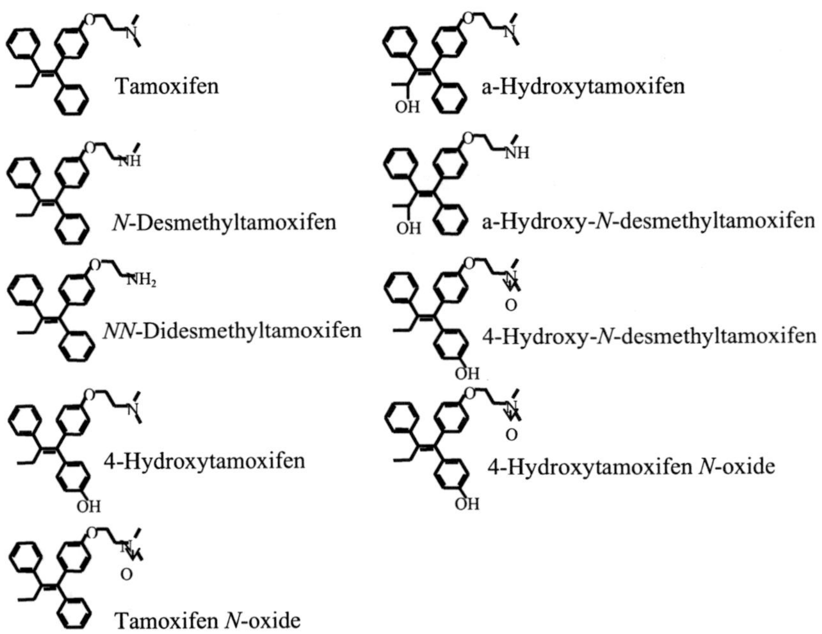


Figure 4. Tamoxifen and its metabolites identified in plasma of breast cancer patients treated with tamoxifen. Data taken from Poon *et al.* [44]

There is a marked species difference in the metabolism and pharmacokinetics of tamoxifen between women, rats and mice. This is reflected by differences in the plasma half-life. In humans, the elimination is biphasic with half-lives of about 7 to 14 h and over 7 days [42, 47, 48], while in rats and mice, half-lives are in the order of 14h and 8h respectively [49]. Comparing rats (Sprague-Dawley), mice (ICR) and human breast cancer patients, it was concluded that rats were more representative than the mouse for toxicology and antitumor studies [37].

Species differences in activation and detoxication of tamoxifen are critical in determining the hepatocarcinogenicity of this drug. In women, levels in the liver of around 8000 ng/g tissue are achieved on a therapeutic dose of 0.3 mg/kg [43], whereas similar levels accumulate in rats given 20mg/kg, nearly a two order of magnitude higher dose [23]. As has been indicated above, 20 mg/kg given long-term to rats can lead to the development of hepatocellular carcinomas. Tamoxifen is now known to be converted in the liver to electrophiles that damage DNA. It was the detection of such damage and the structural identification of the DNA adducts, described below, that led to a mechanistic understanding of the genotoxicity of tamoxifen and has enabled risk assessment to be made.

## Tamoxifen Induced DNA Damage in Rats

The induction of liver tumors in tamoxifen treated rats is mediated through a genotoxic mechanism, involving the generation of hepatic tamoxifen-DNA adducts, which are formed in a dose-dependent manner and accumulate with repeated administration [23, 50]. DNA adducts are a type of damage, arising when a reactive chemical covalently binds to nucleophilic sites on DNA [51]. Often, metabolic activation is a prerequisite for adduct formation, converting a stable parent compound to a reactive electrophilic species. DNA adducts are an early initiating event in the carcinogenic process since if they are not repaired correctly and efficiently prior to DNA replication, they may cause incorporation of an incorrect base or deletions or insertions opposite the lesion, resulting in a mutation. If these mutations are fixed and present in critical genes such as tumor suppressors or proto-oncogenes, then they can ultimately result in cancer [52]. The presence of DNA adducts therefore indicates a drug or chemical is a potential carcinogen.

As many as twelve structurally distinct DNA adducts can be detected in rat liver following tamoxifen treatment, using the $^{32}$P-postlabeling assay in combination with HPLC separation [53]. DNA damage accumulates with long term dosing, reaching around 1600 adducts/$10^8$ nucleotides after 12 weeks in Wistar (Han) rats, by which time approximately one third of animals have developed liver cancer [25]. Total adduct levels differ in various rat strains and generally correlate with susceptibility to liver carcinogenesis, in terms of the time elapsing before development of hepatic tumors [23]. In Wistar (Han) rats, a threshold level of liver DNA damage equivalent to 180 tamoxifen adducts/$10^8$ nucleotides has been reported necessary for the induction of cancer [25].

It is now generally accepted that there is a correlation between the initiation of DNA damage and the subsequent development of liver tumors in rats given tamoxifen. However, when α-hydroxytamoxifen was given to the sensitive Wistar/Han rat strain at doses of 40 or 4 mg/kg for 10 days, DNA damage in the liver was in the order of 3000 and 300 adducts/$10^8$ nucleotides respectively [26]. According to studies with tamoxifen [25], this level of damage should be sufficient to yield liver tumors but surprisingly, in the α-hydroxytamoxifen treated animals, none were found 13 months later even with phenobarbital promotion. It is possible that the hepatic cell population targeted by α-hydroxytamoxifen might not be the same as that seen after tamoxifen administration. Immunohistochemical detection methods have since been developed, sufficiently sensitive to detect the presence of tamoxifen-DNA adducts in the hepatic parenchymal cells of dosed rats [54]. It would be fascinating to establish if the cellular localization of DNA adducts in the liver after dosing with α-hydroxytamoxifen was the same as in tamoxifen dosed animals. There is presently no explanation as to why DNA damage caused by α-hydroxytamoxifen itself does not result in liver tumors in rats.

In extrahepatic organs, tamoxifen DNA adducts are either not formed or present at extremely low levels [31, 50]. It is interesting that in uterine tissues, using $^{32}$P-postlabeling, no significant DNA adducts could be detected after dosing rats with tamoxifen, 4-hydroxytamoxifen or even the reactive metabolite α-hydroxytamoxifen [55, 56]. However, using a more sensitive technique, accelerator mass spectrometry (AMS), a low level of adduct formation was detectable after administration of a single dose of [$^{14}$C]tamoxifen, in rat colon, reproductive tract, spleen, lung and kidney at levels equivalent to 46, 18, 17, 12 and 4% of liver binding respectively [57]. This suggests adduct formation is possible in numerous tissues but levels may be too low to detect using conventional methodology. As an alternative mechanism, one study has also described an enhancement of endogenous uterine DNA damage with tamoxifen treatment, suggesting that tamoxifen could initiate tumor development through an indirect action [58].

## DNA Damage in Rats Caused by Tamoxifen Analogues

Toremifene when given to rats (40 mg/kg/day for 7d) results in little or no DNA adducts in the liver. With prolonged dosing, little DNA damage accumulates in the liver. Even after 18 months exposure (500ppm dietary toremifene) only low levels of DNA damage were detected in liver (13 adducts/$10^8$ nucleotides) and kidney (68 adducts/$10^8$ nucleotides), while no toremifene related DNA damage was seen in the uterus [59]. No DNA adducts have been detected following dosing of rats with droloxifene [31]. Idoxifene that was designed to be resistant to metabolism by the liver CYP system also results in trace levels of DNA damage in the livers of dosed rats [60]. Although there are many steps between initiation and the subsequent development of the hepatocellular tumors, with all of the triphenylethylene drugs tested, initiation of DNA damage above a certain threshold in the liver, offers a plausible explanation for the neoplastic effects of these compounds.

## Characterization of Tamoxifen DNA Adducts

The primary mechanism of tamoxifen metabolic activation in rat liver is now well established and involves α-hydroxylation followed by α-sulfation (Fig. 5). Subsequent loss of the sulfate moiety yields an unstable carbocation, which binds predominantly to deoxyguanosine in DNA and deoxyadenosine to a small extent, when reacted *in vitro* [61, 62]. The major adducts detected in rat liver following tamoxifen treatment have been identified as tamoxifen, or its Phase I metabolite, *N*-desmethyltamoxifen, linked *via* the α-carbon to the exocyclic amino group of deoxyguanosine, forming α-($N^2$-deoxyguanosinyl)-tamoxifen (dG-$N^2$-tam) and α-($N^2$-deoxyguanosinyl)-*N*-desmethyltamoxifen (dG-$N^2$-*N*-desmethyltam) respectively [54, 62-64]. Structural characterization of these adducts was initially achieved by chromatographic comparison to synthesized standards, prepared by reaction of DNA or nucleotides with acetate or sulfate esters of α-hydroxytamoxifen. Subsequently, both adducts have been identified directly by mass spectrometry analysis of hydrolyzed liver DNA from tamoxifen treated rats [65, 66]. Since the α-carbon of α-hydroxytamoxifen is chiral and the resulting carbocation can undergo conversion to the *cis*-isomer, each tamoxifen adduct can exist as four diastereoisomers, with the two *cis* isomers typically formed at much lower levels *in vivo* [67]. Other adducts derived from sequential α-hydroxylation of the major Phase I metabolites of tamoxifen, *N,N*-didesmethyltamoxifen and tamoxifen *N*-oxide have also been identified in rat and mouse liver [63, 68-70]. The metabolite 4-hydroxytamoxifen can also form adducts *in vitro* when oxidised chemically or enzymatically to a quinone, quinone methide or α,4-dihydroxytamoxifen. The major adduct generated by the one electron oxidation product of 4-hydroxytamoxifen, the quinone methide, corresponds to a 4-hydroxylated version of dG-$N^2$-tam, which is also formed when α,4-dihydroxytamoxifen reacts with DNA [71, 72]. Although this adduct has similar chromatographic properties to a minor adduct present in rat liver it has not been characterised directly [53, 56]. 4-Hydroxytamoxifen itself, when administered to rats or incubated with hepatocytes, does not result in significant adduct formation, presumably due to rapid detoxification and excretion [56, 72]. Consequently, there is currently no conclusive evidence to prove that adducts derived from this metabolite are actually formed *in vivo*.

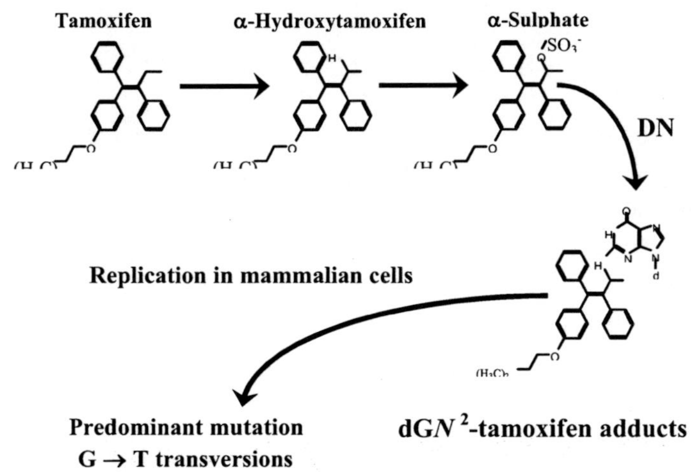


Figure 5. Primary mechanism of tamoxifen metabolic activation responsible for formation of the major DNA adducts in rat liver which induce predominantly G→T transversion mutations in cultured mammalian and human cells. Analogous metabolism of *N*-desmethyltamoxifen results in a second major adduct in rat liver, α-($N^2$-deoxyguanosinyl)-*N*-desmethyltamoxifen.

## TAMOXIFEN ADDUCT FORMATION IN OTHER SPECIES

DNA adducts are detected in mouse liver at levels approximately one-third that observed in rat liver, even though tamoxifen does not cause hepatic tumors in this species [36]. The reason mice are not susceptible to tamoxifen induced liver carcinogenesis may be because there is insufficient total DNA damage, since tamoxifen DNA adducts do not accumulate with long-term administration in mice. In fact, after three months dosing they actually begin to decrease over time. This may be explained by a more rapid clearance, or depletion of tamoxifen and its metabolites in mice, modulating the balance between adduct formation and removal in mice. Another contributing factor could be that mouse DNA repair enzymes are more efficient in excising tamoxifen-modified nucleotides which is consistent with the much shorter adduct half-life in mice relative to rats (several days compared to months) [36].

Following administration of tamoxifen to cynomolgus monkeys for a month, at doses 6-times the human daily therapeutic dose, significant levels of tamoxifen adduct formation were apparent in multiple tissues, using three different detection methods [73, 74]. Highest levels were measured in the liver, in the order of 2-11 adducts/$10^8$ nucleotides and the lowest in the kidney, where they were not detectable by $^{32}$P-postlabeling [73]. Adducts were also detected in the ovary, brain cortex, and uterus of at least one out of the three tamoxifen exposed animals. These findings demonstrate that monkeys, and therefore potentially other primates including humans, are capable of metabolising tamoxifen to genotoxic intermediates that form adducts in multiple tissues.

## TAMOXIFEN DNA ADDUCT FORMATION IN WOMEN

The matter of whether tamoxifen forms DNA adducts in human tissues has attracted much interest and considerable controversy [75]. Limited information is available on the ability of tamoxifen to bind to human liver DNA, partly due to difficulties in obtaining tissue from treated women. One study which examined liver DNA samples from tamoxifen treated (n=7) and control (n=7) women using $^{32}$P-postlabeling with TLC separation, found no significant difference in the levels of detectable damage between patient groups [46] (Table 3). However, analysis of $^{32}$P-postlabeled liver DNA digests using an alternative, more specific HPLC method resulted in the detection of a very low level of tamoxifen adduct formation, in the region of 1-2 adducts/$10^8$ nucleotides, in samples from two out of four women treated with tamoxifen [E. A Martin and K. Hemminki, personal communication]. This level of damage, which according to HPLC analysis seems to be due to formation of the major adducts found in rat liver, dG-$N^2$-tam and dG-$N^2$-*N*-desmethyltam (Fig. 6), is comparable to that reported in endometrial tissue [76].

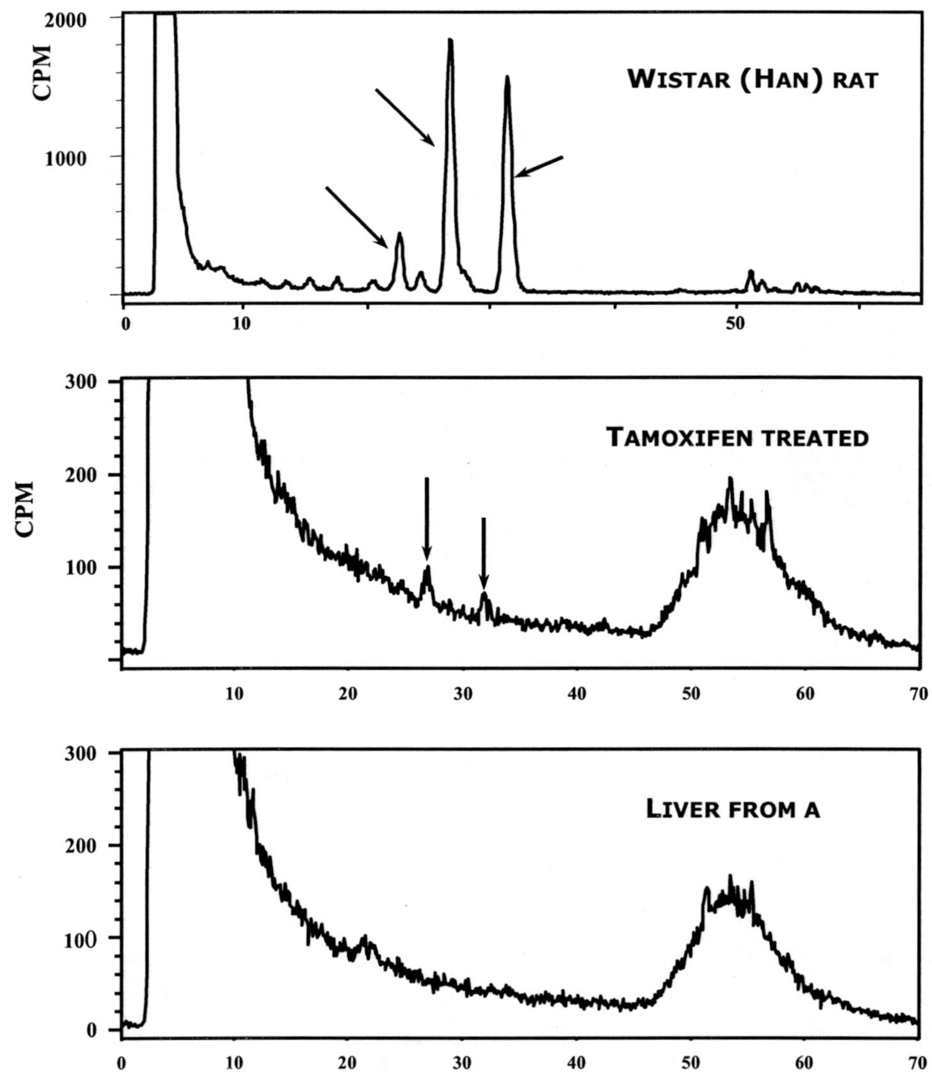


Figure 6. HPLC separation of $^{32}P$-postlabeled rat and human liver DNA digests using the system described in Martin *et al.* [53]. Numerous adduct peaks are detectable in rat liver after dietary treatment with tamoxifen (**A**), of which three have been characterized [70]. Two small peaks, eluting at the same time as the major adducts formed in rat liver were detectable in the liver of a patient on tamoxifen therapy (**B**), whilst no adduct peaks are visible in DNA from a control patient (**C**). Results were communicated by E. A. Martin and K. Hemminki.

**Table 3. Studies investigating the formation of tamoxifen DNA adducts in human tissues.**

| Tissue Type | Adducts Detected | Detection Limit (adducts/$10^9$ nucleotides) | Detection Method | Reference |
|---|---|---|---|---|
| Liver | No | Not reported | $^{32}$P-postlabelling/TLC | [46] |
| Endometrium | No | 1, 0.4 | $^{32}$P-postlabelling/HPLC/TLC | [77, 140] |
| White blood cells | No | 80 | $^{32}$P-postlabelling/TLC | [79] |
| Endometrium | No | 5 | HPLC-MS | [80] |
| Endometrium | Inconclusive | 3 | Immunoassay | [75] |
| | | Adduct Level (adducts/$10^9$ nucleotides) | | |
| Endometrium | Yes | 15-131, 2-180 | $^{32}$P-postlabelling/TLC/HPLC | [76, 81] |
| Leukocytes | Yes | 2.6 | $^{32}$P-postlabelling/HPLC | [75] |
| Endometrium | Yes | 0.24 | AMS | [82] |
| Myometrium | Yes | 0.49 | AMS | [82] |
| Endometrium | Yes | 2.7 | $^{32}$P-postlabelling/HPLC | [84] |
| Leucocytes | Yes | 5.5 | $^{32}$P-postlabelling/HPLC | [83] |

A number of studies conducted in various laboratories using either $^{32}$P-postlabeling, HPLC-mass spectrometry or a chemiluminescence immunoassay for adduct detection have reported an absence of tamoxifen DNA adducts in uterine endometrium or white blood cells from women on long-term tamoxifen treatment (Table 3) [75, 75-84]. Although these methods are sensitive, the inability to detect adducts may be because if formed, they are present at very low levels, close to the limits of detection attainable with these techniques. This is supported by studies using a more sensitive adaptation of the $^{32}$P-postlabeling assay, in which dG-$N^2$-tam adducts were detected in the endometrium of 8 out of 16 patients treated with tamoxifen for periods of one month to six years [76]. The level of DNA damage, ranged from 0.2-18 adducts/$10^8$ nucleotides and no tamoxifen adducts were detected in any untreated control patients.

In an alternative approach to ascertain whether tamoxifen is capable of binding to uterine DNA, ten women were administered a single therapeutic dose of [$^{14}$C]-tamoxifen (20mg, 1.85MBq) 18 hours prior to hysterectomy and DNA extracted from tissue removed at the time of surgery was analyzed by accelerator mass spectrometry (AMS) [82]. This is the most sensitive method available for detecting low levels of DNA adducts, measuring concentrations of rare, long-lived radioisotopes at attomole levels with high precision [85,86].The sensitivity of this method ensures that the radioisotope dose required is low, in this case less than the natural background radiation to which people are exposed in daily life during the course of a month. AMS analysis of endometrial and myometrial DNA demonstrated the presence of irreversibly bound $^{14}$C-tamoxifen in samples from all treated patients as shown in Fig. 7. There was no significant difference between mean adduct levels in the endometrium (237 adducts/$10^{12}$ nucleotides) and myometrium (492 adducts/$10^{12}$ nucleotides). The overall extent of uterine DNA binding was in the region of 10-500 fold lower than that detected in women receiving the drug therapeutically. This is consistent with the fact plasma concentrations of tamoxifen equivalents after a single dose are an order of magnitude lower than steady state levels achieved with chronic treatment [82]. Furthermore, tamoxifen DNA adduct formation in human uterus was at least 10 times lower than that found in the livers of adult rats administered an equivalent single dose of [$^{14}$C]-tamoxifen (0.3mg/kg) and comparable to the levels detected in rat uterus, where tamoxifen-induced tumors do not develop. [82]This study illustrates the potential for tamoxifen to act as a human genotoxic carcinogen, however, in general, the relative role of low levels of DNA damage is unclear and difficult to elucidate. The fact adducts were detectable in the myometrium of women, a tissue in which tamoxifen associated tumors do not arise, signifies that DNA damage alone is insufficient to cause tumor development and a combination of various tissue specific factors along with the precise nature and position of the damage act together to modulate the biological consequences of adducts. Therefore, although tamoxifen adducts have been detected in endometrial and hepatic DNA from treated women the significance of such a low level of DNA damage in the development of human cancers remains to be determined.

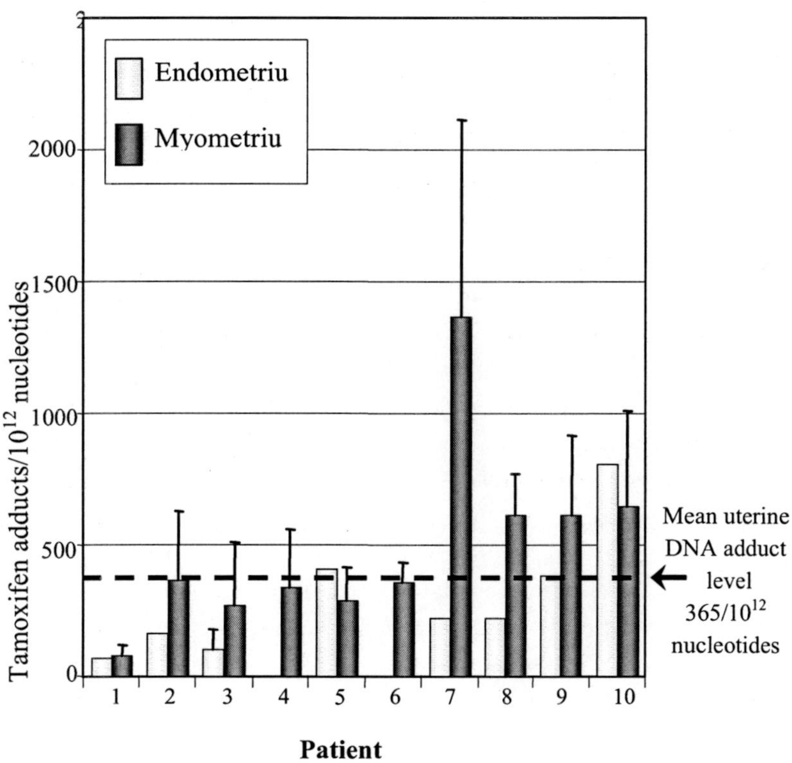


Figure 7. Levels of tamoxifen binding in endometrial and myometrial DNA of women administered a single therapeutic dose of [$^{14}$C]-tamoxifen. Values are the mean + SE of 1 to 6 analyses as described in Martin *et al.* [82]

## TAMOXIFEN MUTAGENICITY

The ability of tamoxifen to induce mutations in hepatic DNA of transgenic animals *in vivo* has been well documented [87, 88]. However, despite inducing an increase in mutation frequency in both the liver *lacI* and *cII* genes in Big Blue transgenic rats [89, 90], neither tamoxifen or the reactive metabolite, α-hydroxytamoxifen, caused an elevated mutation frequency in these genes in the uterus, consistent with a lack of DNA adduct formation and tumor development in this tissue. Furthermore, there was no increase in *Hprt* mutation frequency in spleen T-lymphocytes isolated from Sprague-Dawley rats treated with tamoxifen or α-hydroxytamoxifen [91]. Qualitatively, the mutation spectra induced by tamoxifen and its α-hydroxylated derivative in transgenic animals are similar, with the major alteration being G→T transversions, which differs from the predominant mutation in untreated rats, G→A transitions [87-89]. In contrast to the above studies, which involved dosing for 21 days, shorter treatment with α-hydroxytamoxifen for 10 days, caused a small (1.8 fold) increase in mutation frequency at the *lacI* gene in liver tissue of rats but there was no elevation in the proportion of G→T transversions [26]. This may be attributed to a combination of shorter exposure period and lower doses reaching the systemic circulation due to deactivation in the stomach.

A high frequency (50%) of characteristic *p53* mutations have been reported in hepatocarcinomas formed in rats administered tamoxifen for 12 months [92]. These mutations were clustered at two sites in exon 6-7 and exon 8, however, the specific types of changes detected, A→G and C→T transitions, differ from those typically observed in transgenic animals and caused by the major tamoxifen DNA adduct in mammalian cells *in vitro*. Consequently, there has been some question as to whether amplification of pseudogenes may be responsible for the high incidence of *p53* mutations observed and this remains to be clarified [93, 94].

The mutational effects of specific tamoxifen DNA adducts have been demonstrated by studies in which an individual isomer of dG-$N^2$-tam was incorporated into a single stranded plasmid and replicated in simian kidney (COS-7) cells. One of the *trans* forms of dG-$N^2$-tam promoted preferential incorporation of the correct base opposite, with a small proportion of G→A transitions and G→T transversions. The other three isomers induced a higher degree (~12%) of mutations, predominantly G→T transversions [95]. These adducts have also been shown to be highly miscoding to mammalian DNA polymerases α, β and δ, *in vitro*, resulting in base substitutions and deletions [96]. The observation that dG-$N^2$-tam adducts are repaired with only poor to moderate efficiency, using a reconstituted human nucleotide excision repair system, led to the suggestion that variations in repair capacity may influence an individual's risk of developing tamoxifen induced cancer [97]. The mutagenicity of multiple adducts formed by reactive metabolites of tamoxifen have been investigated in several cellular systems [93, 98, 99]. Interestingly, studies comparing the mutation frequency and spectrum in plasmids reacted with either α-acetoxytamoxifen or 4-hydroxytamoxifen quinone methide and replicated in human cells or *E.coli.*, have illustrated that adducts derived from 4-hydroxytamoxifen are 1-2 orders of magnitude more mutagenic, at least *in vitro* [98, 99]. This implies that even if adducts formed by this metabolite only represent a small proportion of the total DNA damage *in vivo*, they may play a significant role in tamoxifen induced mutagenesis.

Little data is available regarding the mutational effects of tamoxifen in humans, although one preliminary report indicated that endometrial tumors in tamoxifen treated women contained an excess of G→A transitions at non-CpG sites in *p53* and the oncogene *K-ras*. The occurrence of these types of mutations were substantially increased compared to that reported in *p53* of sporadic endometrial tumors [100]. More recently, a high incidence of *K-ras* mutations at codon 12 has been detected in endometrial polyps from tamoxifen treated patients (64%) relative to the occurrence in sporadic endometrial hyperplasias (4.5-23%) [101]. Mutations in *K-ras* are considered an early event in neoplastic progression in the endometrium and these findings support the hypothesis that the polyp-carcinoma sequence plays a role in the development of endometrial carcinomas in tamoxifen treated patients. Conducting such studies to establish mutation patterns in various oncogenes and tumor suppressor genes and subsequently identifying correlations between mutational hotspots and preferential sites for adduct formation is an important approach in determining whether the low levels of tamoxifen adducts detected in human endometrium contribute directly to the initiation of endometrial tumors.

## Inductive Effects of Tamoxifen on Phase I and Phase II liver Enzyme Systems

Tamoxifen treatment alters the levels of expression of a number of Phase I and Phase II enzymes in rat liver but it should be noted that the doses used in rats (20-45 mg/kg day) are generally much higher than the human therapeutic dose. Short term dosing of tamoxifen (45 mg/kg daily for 4 days) leads to a selective 2-3-fold increase in CYP2B1, CYP2B2 and CYP3A1 proteins, relative to controls, without altering total microsomal CYP levels [102]. Gene expression of CYP3A subfamily enzymes, responsible for activation by the α-hydroxylation of tamoxifen, was increased by the tamoxifen treatments for 2 and 12 weeks, whereas after the 52 week treatment, the expression in the induced nodules returned to the control level [20]. Increases in CYP2B1, CYP2B2, CYP3A and microsomal epoxide hydrolase protein levels and mRNA were similarly found in male and female rats. The expression of CYP1A1, CYP1A2 and gamma-glutamyl transpeptidase mRNA were not significantly affected by tamoxifen treatment and it was concluded that tamoxifen was a weak phenobarbital-like inducer of approximately one-tenth the potency [103]. In humans receiving tamoxifen therapeutically, the clinical relevance of CYP induction has not generally been established. For example, pharmacokinetics of the aromatase inhibitor anastrazole (Arimidex$^{TM}$), alone or in combination with tamoxifen, showed the geometric mean steady-state trough plasma concentrations of tamoxifen and *N*-desmethyltamoxifen were statistically equivalent in both groups of patients. However, the mean anastrozole levels were 27% lower in the presence of tamoxifen than with anastrozole alone [104]. It was concluded that this observed reduction in anastrozole levels by tamoxifen was unlikely to be of clinical significance but it was not established whether such a reduction was due to increased metabolism.

Other long-term dosing studies with tamoxifen have examined the effects in F344 rats on Phase II enzymes and has shown a dramatic suppression on the glutathione S-transferase proteins Ya1 and Ya2, at doses directly equivalent to those used for breast cancer treatment [105]. It is only in the preneoplastic nodules of rats that there is a selective upregulation of glutathione S-transferase P. Hepatic UDP-glucuronyltransferase was not altered [105]. On the basis of the assumption that the sulfate ester of α-hydroxytamoxifen is responsible for the hepatocarcinogenic effects of this drug, it might be predicted that the liver tumor incidence in males would be lower than in females, since the expression of rat sulfotransferase a (rHSTa) and other SULT2A forms is substantially lower in male rats than in females. However, liver tumor incidence is similar in both sexes (Table 2). Experimentally, it was found that sulfotransferase activity towards dehydroepiandrosterone, (used as a surrogate for α-hydroxytamoxifen) in male rat liver cytosol was only 17% of the activity of female cytosol after one dose of tamoxifen but increased to 64% after 14 days of exposure. This increase in activity correlated with increases in the levels of SULT2A protein, detected by Western blotting and after prolonged exposure to tamoxifen, DNA adduct formation and rHSTa expression in males are significantly closer to the levels in females than they are after initial exposure. These changes explain the similar susceptibility of male and female rats to tamoxifen carcinogenesis [106].

## Hepatic Metabolism of Tamoxifen in Liver Microsomal Systems

A study by Coller *et al.,* [107] using human liver microsomal preparations from 50 individuals, showed there to be large (~15 fold) inter-individual variations in the rates of formation of α-hydroxytamoxifen, *N*-desmethyltamoxifen and *N,N*-didesmethyltamoxifen from tamoxifen. A comparison of the metabolism of tamoxifen in female rat, mouse and human liver microsomal systems in the presence of NADPH was carried out by Lim *et al.* [108]. The metabolites formed were analysed by reverse phase liquid chromatography-electrospray ionization mass spectrometry. The major metabolites were found to be 4-hydroxytamoxifen, *N*-desmethyltamoxifen and tamoxifen *N*-oxide (Fig. 8). Two additional polar products with an $[M+H]^+$ ion at m/z 388 were identified. At the time, these were claimed to be tamoxifen 3,4-epoxide and 3',4'-epoxide [108]. However, the identities were never substantiated and in the light of our present knowledge, these two components could have been the *trans* and *cis* isomers of α-hydroxytamoxifen [55]. The pattern of the major metabolites was qualitatively similar in the three species. The major difference between rat and human liver microsomes was the lower amounts of hydroxylated metabolites in humans. In contrast, in mice compared to humans, relatively higher levels of both 4-hydroxytamoxifen and tamoxifen *N*-oxide are formed (Fig. 9). This more rapid metabolism of tamoxifen in mouse liver to potentially less toxic water soluble *N*-oxides and 4-hydroxy- metabolites may in part account for the lower levels of hepatic DNA damage and absence of liver tumors seen in mice following tamoxifen treatment.

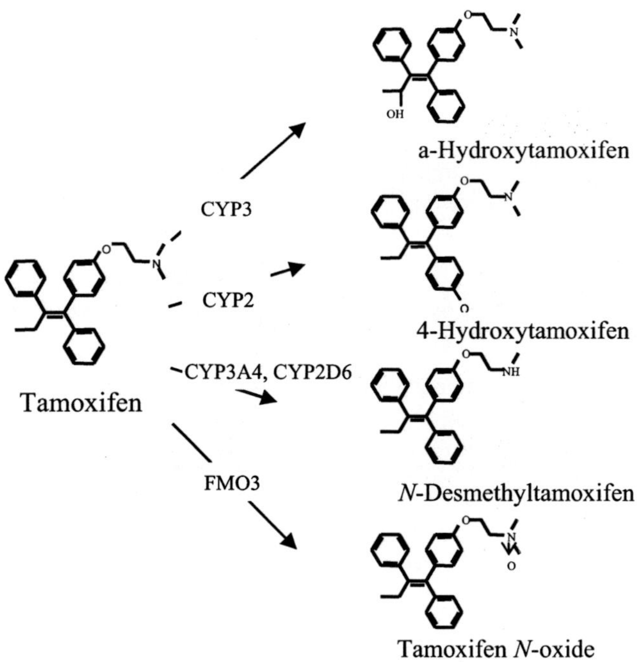


Figure 8. Some liver microsomal Phase I metabolites of tamoxifen. Only the principal CYP forms that catalyse *N*-demethylation and 4-hydroxylation are shown (*see Table 4*).

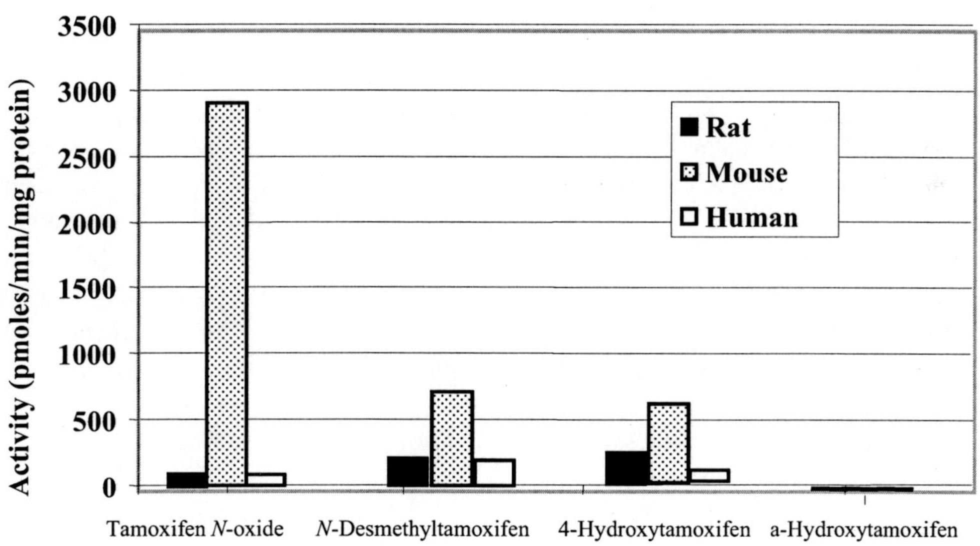


Figure 9. Species differences in the rates of metabolism of tamoxifen to its major Phase 1 metabolites and α-hydroxytamoxifen. Data taken from refs [108, 118]

## Identity of the Active Metabolites of Tamoxifen

A number of potential reactive intermediates have been proposed to account for the genotoxicity of tamoxifen and its ability to form protein adducts. It seems probable, though not proven, that the same active metabolite is involved in both. Proposed electrophiles include those derived from 4-hydroxtamoxifen such as 4-hydroxytamoxifen quinonemethide [109] or 3,4-dihydroxytamoxifen [110]. An additional pathway of activation of 4-hydroxytamoxifen is through peroxidase generated free radical intermediates [111, 112]. Although peroxidases are widely distributed in the body, these reactions have only been demonstrated *in vitro* and there is little evidence to suggest they operate in the liver. It is now generally accepted that the main route of metabolic activation is via α-hydroxytamoxifen (Fig. 8). Strong evidence for this comes from resolution of the identity of the DNA adducts and from studies where deuterium is substituted at the α-position of tamoxifen. Under these circumstances, both oxidative metabolism by rat liver microsomes [113] to give α-hydroxytamoxifen and DNA adduct formation, either in the rat liver or in isolated hepatocytes, show about a 2-fold reduction, due to a kinetic isotope effect retarding metabolism at this site [114, 115]. In contrast, deuteration at the beta position has no effect on metabolism or DNA adduct formation. α-Hydroxytamoxifen possesses a chiral carbon and therefore contains two enantiomers, both of which are formed in equal amounts when tamoxifen is incubated with rat liver microsomes [116]. Interestingly, reaction of individual enantiomers with DNA *in vitro* results in similar levels of covalent binding but in cultured hepatocytes R-(+)- α-hydroxytamoxifen induces at least eight times as many DNA adducts as the S-(-) isomer. This can probably be explained by the R-(+)-isomer being a better substrate for the sulfotransferase enzymes involved in production of α-sulfate tamoxifen. It is perhaps not surprising that since experimental studies in rats and humans have found that higher levels of *N*-desmethyltamoxifen accumulate in the liver than tamoxifen itself [65], this and certain other Phase I metabolites can also undergo further activation by α-hydroxylation to give DNA adducts as described above. Although theoretically 4-hydroxytamoxifen could undergo additional α-hydroxylation and prepared chemically, α,4-dihydroxytamoxifen, reacts more strongly with DNA than α-hydroxytamoxifen [72, 117], there is little evidence to suggest *in vivo* 4-hydroxytamoxifen can undergo activation in the liver by this or other oxidative pathways to give DNA adducts. One reason for this may be that Phase II conjugation reactions, particularly glucuronidation, result in stable products such as 4-hydroxytamoxifen glucuronide that can be excreted via the bile [118].

α-Hydroxytamoxifen can react weakly with DNA *in vitro* at physiological pH values and in some tissues where sulfotransferases are not known to occur, such as the uterine endometrium, this may be the only species that reacts with DNA, forming low adduct levels. However, in the liver, α-hydroxytamoxifen gets conjugated to a chemically more reactive α-sulfate ester. Evidence for this comes from studies that showed when hepatocytes were incubated with tamoxifen either in sulfate free medium, or with a sulfotransferase inhibitor, dehydroisoandrosterone-3-sulfate, the level of DNA damage was reduced and this was restored when sulfate was included in the medium [119]. Prepared chemically, the reactivity of the α-sulfate ester of tamoxifen to DNA is much higher than that of α-hydroxytamoxifen. Similarly, the formation of tamoxifen-DNA adducts induced by α-acetoxytamoxifen is 1100-

fold higher than that of α-hydroxytamoxifen [64, 114]. α-Acetoxytamoxifen is often used as a surrogate for the α-sulfate because of its ease of preparation and greater stability. The α-sulfate ester of tamoxifen has a half-life of a few seconds at physiological pH values and unlike α-hydroxytamoxifen, is not sufficiently stable to be detected in plasma [44]. It seems probable that the sulfate will only be active in cells where it is enzymically generated.

It is fascinating that the formation of α-hydroxytoremifene by human CYP3A4 or rat CYP3A1and CYP3A2 is ~3 to 6 fold *higher* than the equivalent rates of formation of α-hydroxytamoxifen from tamoxifen [120]. These results are in agreement with a much earlier finding, that following metabolic activation by rat liver microsomes (in the absence of sulfotransferases), covalent binding of [$^{14}$C]toremifene is higher than for [$^{14}$C]tamoxifen [57]. Toremifene also results in a dose dependent increase in micronucleus formation in CYP3A4 expressing MCL-5 cells in culture [31]. These results suggest that after Phase I activation *in vitro*, toremifene may have a genotoxicity similar to that of tamoxifen. However, α-hydroxytoremifene is a poor substrate for rat or human hydroxysteroid sulfotransferases and the model electrophile α-acetoxytoremifene reacts less readily with DNA [121]. Thus, where the sulfate ester is the electrophile that reacts with DNA such as in the liver, toremifene is a safer alternative but if α-hydroxytoremifene is involved in damaging DNA, toremifene may offer no advantage over tamoxifen. It will be of great interest to see the outcome of the long-term clinical studies comparing the incidence of uterine tumors in tamoxifen versus toremifene treated patients.

## CYP Forms Involved in the Activation of Tamoxifen

Since the early 1990s it had been known that following incubation of [$^{14}$C]tamoxifen with rat liver microsomes and NADPH, covalent binding of radiolabel to microsomal protein occurred. This binding was decreased by CO, inhibitors of P450, and antibodies to rat NADPH-P450 reductase, indicating catalysis by CYPs [122]. This study also showed by dual-labelling that neither *N*-desmethyltamoxifen nor tamoxifen-*N*-oxide, the principal CYP and flavin monooxygenase-mediated metabolites, respectively, were on the major route responsible for adduct formation. Rats and humans demonstrated low tamoxifen binding activity, ranging from 0.1 to 0.4 nmol bound/mg protein/h. In contrast, hamsters and mice exhibit high binding of 1.2 and 1.6 nmol tamoxifen/mg protein/h respectively. Treatment of male rats with phenobarbital or pregnenolone-16α-carbonitrile markedly elevated the binding of tamoxifen to liver microsomal proteins, while methylcholanthrene treatment had no effect on binding. These findings suggested the involvement of CYP3A in catalysis of the covalent binding [123]. White *et al.*, [124] also investigated species differences between human, female F344 rats and DBA/2 mice with respect to the NADPH-dependent covalent binding of [$^{14}$C]tamoxifen to liver microsomes. Protein binding was used as an index of metabolic activation and as a surrogate for DNA binding. Covalent binding of tamoxifen in rats was 3.8-fold and in mice, 17-fold higher than in human liver microsomal preparations. As found by both groups, the greater potential of mouse liver microsomes to activate tamoxifen under saturating substrate concentrations, relative to rats, does not reflect DNA damage or hepatocarcinogenicity seen following dosing with tamoxifen *in vivo* and further emphasises the importance of pharmacokinetics and detoxication reactions. In human liver microsomes, protein binding of tamoxifen showed a positive correlation with CYP3A4 and CYP2B6 content.

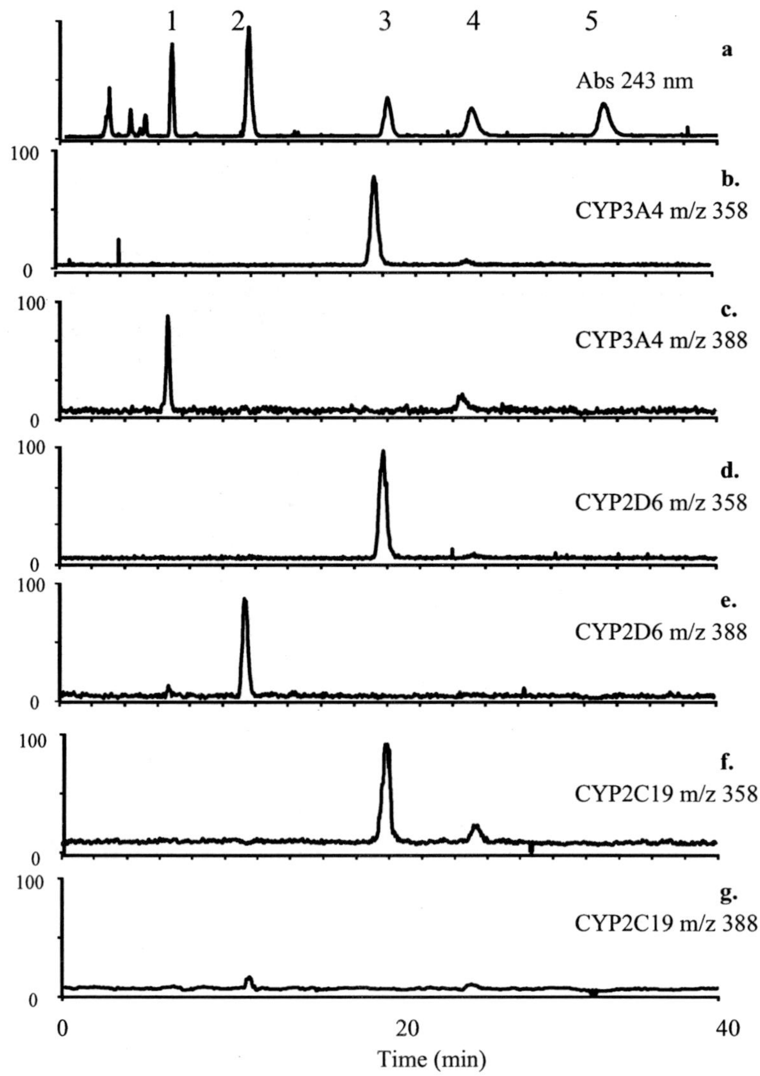


Figure 10. On-line liquid chromatography-electrospray ionisation mass spectrometry analysis of the incubation products of tamoxifen with individual insect baculovirus expressed CYP forms. Trace a, UV absorbance of standards at 243 nm. These were: (1) α-hydroxytamoxifen; (2) 4-hydroxytamoxifen; (3) *N*-desmethyltamoxifen; (4) tamoxifen *N*-oxide; (5) tamoxifen. Traces b, d and f, reaction products with $[M + H]^+$ at m/z 358. Traces c, e and g reaction products with $[M + H]^+$ at m/z 388. Metabolites generated by CYP3A4 (b and c), CYP2D6 (d and e) and CYP2C19 (f and g) are shown. Reproduced from Boocock *et al.* Identification of human CYP forms involved in the activation of tamoxifen and irreversible binding to DNA. *Carcinogenesis*, 2002, 23, 1897-1901 by permission of Oxford University Press. [128]

Mechanistic studies in a human lymphoma cell line, stably transfected with human CYP1A1, CYP1A2, CYP2D6, CYP2E1, CYP3A4 and epoxide hydrolase, using micronucleus formation as an index of metabolic activation showed tamoxifen was clastogenic *in vitro.* Interestingly in this study, toremifene gave a positive result while droloxifene was negative [31]. Using lymphoma cell lines expressing individual CYP forms suggested CYP3A4 and CYP2E1 were responsible for activation [34]. Using recombinant human CYPs co-expressed in *E.coli* with recombinant human NADPH-cytochrome P450 reductase, drug-protein adducts formed specifically with CYP3A4 as well as with purified CYP3A4 and it was suggested that the electrophilic species generated reacted preferentially with this CYP form [125]. Tamoxifen *N*-demethylation was mediated by CYP3A4, CYP2D6, CYP1A1, CYP1A2, CYP1B1, CYP2C9, CYP2C19 and CYP3A5, dependent on the substrate concentration while CYP2D6 and CYP2B6 were the major catalysts of 4-hydroxylation [126]. In a separate study, recombinant human CYP2C8, CYP2C9, CYP2C18, CYP2C19 or CYP2D6 expressed in *E. coli,* and reconstituted with P450 reductase, catalyzed *N*-demethylation to various degrees while only CYP2D6 yielded detectable levels of 4-hydroxytamoxifen [127]. These results suggested *N*-demethylation to be catalysed by many CYP forms whereas 4-hydroxylation was more specific to CYP2D6. Correlation of CYP forms, determined by Western blotting with metabolite formation in microsomal preparations from 50 individuals showed that *a*-hydroxytamoxifen formation, measured by LC-MS, was associated with CYP2B6, CYP2C9 and CYP3A4. The formation of *N*-desmethyltamoxifen and *N,N*-didesmethyltamoxifen was also positively correlated with CYP3A4 [107]. In contrast to the results described below, this group found no association between the levels on CYP2D6 and rates of *N*-demethylation. Using insect baculovirus expressed human CYPs, in combination with liquid chromatography-mass spectrometry analysis, a number of different forms were identified that were capable of carrying out 4-hydroxylation to give the protonated molecular ion $[M + H]^+$ at m/z 388. *N*-Demethylation was detected by the formation of a component with a protonated molecular ion at m/z 358. Only CYP3A4 was able to carry out α-hydroxylation (Table 4). This gave a protonated molecular ion at m/z 388 (Peak #1, Fig. 10a,c) but the product was more polar with a shorter retention time than 4-hydroxytamoxifen (Peak #2, Fig. 10a). With $[^{14}C]$tamoxifen as substrate and employing the highly sensitive technique of accelerator mass spectrometry, only CYP3A4 was able to catalyze the covalent binding of this drug to DNA (Fig. 11) [128]. Although the same human CYP proteins are expressed by *E coli* and insect baculovirus systems, for some reason, the specificity of the latter appears to be higher. Confirming these results, among the 18 human insect baculovirus CYP enzymes, only CYP3A4 generated a significant amount of α-hydroxytamoxifen while with rat CYP forms, CYP3A2 also catalyzed this reaction [120]. As with the clastogenicity assays described above, this group showed that toremifene also undergoes metabolic activation to an electrophile, confirmed by tandem mass spectroscopy to be α-hydroxytoremifene. As with tamoxifen, this reaction was also catalysed by the CYP3A family.

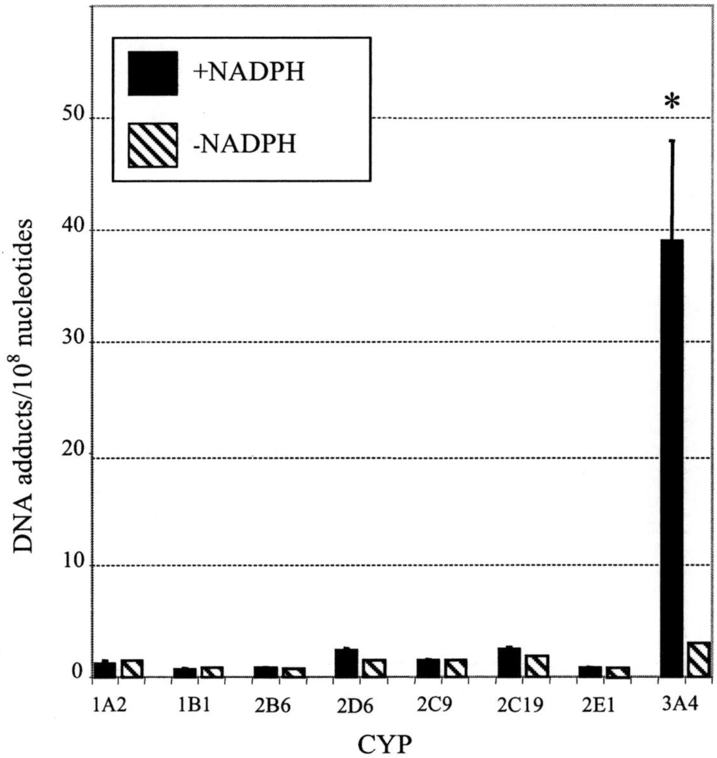


Figure 11. Irreversible binding of [$^{14}$C]tarmoxifen to DNA catalysed by human CYPs. Following incubation of individual CYPS with [$^{14}$CJtamoxifen (100 μM) and salmon sperm DNA, the amount of covalently bound radiolabel was determined by accelerator mass spectrometry. *Significantly higher level of radiolabel bound in the presence of NADPH than in its absence. Reproduced from Boocock *et al.* Identification of human CYP forms involved in the activation of tamoxifen and irreversible binding to DNA. *Carcinogenesis*, 2002, 23, 1897-1901 by permission of Oxford University Press. [128]

**Table 4. Metabolism of tamoxifen metabolites by different human CYP forms using baculovirus-insect cells expressed enzymes[8].**

| CYP form | Tamoxifen metabolites (pmol/2h) | | |
|---|---|---|---|
| | α-Hydroxytamoxifen | 4-Hydroxytamoxifen | *N*-Desmethyltamoxifen |
| CYP1A1 | - | - | 3260 |
| CYP1A2 | - | - | 720 |
| CYP1B1 | - | - | - |
| CYP2A6 | - | - | - |
| CYP2B6 | - | - | 92 |
| CYP2C8 | - | - | 1250 |
| CYP2C9 | - | 300 | 550 |
| CYP2C18 | - | - | 700 |
| CYP2C19 | - | 100 | 660 |
| CYP2D6 | - | **630** | 3500 |
| CYP 2E1 | - | - | - |
| CYP 3A4 | **53** | - | **6170** |
| CYP 3A5 | - | 65 | 1820 |
| CYP 3A7 | - | 97 | 160 |
| CYP 4A11 | - | | |
| CYP 4F2 | - | | |
| CYP 4F3A/B | - | | |

## DETOXICATION PATHWAYS OF α-HYDROXYTAMOXIFEN

In assessing the risks to patients taking tamoxifen therapeutically, it is necessary to consider not only the relative rates of activation of tamoxifen to □-hydroxytamoxifen and subsequently, the□-sulfate ester but also rates of detoxication (Fig. 12). One factor that makes women less sensitive to the genotoxic effects of tamoxifen is that human liver microsomes catalyse □-hydroxylation at approximately half the rate of rat liver microsomes [129]. When [14C]tamoxifen is given to rats, the major radiolabelled biliary metabolite, about 10% of dose, is excreted as the non-toxic glucuronide of 4-hydroxytamoxifen, while only 0.1% of the dose is recovered as α-hydroxytamoxifen [118]. The UDP-glucuronyltransferases involved in these reactions have not been determined, though it seems probable that different ones are involved in 4-hydroxylation and α-hydroxylation (I.N.H. White, unpublished observations). *O*-Glucuronylation will deactivate and compete with sulphonation and this study showed that the rank order of this reaction in liver microsomes was human > > mouse > rat. The UDP-glucuronyltransferase activity in women towards α-hydroxytamoxifen is about 50 fold higher than in rats. In view of the critical role that glucuronidation plays in the detoxication of α-hydroxtamoxifen, it may be prudent for those

[8] Data taken from Kim *et al.*, [120]

women with deficiencies in this group of enzymes, such as UGT1A1 in Gilberts syndrome [130], to exercise caution with tamoxifen therapy. In addition, rates of *O*-sulphonation of α-hydroxytamoxifen in hepatic cytosol, in female CD-1 mice or Sprague-Dawley rats were 4 to 5 fold higher than in women [129]. Finally, as has been pointed out above, the normal human dose of 20mg/day (0.3 mg/kg) is about two orders of magnitude lower than the doses used in rats (~30 mg/kg/day) that result in liver tumors. These factors can be summarised as follows:

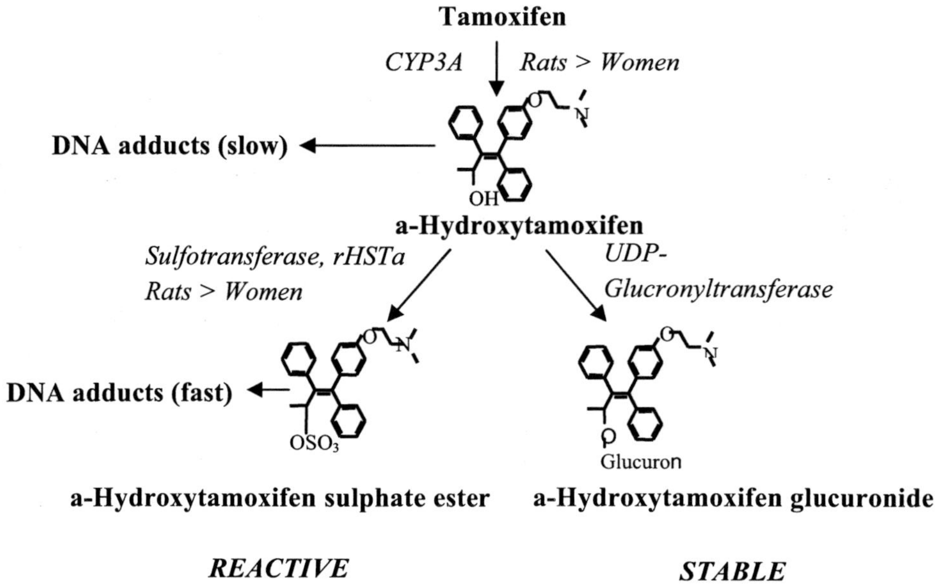


Figure 12. Pathways of activation and detoxication of α-hydroxytamoxifen.

| | | |
|---|---|---|
| **Activation:** | tamoxifen to α-hydroxytamoxifen by liver microsomes: | **women < rats** |
| **Activation:** | Conversion of α-hydroxytamoxifen to sulfate ester: | **women < rats** |
| **Detoxication:** | UDP glucuronyltransferase α-hydroxytamoxifen: | **women >> rats** |
| **Dose:** | | **women < rats** |

## Conclusions

The results of these mechanistic studies clearly show that rats are inappropriate models for tamoxifen hepatocarcinogenicity in women and that tamoxifen treated women are unlikely to develop liver tumors as a result of such treatment [131-133]. Investigations into the reasons for these conclusions, however, have made a significant contribution to our overall understanding of mechanisms of drug metabolism and genotoxicity. Although there is always pressure to use alternatives to animals in toxicity testing, computer-based assessment of potential toxicity, such as the knowledge-based DEREK [134], did not predict the genotoxic potential of this drug. Furthermore, the Ames *Salmonella* mutagenicity assay is used throughout the pharmaceutical industry for genotoxicity testing but tamoxifen steadfastly gave negative results in this test, irrespective of the type of activation mixtures used.

Following the finding that tamoxifen was a powerful hepatocarcinogen in rats [21], mechanistic studies showed that treatment led to DNA damage detectable by $^{32}$P-postlabelling [31, 50]. This enabled the determination of pathways for activation involving α-hydroxylation, enzymic sulphonation in hepatocytes to the sulfate ester [119, 135]. It was only then that *Salmonella* constructs could be made expressing the appropriate sulphotransferase enzyme that gave a positive result in this mutation assay [136]. The discovery of higher rates of glucuronidation of α-hydroxytamoxifen in women relative to rats offered a plausible explanation as why women might not be at risk of forming liver DNA adducts and developing tumors [129]. These theoretical considerations were confirmed by the studies of Martin *et al.* [137] who showed no detectable DNA damage above background levels in the livers of breast cancer patients taking tamoxifen therapeutically, using $^{32}$P-postlabelling.

Tamoxifen is an interesting example in that while mechanistic studies show little risk to women from hepatocellular carcinomas, epidemiological studies in breast cancer patients have shown a clear association with treatment and an increase in the incidence of endometrial cancers. While there is some evidence to suggest a very low level of DNA damage in this tissue [76, 82], it seems more likely that its estrogenic agonist action in this organ is responsible. The precise processes involved are still being investigated but it is only through understanding such mechanisms that the potential risks of other drugs of this class can be established.

## REFERENCES


[1] Shiau, A. K., Barstad, D., Loria, P. M., Cheng, L., Kushner, P. J., Agard, D. A., and Greene, G. L. The structural basis of estrogen receptor/coactivator recognition and the antagonism of this interaction by tamoxifen. *Cell*, 95: 927-937, 1998.

[2] IARC Tamoxifen. IARC Monographs on the Evaluation of Carcinogenic Risks to Humans, *66*: 253-365, 1996.

[3] Powles, T. J. The case for clinical trials of tamoxifen for prevention of breast cancer. *Lancet*, 340: 1145-1147, 1992.

[4] Early Breast Cancer Trialists' Collaborative Group Tamoxifen for early breast cancer: an overview of the randomised trials. *Lancet*, 351: 1451-1467, 1998.

[5] Fisher, B., Dignam, J., Bryant, J., and Wolmark, N. Five versus more than five years of tamoxifen for lymph node- negative breast cancer: Updated findings from the National Surgical Adjuvant Breast and Bowel Project B-14 randomized trial. *J.Natl.Cancer Inst.*, 93: 684-690, 2001.

[6] Peto, R., Boreham, J., Clarke, M., Davies, C., and Beral, V. UK and USA breast cancer deaths down 25% in year 2000 at ages 20-69 years. *Lancet*, 355: 1822, 2000.

[7] Cuzick, J., Powles, T., Veronesi, U., Forbes, J., Edwards, R., Ashley, S., and Boyle, P. Overview of the main outcomes in breast-cancer prevention trials. *Lancet*, 361: 296-300, 2003.

[8] Cuzick, J. Future possibilities in the prevention of breast cancer: breast cancer prevention trials. *Breast Cancer Res.*, 2: 258-263, 2000.

[9] Powles, T. J. Anti-oestrogenic prevention of breast cancer - the make or break point. *Nature Reviews Cancer,* 2: 787-794, 2002.

[10] Gail, M. H., Costantino, J. P., Bryant, J., Croyle, R., Freedman, L., Helzlsouer, K., and Vogel, V. Weighing the risks and benefits of tamoxifen treatment for preventing breast cancer. *J Natl Cancer Inst*, 91: 1829-1846, 1999.

[11] Freedman, A. N., Graubard, B. I., Rao, S. R., McCaskill-Stevens, W., Ballard-Barbash, R., and Gail, M. H. Estimates of the number of US women who could benefit from tamoxifen for breast cancer chemoprevention. *J.Natl.Cancer Inst.*, 95: 526-532, 2003.

[12] IARC Overall Evaluation of Carcinogenicity: An Update of IARC Mongraphs Volumes 1 to 42, Lyon. *IARC Monographs on the Evaluation of Carcinogeic Risks to Humans*, Suppl.7., 272-310, 1987.

[13] Shimomura, M., Higashi, S., and Mizumoto, R. $^{32}$P-postlabeling analysis of DNA adducts in rats during estrogen-induced hepatocarcinogenesis and effect of tamoxifen on DNA adduct level. *Jpn.J Cancer Res,* 83: 438-444, 1992.

[14] Chow, P. K., Tai, B. C., Tan, C. K., Machin, D., Win, K. M., Johnson, P. J., and Soo, K. C. High-dose tamoxifen in the treatment of inoperable hepatocellular carcinoma: A multicenter randomized controlled trial. *Hepatology,* 36: 1221-1226, 2002.

[15] Llovet, J. M. and Bruix, J. Systematic review of randomized trials for unresectable hepatocellular carcinoma: Chemoembolization improves survival. *Hepatology*, 37: 429-442, 2003.

[16] Paganini-Hill, A. and Clark, L. J. Eye problems in breast cancer patients treated with tamoxifen. *Breast Cancer Res Treat*, 60: 167-172, 2000.

[17] Fisher, B., Costantino, J. P., Redmond, C. K., Fisher, E. R., Wickerham, D. L., and Cronin, W. M. Endometrial cancer in tamoxifen-treated breast cancer patients: Findings from the National Surgical Adjuvant Breast and Bowel Project (NSABP) B-14. *J.Natl.Cancer Inst.*, 86: 527-537, 1994.

[18] Rutqvist, L. E., Johansson, H., Signomklao, T., Johansson, U., Fornander, T., and Wilking, N. Adjuvant tamoxifen therapy for early stage breast cancer and second primary malignancies. Stockholm Breast Cancer Study Group. *J.Natl.Cancer Inst.*, 87: 645-651, 1995.

[19] Nyberg, U., Nilsson, B., Travis, L. B., Holm, L. E., and Hall, P. Cancer incidence among Swedish patients exposed to radioactive thorotrast: a forty-year follow-up survey. *Radiat.Res,* 157: 419-425, 2002.

[20] Kasahara, T., Hashiba, M., Harada, T., and Degawa, M. Change in the gene expression of hepatic tamoxifen-metabolizing enzymes during the process of tamoxifen-induced hepatocarcinogenesis in female rats. *Carcinogenesis*, 23: 491-498, 2002.

[21] Greaves, P., Goonetilleke, R., Nunn, G., Topham, J., and Orton, T. Two-year carcinogenicity study of tamoxifen in Alderley Park Wistar-derived rats. *Cancer Res*, 53: 3919-3924, 1993.

[22] Williams, G. M., Iatropoulos, M. J., Djordjevic, M. V., and Kaltenberg, O. P. The triphenylethylene drug tamoxifen is a strong liver carcinogen in the rat. *Carcinogenesis*, 14: 315-317, 1993.

[23] Carthew, P., Rich, K. J., Martin, E. A., De Matteis, F., Lim, C. K., Manson, M. M., Festing, M. F., White, I. N. H., and Smith, L. L. DNA damage as assessed by $^{32}$P-postlabelling in three rat strains exposed to dietary tamoxifen: the relationship between cell proliferation and liver tumor formation. *Carcinogenesis*, 16: 1299-1304, 1995.

[24] Carthew, P., Martin, E. A., White, I. N. H., De Matteis, F., Edwards, R. E., Dorman, B. M., Heydon, R. T., and Smith, L. L. Tamoxifen induces short-term cumulative DNA damage and liver tumors in rats: Promotion by phenobarbital. *Cancer Res.*, 55: 544-547, 1995.

[25] Carthew, P., Lee, P. N., Edwards, R. E., Heydon, R. T., Nolan, B. M., and Martin, E. A. Cumulative exposure to tamoxifen: DNA adducts and liver cancer in the rat. *Arch Toxicol,* 75: 375-380, 2001.

[26] White, I. N. H., Carthew, P., Davies, R., Styles, J., Brown, K., Brown, J. E., Smith, L. L., and Martin, E. A. Short-term dosing of alpha-hydroxytamoxifen results in DNA damage but does not lead to liver tumors in female Wistar/Han rats. *Carcinogenesis*, 22: 553-557, 2001.

[27] Williams, G. M., Iatropoulos, M. J., and Karlsson, S. Initiating activity of the anti-estrogen tamoxifen, but not toremifene in rat liver. *Carcinogenesis,* 18: 2247-2253, 1997.

[28] Hard, G. C., Iatropoulos, M. J., Jordan, K., Radi, L., Kaltenberg, O. P., Imondi, A. R., and Williams, G. M. Major differences in the hepatocarcinogenicity and DNA adduct forming ability between toremifene and tamoxifen in female Crl: CD(BR) rats. *Cancer Res.*, 53: 4534-4541, 1993.

[29] Karlsson, S., Hirsimaki, Y., Mantyla, E., Nieminen, L., Kangas, L., Hirsimaki, P., Perry, C. J., Mulhern, M., Millar, P., Handa, J., and Williams, G. M. A two-year dietary carcinogenicity study of the antiestrogen toremifene in Sprague-Dawley rats. *Drug Chem.Toxicol.*, 19: 245-266, 1996.

[30] Dahme, E. and Rattel, B. Unlike tamoxifen, droloxifene produces no hepatic tumors in the rat. *Onkologie*, 17: 6-16, 1994.

[31] White, I. N. H., De Matteis, F., Davies, A. M., Smith, L. L., Crofton-Sleigh, C., Venitt, S., Hewer, A., and Phillips, D. H. Genotoxic potential of tamoxifen and analogues in

female Fischer F344/N rats, DBA/2 and C57Bl/6 mice and in human MCL-5 cells. *Carcinogenesis*, 13: 2197-2203, 1992.

[32] Sargent, L. M., Dragan, Y. P., Sattler, C., Bahnub, N., Sattler, G., Martin, P., Cisneros, A., Mann, J., Thorgeirsson, S., Jordan, V. C., and Pitot, H. C. Induction of hepatic aneuploidy in vivo by tamoxifen, toremifene and idoxifene in female Sprague-Dawley rats. *Carcinogenesis*, 17: 1051-1056, 1996.

[33] Sargent, L. M., Dragan, Y. P., Bahnub, N., Wiley, J. E., Sattler, C. A., Schroeder, P., Sattler, G. L., Jordan, V. C., and Pitot, H. C. Tamoxifen induces hepatic aneuploidy and mitotic spindle disruption after a single in vivo administration to female Sprague-Dawley rats. *Cancer Res*., 54: 3357-3360, 1994.

[34] Styles, J. A., Davies, A. M., Davies, R., White, I. N. H., and Smith, L. L. Clastogenic and aneugenic effects of tamoxifen and some of its analogues in hepatocytes from dosed rats and in human lymphoblastoid cells transfected with human P450 cDNAs (MCL-5 cells). *Carcinogenesis*, 18: 303-313, 1997.

[35] Marx, J. Medicine. Building better mouse models for studying cancer. *Science*, 299: 1972-1975, 2003.

[36] Martin, E. A., Carthew, P., White, I. N., Heydon, R. T., Gaskell, M., Mauthe, R. J., Turteltaub, K. W., and Smith, L. L. Investigation of the formation and accumulation of liver DNA adducts in mice chronically exposed to tamoxifen. *Carcinogenesis,* 18: 2209-2215, 1997.

[37] Robinson, S. P., Langan-Fahey, S. M., Johnson, D. A., and Jordan, V. C. Metabolites, pharmacodynamics, and pharmacokinetics of tamoxifen in rats and mice compared to the breast cancer patient. *Drug Metab Dispos*., 19: 36-43, 1991.

[38] Liehr, J. G., Sirbasku, D. A., Jurka, E., Randerath, K., and Randerath, E. Inhibition of estrogen-induced renal carcinogenesis in male Syrian hamsters by tamoxifen without decrease in DNA adduct levels. *Cancer Res*, 48: 779-783, 1988.

[39] Coe, J. E., Ishak, K. G., Ward, J. M., and Ross, M. J. Tamoxifen prevents induction of hepatic neoplasia by zeranol, an estrogenic food contaminant. *Proc Natl Acad Sci U S A*, 89: 1085-1089, 1992.

[40] Peyrade, F., Frenay, M., Etienne, M. C., Ruch, F., Guillemare, C., Francois, E., Namer, M., Ferrero, J. M., and Milano, G. Age-related difference in tamoxifen disposition. *Clin Pharmacol Therap*, 59: 401-410, 1996.

[41] Furr, B. J. A. and Jordan, V. C. The pharmacology and clinical uses of tamoxifen. *Pharmacol.Ther.*, 25: 127-205, 1984.

[42] Adam, H. K., Patterson, J. S., and Kemp, J. V. Studies on the metabolism and pharmacokinetics of tamoxifen in normal volunteers. *Cancer Treat.Rep.*, 64: 761-764, 1980.

[43] Lien, E. A., Solheim, E., and Ueland, P. M. Distribution of tamoxifen and its metabolites in rat and human tissues during steady-state treatment. *Cancer Res.*, 51: 4837-4844, 1991.

[44] Poon, G. K., Walter, B., Lonning, P. E., Horton, M. N., and McCague, R. Identification of tamoxifen metabolites in human HEP G2 cell line, human liver homogenate, and patients on long-term therapy for breast cancer. *Drug Metab.Dispos.*, 23: 377-382, 1995.

[45] Poon, G. K., Cui, Y. C., McCague, R., Lonning, P. E., Feng, R., Rowlands, M. G., and Jarman, M. Analysis of phase I and phase II metabolites of tamoxifen in breast cancer patients. *Drug Metab.Dispos.*, 21: 1119-1124, 1995.

[46] Martin, E. A., Rich, K., White, I. N. H., Woods, K. L., Powles, T. J., and Smith, L. L. $^{32}$P-Postlabelled DNA adducts in liver obtained from women treated with tamoxifen. *Carcinogenesis*, 16: 1651-1654, 1995.

[47] Fuchs, W. S., Leary, W. P., van der Meer, M. J., Gay, S., Witschital, K., and von Nieciecki, A. Pharmacokinetics and bioavailability of tamoxifen in postmenopausal healthy women. *Arzneimittelforschung.*, 46: 418-422, 1996.

[48] Fromson, J. M., Pearson, S., and Bramah, S. The metabolism of tamoxifen (I.C.I. 46,474). II. In female patients. *Xenobiotica*, 3: 711-714, 1973.

[49] Fromson, J. M., Pearson, S., and Bramah, S. The metabolism of tamoxifen (I.C.I. 46,474). I. In laboratory animals. *Xenobiotica*, 3: 693-709, 1973.

[50] Han, X. and Liehr, J. G. Induction of covalent DNA adducts in rodents by tamoxifen. *Cancer Res.*, 52: 1360-1363, 1992.

[51] Dipple, A. DNA adducts of chemical carcinogens. *Carcinogenesis*, 16: 437-441, 1995.

[52] Garner, R. C. The role of DNA adducts in chemical carcinogenesis. *Mutat.Res.*, 402: 67-75, 1998.

[53] Martin, E. A., Heydon, R. T., Brown, K., Brown, J. E., Lim, C. K., White, I. N., and Smith, L. L. Evaluation of tamoxifen and alpha-hydroxytamoxifen 32P-post-labelled DNA adducts by the development of a novel automated on-line solid-phase extraction HPLC method. *Carcinogenesis*, 19: 1061-1069, 1998.

[54] Divi, R. L., Osborne, M. R., Hewer, A., Phillips, D. H., and Poirier, M. C. Tamoxifen-DNA adduct formation in rat liver determined by immunoassay and $^{32}$P-postlabeling_. *Cancer Res.*, 59: 4829-4833, 1999.

[55] Brown, K., Brown, J. E., Martin, E. A., Smith, L. L., and White, I. N. H. Determination of DNA damage in F344 rats induced by geometric isomers of tamoxifen and analogues. *Chem.Res.Toxicol.*, 11: 527-534, 1998.

[56] Beland, F. A., McDaniel, L. P., and Marques, M. M. Comparison of the DNA adducts formed by tamoxifen and 4-hydroxytamoxifen *in vivo*. *Carcinogenesis*, 20: 471-477, 1999.

[57] White, I. N. H., Martin, E. A., Vogel, J. S., Mauthe, R. J., Turteltaub, K. W., and Smith, L. L. Comparison of the binding of [$^{14}$C]radiolabelled tamoxifen or toremifene to rat DNA using accelerator mass spectrometry. *Chem.Biol.Interact.*, 106: 149-160, 1997.

[58] Koskinen, M., Rajaniemi, H., and Hemminki, K. Analysis of tamoxifen-induced DNA adducts by 32P-postlabelling assay using different chromatographic techniques. *J.Chromatogr.B Biomed.Sci.Appl.*, 691: 155-160, 1997.

[59] Li, D., Dragan, Y., Jordan, V. C., Wang, M., and Pitot, H. C. Effects of chronic administration of tamoxifen and toremifene on DNA adducts in rat liver, kidney, and uterus. *Cancer Res.*, 57: 1438-1441, 1997.

[60] Osborne, M. R., Hewer, A., Davis, W., Strain, A. J., Keogh, A., Hardcastle, I. R., and Phillips, D. H. Idoxifene derivatives are less reactive to DNA than tamoxifen derivatives, both chemically and in human and rat liver cells. *Carcinogenesis*, 20: 293-297, 1999.

[61] Osborne, M. R., Hardcastle, I. R., and Phillips, D. H. Minor products of reaction of DNA with alpha-acetoxytamoxifen. *Carcinogenesis*, 18: 539-543, 1997.

[62] Osborne, M. R., Hewer, A., Hardcastle, I. R., Carmichael, P. L., and Phillips, D. H. Identification of the major tamoxifen-deoxyguanosine adduct formed in the liver DNA of rats treated with tamoxifen. *Cancer Res.*, 56: 66-71, 1996.

[63] Phillips, D. H., Hewer, A., Horton, M. N., Cole, K. J., Carmichael, P. L., Davis, W., and Osborne, M. R. N-demethylation accompanies alpha-hydroxylation in the metabolic activation of tamoxifen in rat liver cells. *Carcinogenesis*, 20: 2003-2009, 1999.

[64] Dasaradhi, L. and Shibutani, S. Identification of tamoxifen-DNA adducts formed by α-sulfate tamoxifen and α-acetoxytamoxifen. *Chem.Res.Toxicol.*, 10: 189-196, 1997.

[65] Rajaniemi, H., Rasanen, I., Koivisto, P., Peltonen, K., and Hemminki, K. Identification of the major tamoxifen-DNA adduct in rat liver by mass spectrometry. *Carcinogenesis*, 20: 305-309, 1999.

[66] Gamboa, d. C., Marques, M. M., Beland, F. A., Freeman, J. P., Churchwell, M. I., and Doerge, D. R. Quantification of tamoxifen DNA adducts using on-line sample preparation and HPLC-electrospray ionization tandem mass spectrometry. *Chem.Res.Toxicol.*, 16: 357-366, 2003.

[67] Umemoto, A., Komaki, K., Monden, Y., Suwa, M., Kanno, Y., Kitagawa, M., Suzuki, M., Lin, C. X., Ueyama, Y., Momen, M. A., Ravindernath, A., and Shibutani, S. Identification and quantification of tamoxifen-DNA adducts in the liver of rats and mice. *Chem.Res.Toxicol.*, 14: 1006-1013, 2001.

[68] Gamboa, d. C., Marques, M. M., Freeman, J. P., and Beland, F. A. Synthesis and investigation of alpha-hydroxy-N,N-didesmethyltamoxifen as a proximate carcinogen in the metabolic activation of tamoxifen. *Chem.Res.Toxicol.*, 16: 1090-1098, 2003.

[69] Umemoto, A., Monden, Y., Komaki, K., Suwa, M., Kanno, Y., Suzuki, M., Lin, C. X., Ueyama, Y., Momen, M. A., Ravindernath, A., and Shibutani, S. Tamoxifen-DNA adducts formed by alpha-acetoxytamoxifen N-oxide. *Chem.Res.Toxicol.*, 12: 1083-1089, 1999.

[70] Brown, K., Heydon, R. T., Jukes, R., White, I. N., and Martin, E. A. Further characterization of the DNA adducts formed in rat liver after the administration of tamoxifen, N-desmethyltamoxifen or N, N-didesmethyltamoxifen. *Carcinogenesis*, 20: 2011-2016, 1999.

[71] Marques, M. M. and Beland, F. A. Identification of tamoxifen-DNA adducts formed by 4-hydroxytamoxifen quinone methide. *Carcinogenesis*, 18: 1949-1954, 1997.

[72] Osborne, M. R., Davis, W., Hewer, A. J., Hardcastle, I. R., and Phillips, D. H. 4-Hydroxytamoxifen gives DNA adducts by chemical activation, but not in rat liver cells. *Chem.Res.Toxicol.*, 12: 151-158, 1999.

[73] Shibutani, S., Suzuki, N., Laxmi, Y. R., Schild, L. J., Divi, R. L., Grollman, A. P., and Poirier, M. C. Identification of tamoxifen-DNA adducts in monkeys treated with tamoxifen. *Cancer Res.*, 63: 4402-4406, 2003.

[74] Schild, L. J., Divi, R. L., Beland, F. A., Churchwell, M. I., Doerge, D. R., Gamboa, d. C., Marques, M. M., and Poirier, M. C. Formation of tamoxifen-DNA adducts in multiple organs of adult female cynomolgus monkeys dosed with tamoxifen for 30 days. *Cancer Res.*, 63: 5999-6003, 2003.

[75] Poirier, M. C. and Schild, L. J. The genotoxicity of tamoxifen: extent and consequences, Kona, Hawaii, January 23, 2003. *Mutagenesis*, 18: 395-399, 2003.

[76] Shibutani, S., Ravindernath, A., Suzuki, N., Terashima, I., Sugarman, S. M., Grollman, A. P., and Pearl, M. L. Identification of tamoxifen-DNA adducts in the endometrium of women treated with tamoxifen. *Carcinogenesis*, 21: 1461-1467, 2000.

[77] Carmichael, P. L., Sardar, S., Crooks, N., Neven, P., Van, H., I, Ugwumadu, A., Bourne, T., Tomas, E., Hellberg, P., Hewer, A. J., and Phillips, D. H. Lack of evidence from HPLC 32P-post-labelling for tamoxifen-DNA adducts in the human endometrium. *Carcinogenesis*, 20: 339-342, 1999.

[78] Bartsch, H., Phillips, D. H., Nair, J., Hewer, A., Meyberg-Solomeyer, G., and Grischke, E. M. Lack of evidence for tamoxifen- and toremifene-DNA adducts in lymphocytes of treated patients. *Carcinogenesis,* 21: 845-847, 2000.

[79] Phillips, D. H., Hewer, A., Grover, P. L., Poon, G. K., and Carmichael, P. L. Tamoxifen does not form detectable DNA adducts in white blood cells of breast cancer patients. *Carcinogenesis*, 17: 1149-1152, 1996.

[80] Beland, F. A., Churchwell, M. I., Doerge, D. R., Malejka-Giganti, D., Zhang, X., Divi, R. L., Poirier, M. C., Gamboa da Costa, G., and Marques, M. M. High performance liquid chromatography electrospray ionization tandem mass spectrometry analysis of DNA adducts in rats, monkeys and humans. *Proc.Am.Assoc.Cancer Res.*, 43: 343, 2002.

[81] Shibutani, S., Suzuki, N., Terashima, I., Sugarman, S. M., Grollman, A. P., and Pearl, M. L. Tamoxifen-DNA adducts detected in the endometrium of women treated with tamoxifen. *Chem.Res.Toxicol.*, 12: 646-653, 1999.

[82] Martin, E. A., Brown, K., Gaskell, M., Al Azzawi, F., Garner, C., Boocock, D. J., Mattock, E., Pring, D. W., Dingley, K., Turteltaub, K. W., Smith, L. L., and White, I. N. H. Tamoxifen DNA damage detected in human endometrium using accelerator mass spectrometry. *Cancer Res.*, 63: 8461-8465, 2003.

[83] Hemminki, K., Rajaniemi, H., Koskinen, M., and Hansson, J. Tamoxifen-induced DNA adducts in leucocytes of breast cancer patients. *Carcinogenesis*, 18: 9-13, 1997.

[84] Hemminki, K., Rajaniemi, H., Lindahl, B., and Moberger, B. Tamoxifen-induced DNA adducts in endometrial samples from breast cancer patients. *Cancer Res.*, 56: 4374-4377, 1996.

[85] Turteltaub, K. W., Felton, J. S., Gledhill, B. L., Vogel, J. S., Southon, J. R., Caffee, M. W., Finkel, R. C., Nelson, D. E., Proctor, I. D., and Davis, J. C. Accelerator mass spectrometry in biomedical dosimetry: relationship between low-level exposure and covalent binding of heterocyclic amine carcinogens to DNA. *Proc.Natl.Acad.Sci.U.S.A*, 87: 5288-5292, 1990.

[86] Turteltaub, K. W. and Vogel, J. S. Bioanalytical applications of accelerator mass spectrometry for pharmaceutical research. *Curr.Pharm.Des*, 6: 991-1007, 2000.

[87] Davies, R., Gant, T. W., Smith, L. L., and Styles, J. A. Tamoxifen induces G:C-->T:A mutations in the cII gene in the liver of lambda/lacI transgenic rats but not at 5'-CpG-3' dinucleotide sequences as found in the lacI transgene. *Carcinogenesis*, 20: 1351-1356, 1999.

[88] Davies, R., Oreffo, V. I., Martin, E. A., Festing, M. F., White, I. N., Smith, L. L., and Styles, J. A. Tamoxifen causes gene mutations in the livers of lambda/lacI transgenic rats. *Cancer Res.*, 57: 1288-1293, 1997.

[89] Chen, T., Gamboa, d. C., Marques, M. M., Shelton, S. D., Beland, F. A., and Manjanatha, M. G. Mutations induced by alpha-hydroxytamoxifen in the lacI and cII genes of Big Blue transgenic rats. *Carcinogenesis*, 23: 1751-1757, 2002.

[90] da Costa, G. G., Manjanatha, M. G., Marques, M. M., and Beland, F. A. Induction of lacI mutations in Big Blue rats treated with tamoxifen and alpha-hydroxytamoxifen. *Cancer Lett.*, 176: 37-45, 2002.

[91] da Costa, G. G., McDaniel-Hamilton, L. P., Heflich, R. H., Marques, M. M., and Beland, F. A. DNA adduct formation and mutant induction in Sprague-Dawley rats treated with tamoxifen and its derivatives. *Carcinogenesis*, 22: 1307-1315, 2001.

[92] Vancutsem, P. M., Lazarus, P., and Williams, G. M. Frequent and specific mutations of the rat p53 gene in hepatocarcinomas induced by tamoxifen. *Cancer Res.*, 54: 3864-3867, 1994.

[93] Yadollahi-Farsani, M., Davies, D. S., and Boobis, A. R. The mutational signature of alpha-hydroxytamoxifen at Hprt locus in Chinese hamster cells. *Carcinogenesis,* 23: 1947-1952, 2002.

[94] Wogan, G. N. Review of the toxicology of tamoxifen. *Semin.Oncol.*, 24: S1, 1997.

[95] Terashima, I., Suzuki, N., and Shibutani, S. Mutagenic potential of alpha-(N2-deoxyguanosinyl)tamoxifen lesions, the major DNA adducts detected in endometrial tissues of patients treated with tamoxifen. *Cancer Res.*, 59: 2091-2095, 1999.

[96] Shibutani, S. and Dasaradhi, L. Miscoding potential of tamoxifen-derived DNA adducts: alpha-(N2-deoxyguanosinyl)tamoxifen. *Biochemistry*, 36: 13010-13017, 1997.

[97] Shibutani, S., Reardon, J. T., Suzuki, N., and Sancar, A. Excision of tamoxifen-DNA adducts by the human nucleotide excision repair system. *Cancer Res.*, 60: 2607-2610, 2000.

[98] Lowes, D. A., Brown, K., Heydon, R. T., Martin, E. A., and Gant, T. W. Site-specific tamoxifen-DNA adduct formation: lack of correlation with mutational ability in Escherichia coli. *Biochemistry*, 38: 10989-10996, 1999.

[99] McLuckie, K. I., Routledge, M. N., Brown, K., Gaskell, M., Farmer, P. B., Roberts, G. C., and Martin, E. A. DNA adducts formed from 4-hydroxytamoxifen are more mutagenic than those formed by alpha-acetoxytamoxifen in a shuttle vector target gene replicated in human Ad293 cells. *Biochemistry*, 41: 8899-8906, 2002.

[100] Welsh, J. A., Moberger, B., Fornander, T., Malfetano, J. H., Ambros, R. A., Weed, J. C., Doligdisch, L., Cohen, C. J., Silva, E. G., Vincent, F., Jones, R. T., and Bennett, W. P. Tamoxifen has a characteristic mutation spectrum in human endometrial cancers. *Proc.Am.Assoc.Cancer Res.*, 38: 450, 1997.

[101] Hachisuga, T., Miyakawa, T., Tsujioka, H., Horiuchi, S., Emoto, M., and Kawarabayashi, T. K-ras mutation in tamoxifen-related endometrial polyps. *Cancer*, 98: 1890-1897, 2003.

[102] White, I. N. H., Davies, A. M., Smith, L. L., Dawson, S., and De Matteis, F. Induction of CYP2B1 and 3A1, and associated monooxygenase activities by tamoxifen and certain analogues in the livers of female rats and mice. *Biochem.Pharmacol.*, 45: 21-30, 1993.

[103] Nuwaysir, E. F., Dragan, Y. P., Jeffcoate, C. R., Jordan, V. C., and Pitot, H. C. Effects of tamoxifen administration on the expression of xenobiotic metabolizing enzymes in rat liver. *Cancer Res.*, 55: 1780-1786, 1995.

[104] Baum, M., Dowsett, M., Coibion, M., Bianco, A. R., Cuzick, J., George, W. D., Gray, J., Howell, A., Houghton, J., Williams, N., Sloane, J., Tobias, J., Buzdar, A., Anderson, M. D., Jackson, I., Sahmoud, T., Gallagher, J., Webster, A., Gangji, D., Petrakova, K., Konopasek, B., Mares, P., Vodvarka, P., Alcazar, A., Campos, O., Maxwell, A., Goedhals, Hacking, D., Landers, G., Smith, L., Vorobiof, D. A., Werner, I. D., Blamey, R., Coleman, R., Grieve, R. J., Hickish, T., Howell, A., Nicholls, J. C., Nicholson, S., Raymond, S., Salman, A., Blum, J., Clark, R., Lyss, A., Miletello, G., Sternberg, J., Forbes, J., Coibion, M., Nabholtz, J. M., Guastalla, J. P., Distler, W., Klijn, J. G. M., Nagykalnai, T., Nicolucci, A., Bianco, A. R., Constenla, M., Nylen, U., Howell, A., Sainsbury, R., Mansel, R. E., Goerge, D., Buzdar, A. U., Locker, G. Y., Gallagher, J., Jackson, I., Sahmoud, T., Houghton, J., Williams, N., Nicolucci, A., Pollard, S., Stroner, P., Buyse, M., Margolese, R., and Northover, J. M. A. Pharmacokinetics of

anastrozole and tamoxifen alone, and in combination, during adjuvant endocrine therapy for early breast cancer in postmenopausal women: a sub-protocol of the 'Arimidex (TM) and Tamoxifen Alone or in Combination' (ATAC) trial. *Br.J.Cancer*, 85: 317-324, 2001.

[105] Nuwaysir, E. F., Daggett, D. A., Jordan, V. C., and Pitot, H. C. Phase II enzyme expression in rat liver in response to the antiestrogen tamoxifen. *Cancer Res.*, 56: 3704-3710, 1996.

[106] Davis, W., Hewer, A., Rajkowski, K. M., Meinl, W., Glatt, H., and Phillips, D. H. Sex Differences in the Activation of Tamoxifen to DNA Binding Species in Rat Liver in Vivo and in Rat Hepatocytes in Vitro: Role of Sulfotransferase Induction. *Cancer Res.*, 60: 2887-2891, 2000.

[107] Coller, J. K., Krebsfaenger, N., Klein, K., Wolbold, R., Nussler, A., Neuhaus, P., Zanger, U. M., Eichelbaum, M., and Murdter, T. E. Large interindividual variability in the in vitro formation of tamoxifen metabolites related to the development of genotoxicity. *British Journal of Clinical Pharmacology,* 57: 105-111, 2004.

[108] Lim, C. K., Yuan, Z. X., Lamb, J. H., White, I. N., De Matteis, F., and Smith, L. L. A comparative study of tamoxifen metabolism in female rat, mouse and human liver microsomes. *Carcinogenesis*, 15: 589-593, 1994.

[109] Moorthy, B., Sriram, P., Pathak, D. N., Bodell, W. J., and Randerath, K. Tamoxifen metabolic activation: Comparison of DNA adducts formed by microsomal and chemical activation of tamoxifen and 4-hydroxytamoxifen with DNA adducts formed in vivo. *Cancer Res.*, 56: 53-57, 1996.

[110] Dehal, S. S. and Kupfer, D. Evidence that the catechol 3,4-dihydroxytamoxifen is a proximate intermediate to the reactive species binding covalently to proteins. *Cancer Res.*, 56: 1283-1290, 1996.

[111] Davies, A. M., Malone, M. E., Martin, E. A., Jones, R. M., Jukes, R., Lim, C. K., Smith, L. L., and White, I. N. H. Peroxidase activation of 4-hydroxytamoxifen to free radicals detected by EPR spectroscopy. Free Radical Biol & Med, 22: 423-431, 1997.

[112] Davies, A. M., Martin, E. A., Jones, R. M., Lim, C. K., Smith, L. L., and White, I. N. H. Peroxidase activation of tamoxifen and toremifene resulting in DNA damage and covalently bound protein adducts. *Carcinogenesis*, 16: 539-545, 1995.

[113] Jarman, M., Poon, G. K., Rowlands, M. G., Grimshaw, R. M., Horton, M. N., Potter, G. A., and McCague, R. The deuterium isotope effect for the alpha-hydroxylation of tamoxifen by rat liver microsomes accounts for the reduced genotoxicity of [D5-ethyl]tamoxifen. *Carcinogenesis*, 16: 683-688, 1995.

[114] Phillips, D. H., Carmichael, P. L., Hewer, A., Cole, K. J., and Poon, G. K. Alpha-hydroxytamoxifen, a metabolite of tamoxifen with exceptionally high DNA-binding activity in rat hepatocytes. *Cancer Res.*, 54: 5518-5522, 1994.

[115] Phillips, D. H., Potter, G. A., Horton, M. N., Hewer, A., Crofton-Sleigh, C., Jarman, M., and Venitt, S. Reduced genotoxicity of [D5-ethyl]-tamoxifen implicates à-

hydroxylation of the ethyl group as a major pathway of tamoxifen activation to a liver carcinogen. *Carcinogenesis*, 15: 1487-1492, 1994.

[116] Osborne, M. R., Hewer, A., and Phillips, D. H. Resolution of alpha-hydroxytamoxifen; R-isomer forms more DNA adducts in rat liver cells. *Chem.Res.Toxicol.*, 14: 888-893, 2001.

[117] Hardcastle, I. R., Horton, M. N., Osborne, M. R., Hewer, A., Jarman, M., and Phillips, D. H. Synthesis and DNA reactivity of alpha-hydroxylated metabolites of nonsteroidal antiestrogens. *Chem.Res.Toxicol.*, 11: 369-374, 1998.

[118] Boocock, D. J., Maggs, J. L., White, I. N., and Park, B. K. Alpha-hydroxytamoxifen, a genotoxic metabolite of tamoxifen in the rat: identification and quantification in vivo and in vitro. *Carcinogenesis*, 20: 153-160, 1999.

[119] Davis, W., Venitt, S., and Phillips, D. H. The metabolic activation of tamoxifen and alpha-hydroxytamoxifen to DNA-binding species in rat hepatocytes proceeds via sulphation. *Carcinogenesis*, 19: 861-866, 1998.

[120] Kim, S. Y., Suzuki, N., Laxmi, Y. R. S., Rieger, R., and Shibutani, S. alpha-hydroxylation of tamoxifen and toremifene by human and rat cytochrome P450 3A subfamily enzymes. *Chem.Res.Toxicol., 16*: 1138-1144, 2003.

[121] Shibutani, S., Ravindernath, A., Terashima, I., Suzuki, N., Laxmi, Y. R. S., Kanno, Y., Suzuki, M., Apak, T. I., Sheng, J. J., and Duffel, M. W. Mechanism of lower genotoxicity of toremifene compared with tamoxifen. *Cancer Res.*, 61: 3925-3931, 2001.

[122] Mani, C. and Kupfer, D. Cytochrome P450 mediated action and irreversible binding of the antiestrogen tamoxifen to proteins in rat and human liver: possible involvement of the flavin-containing monooxygenases in tamoxifen activation. Cancer Res., 51: 6052-6058, 1991.

[123] Mani, C., Pearce, R., Parkinson, A., and Kupfer, D. Involvement of cytochrome P4503A in catalysis of tamoxifen activation and covalent binding to rat and human liver microsomes. *Carcinogenesis*, 15: 2715-2720, 1994.

[124] White, I. N. H., De Matteis, F., Gibbs, A. H., Lim, C. K., Wolf, C. R., Henderson, C., and Smith, L. L. Species differences in the covalent binding of [$^{14}$C]tamoxifen to liver microsomes and the forms of cytochrome P450 involved. *Biochem.Pharmacol.*, 49: 1035-1042, 1995.

[125] Notley, L. M., De Wolf, C. J., Wunsch, R. M., Lancaster, R. G., and Gillam, E. M. Bioactivation of tamoxifen by recombinant human cytochrome p450 enzymes. *Chem.Res.Toxicol.*, 15: 614-622, 2002.

[126] Crewe, H. K., Notley, L. M., Wunsch, R. M., Lennard, M. S., and Gillam, E. M. J. Metabolism of tamoxifen by recombinant human cytochrome P450 enzymes: Formation of the 4-hydroxy, 4 '-hydroxy and N- desmethyl metabolites and isomerization of trans-4- hydroxytamoxifen. *Drug Metab.Dispos.*, 30: 869-874, 2002.

[127] Dehal, S. S. and Kupfer, D. CYP2D6 catalyzes tamoxifen 4-hydroxylation in human liver. *Cancer Res*., 57: 3402-3406, 1997.

[128] Boocock, D. J., Brown, K., Gibbs, A. H., Sanchez, E., Turteltaub, K. W., and White, I. N. H. Identification of human CYP forms involved in the activation of tamoxifen and irreversible binding to DNA. *Carcinogenesis*, 23: 1897-1901, 2002.

[129] Boocock, D. J., Maggs, J. L., Brown, K., White, I. N. H., and Park, B. K. Major inter-species differences in the rates of *O*-suphonation and *O*-glucuronylation of α-hydroxytamoxifen *in vitro*: a metabolic disparity protecting human liver from the formation of tamoxifen-DNA adducts. *Carcinogenesis*, 21: 1851-1858, 2000.

[130] Raijmakers, M. T. M., Jansen, P. L. M., Steegers, E. A. P., and Peters, W. H. M. Association of human liver bilirubin UDP-glucuronyltransferase activity with a polymorphism in the promoter region of the UGT1A1 gene. Journal of *Hepatology*, 33: 348-351, 2000.

[131] Brown, K. Breast cancer chemoprevention: risk-benefit effects of the anti-oestrogen tamoxifen. *Expert Opin.Drug Saf*., 1 : 253-267, 2002.

[132] White, I. N. H. The tamoxifen dilemma. *Carcinogenesis*, 20: 1153-1160, 1999.

[133] White, I. N. H. Tamoxifen: Is it Safe? Comparison of Activation and Detoxication Mechanisms in Rodents and in Humans. *Curr.Drug Metab*, 4: 223-239, 2003.

[134] Ridings, J. E., Barratt, M. D., Cary, R., Earnshaw, C. G., Eggington, C. E., Ellis, M. K., Judson, P. N., Langowski, J. J., Marchant, C. A., Payne, M. P., Watson, W. P., and Yih, T. D. Computer prediction of possible toxic action from chemical structure: an update on the DEREK system. *Toxicology,* 106: 267-279, 1996.

[135] Potter, G. A., McCague, R., and Jarman, M. A mechanistic hypothesis for DNA adduct formation by tamoxifen following hepatic oxidative metabolism. *Carcinogenesis*, 15: 439-442, 1994.

[136] Glatt, H., Davis, W., Meinl, W., Hermersdorfer, H., Venitt, S., and Phillips, D. H. Rat but not human sulfotransferase activates a tamoxifen metabolite to produce DNA adducts and gene mutations in bacteria and mammalian cells in culture. *Carcinogenesis*, 19: 1709-1713, 1998.

[137] Martin, E. A., Turteltaub, K. W., Heydon, R., Davies, A. M., White, I. N. H., and Smith, L. L. Characterisation of tamoxifen induced-DNA adducts formed in rat liver. *The Toxicologist*., 15: 152-Abstract, 1995.

[138] Curtis, R. E., Boice, J. D., Jr., Shriner, D. A., Hankey, B. F., and Fraumeni, J. F., Jr. Second cancers after adjuvant tamoxifen therapy for breast cancer. *J.Natl.Cancer Inst.*, 88: 832-834, 1996.

[139] Fisher, B., Costantino, J. P., Wickerham, D. L., Redmond, C. K., Kavanah, M., Cronin, W. M., Vogel, V., Robidoux, A., Dimitrov, N., Atkins, J., Daly, M., Wieand, S., Tan-Chiu, E., Ford, L., and Wolmark, N. Tamoxifen for prevention of breast cancer: report of the National Surgical Adjuvant Breast and Bowel Project P-1 Study. *J Natl.Cancer Inst.*, 90: 1371-1388, 1998.

[140] Carmichael, P. L., Ugwumadu, A. H., Neven, P., Hewer, A. J., Poon, G. K., and Phillips, D. H. Lack of genotoxicity of tamoxifen in human endometrium. *Cancer Res.*, 56: 1475-1479, 1996.

In: Liver Cancer: New Research
Editor: Felix Lee, pp. 161-184
ISBN 1-59454-182-5


*Chapter VII*

# Immunotherapy in Metastatic Liver Disease

***Jannis Kountouras[9], Christos Zavos and Dimitrios Chatzopoulos***
Department of Gastroenterology, Second Medical Clinic, Ippokration Hospital of Thessaloniki, Aristotle University of Thessaloniki, Greece

## Abstract

Metastatic liver cancer is about 20 times as common as primary liver cancer, and its treatment by surgery or conventional chemotherapy is still limited and most patients die. Thus, a broad spectrum of recent novel treatments, including innovative molecular therapies, such as gene and active immunotherapy or replication-competent viral therapeutic strategies, is under preclinical investigation, and numerous clinical trials are in progress in order to combat this lethal disease. Active immunotherapy, intended to induce antigen-specific T-lymphocyte responses to tumor-associated or tumor-specific antigens, has reemerged as a promising approach for the treatment of metastatic liver malignancies, combined with other therapies, and, moreover, as a modality to prevent cancer metastases or recurrence. Locoregional immunotherapy appears to be an attractive and rational approach for the management of metastatic liver disease, offering several advantages over systemic immunotherapy. Locoregional immunological strategies include intrahepatic infusion of anti-tumor cytokines combined with chemotherapy, adoptive immunotherapy by using lymphokine-activated killer cells or activated tumor-infiltrated lymphocytes, embolization of liver tumors with immunostimulants and gene immunotherapy. New-fangled strategies in the immunotherapy of metastatic liver disease, to further improve the outcome of locoregional chemo-immunotherapy, are reviewed briefly, such as the use of granulocyte-macrophage colony-stimulating factor,

[9] Correspondence: Jannis Kountouras, MD, PhD, Gastroenterologist, Associate Professor of Medicine 8 Phanariou St, Byzantio Thessaloniki, 55 133, Macedonia, Greece Tel: +30-2310-892238, FAX: +30-2310-992794 E-mail: jannis@med.auth.gr

tumor growth factors-beta antagonists, various monoclonal antibodies including vascular endothelial growth factor antibodies, costimulatory molecules, vaccines, transfection of syngeneic major histocompatibility complex class II genes, a variety of immunotherapeutic strategies based on dendritic cell-induced T-cell mediated anti-tumor immunity, Newcastle Disease Virus, intralesional gene therapy and suicide genes. Our challenge is to estimate the effectiveness of these immunotherapeutic approaches and to optimize their application in the clinical practice.

**Keywords:** Immunotherapy, Liver cancer, Metastatic, Locoregional, Systemic, Chemotherapy, Gene therapy

## INTRODUCTION

The liver is second only to lymph nodes as a common site of metastasis from other solid cancers, especially abdominal cancer [1].It is not uncommon for the liver to be the only site of metastatic disease, particularly in patients with colorectal adenocarcinoma [2].Metastatic liver cancer is about 20 times as common as primary liver cancer and, despite the progress made during the last decades, this disease still caries a dismal prognosis.

Today, treatment of metastatic liver cancer by surgery or conventional chemotherapy is limited and most patients die. Indeed, although liver resection, with several ancillary techniques, has acceptable rates of early morbidity and mortality, even for older patients, however, at the time of diagnosis only 20% to 25% of patients with metastatic liver disease are eligible for liver resection and, after surgical resection, 65% to 70% of patients will develop recurrence, with low overall survival rate (30%) [3-5]. In addition, because of the numerous functions of the liver: synthesis of the majority of serum proteins, metabolism of drugs and nutrients, excretion and detoxification of exogenous agents and endogenous toxins, and filtering of portal venous blood, assessing the risks of liver resection in patients with liver disease is a complex serious problem [6]. Besides, although conventional chemotherapy has shown much promise in the treatment of several other malignancies, common systemic chemotherapy does not offer considerably increased survival and is associated with severe side effects and sequela. Hoping to improve the management of metastatic liver disease, a number of investigators have introduced locoregional chemotherapy, but their results were rather disappointing, as survival did not improve and serious sequela remained [4, 5, 7].

Therefore, since only a minority of patients with metastatic liver disease would be candidates for complete surgical resection while the majority of these patients will subsequently develop local or systemic recurrences after conventional chemotherapies of liver metastases, new treatment modalities to control malignant disease and to prevent systemic progression are needed. In this regard, a broad spectrum of recent novel treatments, including innovative molecular therapies, such as gene and active immunotherapy or replication-competent viral therapeutic strategies, is under preclinical investigation, and numerous clinical trials are in progress to combat this lethal disease [8].

In general, immune modulatory therapies, through induction of systemic anti-tumor responses against disseminated cancer cells, are mainly used in advanced diseases, which have failed to respond to conventional therapy [4]. Accordingly, active immunotherapy, intended to induce antigen-specific T-lymphocyte responses to tumor-associated or tumor-specific antigens, has reemerged as a promising approach for the treatment of metastatic liver malignancies, combined with other therapies, and, moreover, as a modality to prevent cancer metastasis or recurrence [9].

## IMMUNOTHERAPEUTIC APPROACHES IN METASTATIC LIVER CANCER

There are two ways to introduce immunotherapy: locoregionally and systemically. An initial important question concerning locoregional immunotherapy for metastatic liver disease is whether immunological responses can be induced in the liver. In this respect, the liver is the largest organ of the reticuloendothelial system and would be suitable target for immunotherapy. The liver contains 80% to 90% of resident macrophages (Kupffer cells) in the entire body. The main function of Kupffer cells is phagocytosis and elimination of pathogens, including bacteria, endotoxins, tumor cells, immune complexes, lipid assemblies and other particulate matter and foreign bodies from circulation [10, 11]. The liver responds rapidly to inflammation, as a secondary response to proinflammatory cytokines, including interleukin (IL)-1, IL-6 and tumor necrosis factor (TNF)-α. Moreover, the liver contains lymphoid cells that provide the liver with innate immunity in the site that encounters a numerous of gut-derived and circulating antigens. Three types of lymphoid cells are present in the liver: pit cells that make up 50% of the total population of lymphocytes, CD4 and CD8 T lymphocytes, and natural killer (NK) T lymphocytes. Pit cells are sinusoidal (vascular side) large granular lymphocytes functioning as natural killer cells with tumoricidal capabilities[12]. $CD3^{+}$ γδ T lymphocytes are also present in the liver, and T lymphocytes expressing the γδ T cell antigen receptor (γδTCR) chains display strong major histocompatibility complex (MHC)-unrestricted cytotoxicity against cancer cells when activated *in vitro* by IL-2. The cytotoxic activity of γδTCR cells are reminiscent of NK cells, which preferentially lyse target cells that have lost MHC class I alleles, a frequent occurrence in cancer progression [13]. These hepatic immune cells can be activated by various cytokines, including IL-2 and intereferon (IFN)-γ, and display anti-tumor activity [10, 11]. Thus, considering the immunological responses induced in the liver, locoregional immunotherapy appears to be an attractive and rational approach for the management of metastatic liver disease [10].

Locoregional immunotherapy for metastatic liver disease offers several advantages over systemic immunotherapy for the following 3 main reasons: (1) direct administration of immune cells or immunostimulants into the tumor burden alters the environment within the tumor and might break immunotolerance elicited by cancer cells; (2) local administration of anti-tumor cytokines, such as IL-2, IFNs, or TNF-α, minimizes their systemic toxicity, and finally (3) destruction of tumor cells *in situ* provides tumor antigens to the host immune system, which may result in a systemic immune response against the tumor cells (*in situ* cancer vaccine) [10].

Several locoregional immunological strategies have been applied, including intrahepatic infusion of anti-tumor cytokines combined with chemotherapy, adoptive immunotherapy by using lymphokine-activated killer (LAK) cells or activated tumor infiltrated lymphocytes (TILs), embolization of liver tumors with immunostimulants and gene immunotherapy; all of these strategies are particularly useful in local control of unresectable, chemotherapy-resistant liver metastases from gastrointestinal malignancies, melanoma, or breast cancer.

The following preliminary immunological consideration and strategy can be introduced by the surgeon, who intends to remove metastatic liver tumors by a major surgery [14]. It is known that the existence of micrometastases is the major reason responsible for distant organ recurrence in patients with malignancies treated with macroscopically radical surgery. It is also recognized that immunosuppression and activation of angiogenesis are important risk factors for cancer cell proliferation and dissemination with the subsequent stimulation to the growth of eventual micrometastases already existing at the time of surgical removal of the primary tumor. In this respect, a major surgery may induce stimulation of angiogenesis and immunosuppression consisting of lymphocytopenia, reduction of the blood levels of anti-tumor cytokines, including IL-2 and IL-12, and increase of immunosuppressive cytokines, namely IL-6. On the other hand, according to clinical trials, preoperative administration of IL-2, subcutaneously, prevents surgery-induced immunosuppression, and, moreover, counteracts surgery induced-stimulation of angiogenesis by either reducing the increased levels of angiogenic vascular endothelial growth factor (VEGF) observed during surgery or opposing the decline of anti-angiogenic and anti-tumor IL-12 blood levels. In addition, IL-2 is well tolerated in all patients and in particular no cardiovascular complications occur in the perioperative period. Therefore, surgeons may consider introducing this preoperative immunotherapeutic approach. However, it is important to note that the systemic use of IL-2 is limited by dose-dependent toxicity characterized by weight gain, dyspnea, ascites, and pulmonary edema [15]. Such toxicity results from increased capillary leak, also known as vascular leak syndrome (VLS). The exact mechanism of induction of VLS is not known. Several recent studies have suggested that VLS may result from actual damage to the endothelial cells caused by cytotoxic T lymphocytes (CTLs) [16, 17]. In patients who develop VLS, systemic administration of IL-2 triggers severe side effects resulting in anasarca and multiorgan system dysfunction [18, 19]. On the other hand, it has been demonstrated that immunosuppression of mice by pretreatment with irradiation or injection of cyclophosphamide or cortisone markedly reduces or eliminates the development of IL-2-induced VLS [20]. Also, the toxicity associated with IL-2 therapy has been shown to decrease after depletion of NK cells *in vivo* [21].

The above mentioned anti-tumor cytokines (IL-2, IL-12) and other relative cytokines [IFN-γ, granulocyte-macrophage colony-stimulating factor (GM-CSF)] are now recognized as predominant T helper (Th) 1 cytokines, promoting the development of cellular immunity important for the anti-tumor response [22, 23]. Although noticeably efficacious in some cases, this approach has limited use systemically, due to observed significant toxicity and limited response rates. Because regionally applied cytokines have been shown to augment the cytolytic activity of killer cells, they might be considered for cellular activation of locoregional immunotherapy in metastatic liver disease. Undoubtedly, transplenic and transtumoral administration of these multiple cytokines for *in vivo* immunostimulation is based on their well-known dynamic synergism. Indeed, IL-2, IFN-γ, and IL-12 induce cytolytic activity of LAK and NK cells and are considered for cellular activation to locoregional immunotherapy before, after resection or even in unresectable liver malignancies. There is no doubt that IL-2 induces both generation of LAK cells, and an immune amplification cascade causing a potent anti-tumor response. Continuous attempts to reduce toxicity have led to several strategies, including lowering of IL-2 doses, combining IL-2 with other cytokines, or providing IL-2 directly to the tumor burden. IL-2 has also been administered directly into accessible tumor sites by a slow release form and this strategy is now being attempted in humans through infusion of liposomal IL-2 [24]. In addition, fusing cytokines, e.g. IL-2, to recombinant antibodies ("immunocytokines") appear to be an effective approach to focus cytokine activity to cancer tissue [25]. Moreover, it has been shown that IL-2 modulates 5-fluorouracil (5-FU) metabolizing enzymes and also increases the effectiveness of 5-FU. In this respect, levamisole (a non-specific immune modulator), combined with 5-FU, was used in adjuvant treatment [26].

IL-12 (a growth factor for pre-activated NK cells) is also among the most potent cytokines at stimulating anti-tumor immunity. IL-12 acts by (a) induction of a Thl type of response, (b) activation of NK cells (300 times more potent than IL-2 in promoting NK cytotoxicity) and CTLs, (c) enhanced expression of adhesion molecules on endothelial cells, thus facilitating the traffic of lymphocytes to the tumor, and (d) induction of a potent anti-angiogenic effect. The anti-angiogenic effect of IL-12 is mediated by IFN-γ, which, in turn, stimulates the production of the chemokine IFN-inducible protein-10 that, in addition to acting as a chemoattractant for lymphocytes, has a potent inhibitory effect on the proliferation and differentiation of endothelium. Furthermore, IL-12 stimulated NK cells are cytotoxic for activated endothelial cells, thereby contributing to block the creation of new cancer vasculature [27]. Although IL-12 is a potent anti-tumoral substance, its use is also liable to cause systemic toxic effects mainly derived from the ability of this cytokine to induce IFN-γ production. In order to enhance the anti-tumoral activity of IL-12 while reducing the risk of toxicity, the therapeutic effect of a suboptimal dose of AdIL-12 in combination with an adenovirus expressing the chemokine IP-10 (AdIP-10) has been tested. The rationale was to attract immunoeffector cells to the neoplasm through IP-10 and to activate the attracted lymphocytes with IL-12. It has been shown that this combined therapy allows reduction of the dose of AdIL-12 without loss of anti-tumoral efficacy, but with less risk of toxicity [28]. As activation of dendritic cells (DCs), the most efficient antigen presenting cells (APCs), is critical for induction of anti-tumoral immunity, another possible way to enhance the anti-tumoral effect of low doses of IL-12 is to infect DCs with AdIL-12 *ex vivo* and to inject these engineered DCs into the tumor [29].

Summarizing, such cytokine-based therapeutic strategies induce cytolytic activity of LAK and NK cells and are considered for cellular activation to locoregional immunotherapy in liver metastases.

Regarding the LAK and NK cells together with circulating T lymphocytes and activated macrophages, this heterogeneous army of cells is capable to detect antigenic changes on the surface of cancer cells, and this recognition leads to elimination of malignant cells and generation of memory T lymphocytes, able to recognize the same antigen at reencounter [30]. LAK and NK cells can be generated by incubating lymphoid cells with IL-2 in tumor-bearing patients and in normal donors. They are found in all normal donors and are believed to play an important role in the defense mechanism against a variety of malignant tumor cells. In particular, LAK cells have been shown to lyse fresh NK-resistant tumor cells, but not normal cells. There is evidence suggesting that adoptive transfer of LAK cells plus rIL-2 could mediate regression of pulmonary and hepatic metastases and also original cancers in a variety of experimental and human neoplams [31]. Some studies reported complete or partial responses preferentially in renal cancer, melanoma, Hodgkin's or non-Hodgkin's lymphomas and lung cancers, although severe side effects due to the toxicity of IL-2 were also observed.[31] NK cells also play a role in the defense against tumor cells, functioning either as a form of surveillance against newly arising malignant clones, or as a mechanism by which the accessible cells of established tumors are destroyed [32]. Adoptively transferred IL-2-activated NK cells in a syngeneic rat colorectal cancer liver and lung metastasis model were shown to selectively infiltrate the tumors [33]. Specifically, more NK cells were found in tumors when the NK cells were directly injected into tumor-draining blood vessels than when the cells were injected in systemic blood vessels. It is possible that, after reaching the stroma surrounding the tumor cell nodules, where they are found predominantly, the NK cells may initiate elimination of tumor cells by activating other effector cells, whereas some may eliminate tumor cells by direct cell-to-cell contact. Recent evidence suggests that activated TILs and NK cells by IL-2 and IL-12 can, in turn, kill tumor cells in an apoptotic fashion via Fas/Fas Ligand (FasL) apoptotic pathway, indicating that apoptotic procedure plays an important role in eliminating tumor cells [34]. In particular, NK cells and CTLs can kill cancer cells by two apoptotic mechanisms: a) by engagement and crosslinking of the Fas receptor on tumor cells with its ligand FasL on T lymphocytes (Fas/FasL pathway), and b) by the combined action of the pore-forming proteins (perforins) and the serine protease granzyme B, exocytosed from their cytoplasmic granules. Perforins act by inducing lytic defects in the target cell membrane. Granzyme B enters the target cell independent of perforin, while perforin facilitates granzyme B's rapid access to cytoplasmic and nuclear pre-apoptotic molecules by disrupting endosomes containing the granzymes [13, 34-37].

Considering the LAK cell generation for practical treatment, these nonspecific killer cells are easily induced by activation of human peripheral blood lymphocytes (PBLs) in culture with IL-2 [38]. However, it is difficult to obtain enough cells by the method of harvesting PBLs from cancer patients and adoptively transfer the induced LAK cells back to those patients [38]. On the other hand, spleen is a suitable organ for LAK cell induction, because it has densely packed lymphocytes, and LAK cells generating from tumor-bearer splenocytes are cytotoxic for cancer cells and have effects equal to those from PBLs [38]. Doses of about $2.4 \times 10^9$ LAK cells, generated from the autologous spleen, were adoptively transferred via hepatic arterial catheter for treatment of unresectable liver tumors [38]. Transplenic immunostimulation by IL-2 and IFN-γ (through the splenic artery) activates lymphocytes and monocyte macrophages harbored in the vascular network of the spleen. IFN-γ induces IL-2 receptors in Th1 lymphocytes which are then activated by IL-2. Equally, IFN-γ activates Fc receptors in the monocyte macrophages. The activated Th1 lymphocytes and monocyte macrophages are well known for their cytolytic activities (LAK). Besides, activated macrophages also secrete free oxygen radicals, nitric oxide (NO) and develop an advanced degree of tumor necrosis. It is important to note that the efficacy of LAK cells against lung and liver malignant metastatic lesions is suggested by their interesting trafficking pattern; activated killer cells injected intravenously (i.v.) into humans appeared in the lung early and were subsequently rapidly redistributed to the liver and spleen. The same trafficking patterns were observed regardless of whether injected cells were CTLs cells or LAK cells [38]. As mentioned earlier, adoptive transfer of LAK cells plus rIL-2 could mediate regression of hepatic and pulmonary metastases, as well as original tumors in experimental models and in humans [31]. Therefore, particularly for patients with liver metastases, this characteristic of cytotoxic effectors is suitable for tumor treatment.

A second interesting trafficking pattern concerns NK cells. NK cells in the peripheral blood could become depleted due to selective recruitment or entrapment of these cells at the tumor site, in which case NK cell activity of tumor infiltrating lymphocytes should be high. However, the TILs have been shown to have low NK activity. The defective NK activity could be explained by the following reasons: NK activity could be depressed by factors released from the cancer or by suppressor cells of NK cells, such as those observed in the spleens of *C. parvum* treated mice. Alternatively, it is possible that NK cell activity requires constant priming by IFN, a process that could be disturbed in malignant disease [32]. In fact, TILs show poor effector function, because they produce low cytokine levels, defined as "split anergy" [24]. On the other hand, transtumoral administration of IL-2 and IFN-γ through hepatic artery stimulate TILs to overcome anergy and express activation markers like IL-2r and HLA-DR expression, which, in turn, promote them to mount effector immune responses against the existing tumor [24]. Indeed, according to our findings [24], transplenic and transtumoral administration of IL-2 and IFN-γ combined immunotherapy in patients with advanced unresectable liver and pancreatic malignant disease exert a beneficial immunopotentiating effect on T-lymphocyte populations (CD3+, CD4+, CD8+ T lymphocytes), IL-2r and HLA-DR expression, thereby appearing to be a promising mode of action in the management of malignant metastatic disease. In this respect, human leukocyte IFN causes considerable enhancement of NK cell activity in patients with liver malignant disease. Although the reasons of this increment are not clear, a number of possibilities have been suggested, the conventional view being that IFN 'activates' NK cells in the similar way as lymphokines activate macrophages. Some authors suggest that IFN binds to receptors on NK or pre-NK cells, thereby triggering new messenger RNA production, and then new proteins are involved in the cytotoxic activity of the NK cells. Alternatively, IFN could activate NK cell precursors leading to the maturation of these cells; it has been shown that human mononuclear cells, depleted of functional NK activity by selective adsorption to target cells, could be induced to become cytolytic after IFN administration. Another possibility is that IFN might mediate its effect by acting on various regulatory cells of NK activity, although IFN has been shown to be effective even in the functional lack of T- and B-cells or macrophages. However, there is some evidence to indicate that NK activity is under the control of regulatory lymphocytes; it is possible that IFN, as well as levamisole, which improves the killing of lymphocytes from patients with liver malignant disease, may mediate their effects on NK cell activity via these cells [32].

Another interesting trafficking pattern is the administration of the Lipiodol-Urografin emulsion [an ethiodized oil (Lipiodol) and diatrizoate (Urografin) mixture], because of its unique function to be retained in the vascular network of the spleen and cancer burden[24,39]. In particular, Lipiodol has been shown to have a preferential and prolonged malignant liver neoplasm uptake, following administration directly into the hepatic artery.

The following mechanisms may be involved in this selective localization: 1) selective Lipiodol flow into the tumor due to a siphoning effect, caused by the increased blood flow into the hypervascular tumor mass; 2) selective deposition of Lipiodol in the irregular neoplastic neovasculature; 3) extravascular distribution associated with increased permeability of the neoplasm neovasculature, and 4) decreased rate of the oil elimination from the tumor mass, due to the slow blood flow in the irregular microvasculature and the lack of lymphatic or reticuloendothelial clearance mechanisms in the neoplastic tissue [24]. Therefore, Lipiodol has a dual effect regarding its anti-tumor identities: the oil emulsion, forming small droplets, occludes the small feeding arterioles of the neoplasm, and, on the other hand, decreases the clearance rate of chemotherapy from the neoplastic vasculature. Consequently, apart of the ischemia induction in the tumor mass due to embolism, increased intraneoplastic and decreased systemic levels of the chemotherapeutic agents are achieved. Moreover, the oil seems to have another advantage regarding its distribution: it is not confined to the arterial microvasculare only, but it can reach the nearby sinusoids, where daughter neoplastic nodules or infiltrative lesions can develop, supplied by portal blood as well. This emulsion is retained in the lymphatic system around the portal vein and in metastatic lymph nodes, thereby ensuring its drug effect in malignant lymph nodes. One day after intraarterial infusion of $^{131}$I-labeled Lipiodol, the presence of at least 75% of the radioactivity was demonstrated in the liver and was at least 5 times higher in the liver malignant mass than the surrounding normal hepatic parenchyma. Following this finding, administration of highly radioactive $^{131}$I-labeled Lipiodol has shown to possess a positive effect in terms of tumor size reduction. Similar selective therapeutic Lipiodol deposition has been confirmed in cases of intraarterial Lipiodol chemotherapy. In these cases, the peripheral blood doxorubicin levels are 10 times lower in comparison with plain intraarterial infusion, and the tumor levels remain high up to 1 month later. Clinical trials have shown that Lipiodol chemoembolization can result in a 2-year survival of 33% to 50%, whereas plain arterial embolization leads to a 2-year survival of 15% to 40% [24]. From an additional viewpoint, the effect of Lipiodol-Urografin emulsion of IL-2 and IFN-γ, carried via the transplenic route, is remarkable. After overloading the spleen, the emulsion floods the area of the organ occupied by the neoplasm. The selective retention of the emulsion in the vascular network of the organ space occupied by the neoplasm is identical to the retention seen in the spleen. This is a unique function of the emulsion of the chemo-immunotherapeutical drugs bound to Lipiodol-Urografin droplets [40]. Recent data indicate that IL-2 administration via hepatic artery, suspended in Lipiodol-Urografin droplets, leads to activation of regional antigen-presenting cells, such as Kupffer cells, and endothelial cells known for their cytolytic and phagocytic identities, thereby achieving prolongation of patients' survival. In summary, Lipiodol-Urografin emulsion is probably an ideal cytokine/anti-cancer drug carrier, suitable for the combined locoregional chemo-immunotherapy, because, during Lipiodol retention, a gradual release of both immuno- and chemo-therapeutical drugs is achieved, ensuring a prolonged half-life for these drugs.

## IMMUNOTHERAPY: WITH OR WITHOUT CHEMOTHERAPY?

A further question has been raised concerning the use of immunotherapy alone or combined with chemotherapy. It has been established that regional infusion of IL-2 or other cytokines (TNF-α, IFN-γ) through the hepatic artery or portal vein combined with chemotherapy yield better results than chemotherapy alone [10]. The reason may be due to the fact that the combination of regional application of chemotherapy and immunotherapy contributes to an augmentation of penetration of chemotherapeutical drugs to the surrounding tissues due to the VLS induced by IL-2 regional application resulting in an enhanced effectiveness of regional chemotherapy [41-43]. IL-2 upregulates perforin and FasL activity and these molecules do participate in the induction of VLS, leading to an increased effectiveness of regional chemotherapy [44]. In fact, regionally delivered drugs, being entrapped within the regional capillary network of the organ space occupied by the tumor, lead to a higher concentration of the drug within the tumor itself, which is expected to improve the response rate regarding the extent of tumor necrosis. Moreover, modulation of 5-FU metabolizing enzymes by IL-2 leads to enhanced effectiveness of this chemothepapeutic agent [42].

## LOCOREGIONAL VS. SYSTEMIC IMMUNOTHERAPY

Considering locoregional versus systemic immunotherapy, our recent meta-analysis study [45] indicates that locoregional immunotherapy is superior in terms of response and recurrence rates, thereby resulting in significant prolongation of the overall and of disease-free survival rates. As shown in Table 1, 65 out of 98 (66.3%) patients with metastatic liver disease, who received combined locoregional chemo-immunotherapy prior to or after resection of the tumor, responded completely or partially, whereas only 4 out of 26 (15.4%) control patients received systemic chemo-immunotherapy responded to the treatment ($P \leq 0.001$) [7, 46-53]. There were no significant differences in the response rate between the patients with resectable and unresectable tumors, although the last ones were rather less likely to respond, regardless of the treatment they received. There was noteworthy difference in survival rate in favor of the patients who received combination locoregional therapy (21.0 months, range 3-30 months) compared with controls (10.5 months, range 3.6-25 months), a finding that was clearly stated by all authors. Although a twofold survival rate was noticed in the patients received combined locoregional chemo-immunotherapy compared with the control patients, a P value could not be established, because the standard deviations were not provided by the authors. Tumor recurrence was observed in 29 out of 119 (24.37%) patients received combined locoregional chemo-immunotherapy, and in 39 out of 80 (48.75%) control patients received only systemic chemo-immunotherapy ($P \leq 0.001$).

Side effects of the adjuvant chemotherapy included neutropenia, diarrhea, vomiting, and nausea in 5-25% of the patients, and fever and chills in 70-100% of the patients. There was also a low incidence of jaundice reported. Contrary to the patients received locoregional chemo-immunotherapy, about half of the patients received systemic chemo-immunotherapy were hospitalized due to side effects [47].

**Table 1. Results in Response, Survival and Recurrence Rates in Patients Received Combined Locoregional Chemo-Immunotherapy Versus Control Patients Received Systemic Chemo-Immunotherapy or Chemotherapy**

| Metastatic liver disease | | | | | | | | | | |
|---|---|---|---|---|---|---|---|---|---|---|
| **Author** | **Patients** | | **Response (CR/PR)** | | | **Survival (months)** | | **Recurrence** | | |
| | **LR** | **C** | **LR** | **C** | **P** | **LR** | **C** | **LR** | **C** | **P** |
| Toh U (46) | 2 | - | 2 | - | | - | - | - | - | |
| Lygidakis NJ (47) | 62 | 60 | - | - | | 57 pat/2 yr | 36 pat/2 yr | 21 | 31 | |
| Ueda Y (48)* | 7 | 11 | 3 | 2 | | - | - | - | - | |
| Lygidakis NJ (49) | 19 | - | 12 | - | | - | - | 4 | - | |
| Lygidakis NJ (7) | 33 | 15 | 21 | 2 | | 20.3 (13-29) | 9.9 (3.6-22.5) | - | - | |
| Okuno K (50) | 18 | - | 14 | - | | 28.5 | - | 4 | - | |
| Lygidakis NJ (51) | 20 | 20 | - | - | | 20 (3-30) | 11 (4-25) | 0 | 8 | |
| Lygidakis NJ (52) | 10 | - | 10 | - | | 12 (6-19) | - | - | - | |
| Keilholz U (53)[10] | 9 | - | 3 | - | | - | - | - | - | |
| Total | 180 | 106 | 65/98 (66.3%) | 4/26 (15.4%) | ≤0.001 | 21.0 (3-30) | 10.5 (3.6-25) | 29/119 (24.37%) | 39/80 (48.75%) | ≤0.001 |

LR: combined locoregional chemo-immunotherapy; C: control cases received only systemic chemo-immunotherapy; CR: complete response; PR: partial response; P: statistical significance

The available data, however, have a number of limitations possibly based on the following initial and general consideration: with regard to primary liver cancer, an enhanced LAK activity is observed in approximately 11% of patients with massive hepatocellular carcinomas (HCCs), thereby suggesting that LAK activity in some cases may be enhanced progressively by tumor growth. Therefore, primary and possibly metastatic neoplasms could grow even if the host has intact or enhanced immune function, because the efficacy of immune surveillance depends on recognition of tumor cells, delivery of immune cells and tumoricidal activity [54, 55]. This might partially explain why the efficacy of adoptive immunotherapy with LAK cells for metastatic liver disease is not yet generally established, although striking therapeutic effects have been noted in the observational studies.

The available studies use various methodological strategies, comprising the inclusion criteria, the type of combined therapy, the response, the recurrence or tumor progression and the survival rates, thereby creating some limitations for a uniform meta-analysis of the available data. For example, some of the series included in our meta-analysis [52, 53] account for patients diagnosed, staged and treated at least 10 years ago, when regular screening was rather uncommon, the imaging techniques were less accurate, and the medical management of patients with impairment liver function was less effective. In addition, series of untreated patients also include patients with advanced malignant disease when prognosis is serious, thereby leading to a false-negative estimation of the expected survival. Therefore, candidates to enter the studies investigating the usefulness of new therapeutic options are often individuals who do not fulfill the restrictive criteria to benefit from radical interventional therapies (surgical resection, liver transplantation), and also patients diagnosed at a terminal

[10] Cases reported were unresectable hepatocellular carcinomas

stage. Moreover, survival was infeasible to calculate and compare, because: a) in some papers there were not mentioned the exact mean values and standard deviations, b) the authors have used various follow-up periods, and c) survival did not always correlate with the stage of the disease in which therapy was initiated, because some of the studies had recruited their subjects retrospectively. Furthermore, some authors have used 1-, 2-, and 3-year survival rates, while others have just mentioned the median and survival range in months over a limited follow-up period.

Another limitation is that the patients did not receive a uniform treatment. Moreover, the most recent paper in our meta-analysis [47] compared locoregional chemo-immunotherapy plus systemic chemotherapy versus systemic chemo-immunotherapy in patients with metastatic liver disease of colorectal origin, thereby not actually "fitting" in any of the previously published categories. However, this paper provides opportunities for the introduction of combined locoregional plus systemic therapy in order to possibly offer more promising results, although there are still concerns about the adverse effects from the administration of systemic immunotherapy.

Response to treatment and recurrence of the disease was not clearly mentioned by some authors. Thus, there is need for application of uniform inclusion criteria by the future multicenter and international studies, in order to provide more definite answers concerning the effectiveness of locoregional therapy in patients with metastatic liver cancer.

With regard to the primary sites of metastatic liver cancer, they were focused mainly on the digestive tract (colorectal carcinoma, esophageal cancer), and moreover melanoma (cutaneous and ocular) [45]. None of these studies could predict response or survival in relation to the stage of primary site of cancer prior to treatment, and therefore they could not indisputably establish whether the locoregional chemo-immunotherapeutic option, applied at a later stage, had any effect on improving response and prolonging survival rate. These arising considerations also require further elucidation in future studies.

## Novel Strategies in Immunotherapy of Metastatic Liver Disease

The following innovative approaches have been tested in order to improve the outcome of locoregional chemo-immunotherapy.

### GM-CSF

GM-CSF was used to stimulate antigen-presenting cells in liver metastases. In particular, embolization of melanoma metastatic to the liver with a GM-CSF/ethiodized oil emulsion resulted in control of liver metastases, as well as development of significant immune responses in remote extrahepatic metastases [10]. Moreover, GM-CSF increases the number of patients with stable disease.[8]

## Tumor Growth Factor (TGF)-Beta

TGF-betas play diverse and complex roles in several biological processes. In tumorigenesis, they can function either as tumor suppressors or as pro-oncogenic factors, depending on the stage of the disease. Recent experimental data suggest that *in vivo* TGF-beta antagonist of the soluble type II TGF-beta receptor may selectively neutralize the undesirable TGF-beta associated with metastasis, while sparing the regulatory roles of TGF-betas in normal tissues [56]. Therefore, this soluble TGF-beta antagonist has potential for long-term clinical use in the prevention of metastases.

## Monoclonal Antibodies

A new modality in the management of metastatic disease includes administration of monoclonal antibodies directed against cancer antigens and has proved to be a rational approach in metastatic liver disease. Several groups reported clinical radio-immunotherapy studies, using radioactive iodine labeled anti-carcinoembryonic antigen (CEA) antibody, TAG 72, or A33 murine or chimeric antibodies, to treat metastatic liver disease. In the majority of clinical studies successful tumor targeting and, in some cases, decreased CEA levels or stabilization of disease was observed [8]. Besides, clinical trials have shown that the monoclonal antibody 17-1A, a receptor on the surface of colon cancer cells, is effective in increasing the survival following resection of Dukes C primary colorectal tumors, and can also be used as an adjuvant treatment prior to or after liver resection for liver metastases of colorectal origin [57]. Recent data also indicate that 17-1A is widely expressed on liver metastases of patients with colorectal carcinoma. Therefore, patients with completely resected liver metastases might be suitable candidates for adjuvant therapy with the antibody 17-1A, since only a few of these lesions show coexpression of complement resistance factors[58].

## VEGF

VEGF is a secreted polypeptide and acts as a strong angiogenic factor in both normal and pathologic angiogenesis, mainly through binding to receptor tyrosine kinases on endothelial cells. Some authors demonstrated, in an *in vivo* model, suppression of tumor growth by inhibition of VEGF-angiogenesis [59]. Tumor growth inhibition was observed in nude mice injected with human glioblastoma or sarcoma cells and subsequently treated with an anti-VEGF antibody. In particular, VEGF gene expression has been noticed in surgically resected hepatic tumors from colorectal cancer. Furthermore, mice with liver metastases treated with antibodies against VEGF were associated with significant reduction in the number and volume of malignant liver disease [60]. Recognizing that, even after transarterial chemoembolization, both the development of neovascularization and the expression of VEGF play important roles in establishment of collateral circulation and reconstruction of blood supply of residual cancer tissue, blockade of VEGF receptor signaling combined with chemotherapy provides an effective approach to cancer treatment.

## Costimulatory Molecules

Another important obstacle in generating anti-tumor immune responses is overcoming tolerance or tumor-associated antigens. Modulation of costimulatory interaction, in the context of sensitization to the tumor-associated antigens, may be a way by which tolerance can be overcome, and a productive anti-tumor immune response can be elicited [61]. Transfection of genes encoding B7 costimulatory molecule in combination with suitable cytokines (IL-2, IL-12) resulted in efficient tumor regression of established cancers in experimental models. This is particularly attractive in the light of current understanding of the mode of action of these factors, namely IL-2 as a second signal for T lymphocyte activation, as well as an inhibitor of tumor-induced anergy, and B7 as an inhibitor of T lymphocyte receptor induced apoptosis [61].

## Vaccines

### *Vaccines with Cancer Antigens*

It was only after the recognition of the first human tumor-associated antigen (TAA) that development of specific vaccination trial for cancer patients became possible. Tumor-associated antigens recognized by CD8+ CTLs have been recognized, and antigen-specific vaccines are being designed with recombinant proteins or vectors. Published data concerns phase I/II clinical trials using tumor synthetic peptides presented by common human MHC class I alleles. When using this method it is essential to demonstrate that the immune response is focused on the immunogenic epitopes. CTLs are activated against these peptides and recognize cells endogenously expressing the tumor protein, providing specificity to the anti-tumor response [25]. Another successful approach termed SEREX (serological identification of antigens by recombinant expressing cloning) uses the antibody repertoire of cancer patients to identify tumor antigens. This strategy has revealed tumor antigens and a variety of well-defined tumor antigen peptides are used to specifically activate CTLs *in vivo*. For example, metastatic melanoma patients have received subcutaneous injections of MAGE-3-derived peptide, or MelanA/MART-1 in peptide vaccination trials and the therapeutic effect was considered significant [62].

### *Cytokine-Secreting Tumor Cell Vaccines*

The application of gene transfer techniques for the engineering of cancer cells to express immunostimulatory gene products led to an enhanced delivery of cytokines into the cancer microenvironment. Particular consideration has been devoted to experiments involving GM-CSF and IL-12, as these molecules elicit overlapping but distinct effector mechanisms. Both cytokines promote innate immunity and Th1 responses [63].

### *Genetic Vaccination*

To prevent cancer growth, genetic vaccination has also been applied. In a murine model of subcutaneous HCC it has been shown that DNA vaccination with a cDNA encoding murine AFP induced cancer regression and prolonged animal survival. The anti-tumoral effect was mediated by CTLs, and protective anti-tumoral immunity was shown to depend on both CD4+ and CD8+ T lymphocytes [64]. Recently, improved immunization protocols, such as hepatic arterial administration of adenovirus with wild-type p53 or intra-tumoral injection of adenoviral vectors encoding suicide gene HSV/tk or IL-12 have been applied [65], or are at present been tested, in HCC patients in phase I/II clinical trials. However, clinical trials should determine whether human patients with primary or metastatic liver disease could be treated safely and effectively by such strategies.

## Transfection of Syngeneic MHC Class II Genes

Several approaches are being developed based on the knowledge of the importance of help provided by CD4+ T lymphocytes. Because there is a strong correlation between the anti-tumor immunity and the ability to endogenously synthesize MHC antigens, transfection of syngeneic MHC class II genes is thought to increase immunogenicity and enable the transfected cell to present directly endogenously encoded tumor peptides to CD4+ T helper cells, thereby facilitating the activation of cancer-specific CD8+ CTLs. Clinical trials have provided evidence of tumor regression in patients with melanoma and renal cell carcinoma[13].

## Gene Therapy Studies in Animal Tumor Models and in Humans

A variety of gene therapy-based anticancer strategies have been effective in animal tumor models, including replacement of tumor suppressor genes, selective activation of prodrugs, genetic immunotherapy, and anti-angiogenic actions [66]. Genetic immunotherapy means direct delivery of genes that stimulate immune system. Adenoviral vectors can very efficiently transduce a wide variety of malignant epithelial cells, both *in vitro* and *in vivo*, and gene therapy strategies have been effective against animal models of gastrointestinal tumors[67]. Different cytokines (IL-2, IL-4, IL-6, IL-7, IL-12, IFN-γ, TNF-α, GM-CSF) have been used to modulate the host's immune response by either *ex vivo* or *in vivo* gene transfer. In the past few years, gene therapy has emerged as an appealing treatment option for malignant liver disease, because, despite the fact that resection is currently the only curative approach for metastatic liver cancer, only a small number of cases are suitable for this procedure. Various phase I and II clinical trials in patients with metastatic liver cancer showed that gene therapy has been well tolerated and toxicity has been low, but the clinical benefit was marginal [67]. Therefore, although gene therapy in humans (including tumor-suppressor gene p53, suicide genes, immune genes, and replication-competent oncolytic adenoviruses) is of limited use as a definitive treatment for liver metastases, it may be useful as an adjuvant treatment in combination with radiotherapy, chemotherapy, and/or surgery to achieve disease-free survival.

In animal models with orthotopic HCC intratumoral administration of recombinant adenovirus encoding IL-12 (AdIL-12) caused complete tumor eradication in most animals and increased long-term survival [27]. Interestingly, a proportion of the adenovirus injected into a neoplastic nodule escapes to the general circulation and, because of the strong adenoviral hepatotropism, infects the whole liver. IL-12, produced by the tumor and by hepatocytes surrounding the neoplastic nodules, strongly activates NK cells, induces specific anti-tumoral immunity and enhanced expression of adhesion molecules in the tumoral vessels, and displays a powerful anti-angiogenic effect with resulting tumor regression. AdIL-12 given by the intrahepatic arterial route has also been shown to be efficient in the treatment of a very aggressive model of multifocal HCC in rats, causing a significant reduction in tumor burden and prolongation of survival [27], strategy that may also be applied in metastatic liver disease. In this respect, eradication of murine hepatic metastatic colon carcinomas is achieved using a combination therapy with adenovirus-mediated gene delivery of IL-12 and agonistic antibody anti-4-1BB, a costimulatory molecule expressed on activated TLs [68, 69].

Recent data suggest that the addition of anti-OX40 agonistic antibodies may provide a better treatment modality for advanced cancers. Indeed, the combination therapy of IL-12 plus anti-4-1BB plus anti-OX40 resulted in a significantly higher survival rate in treated mice, compared with IL-12 plus anti-4-1BB treatment. More remarkably, long-term surviving mice from the combination therapy with IL-12 plus anti-4-1BB plus anti-OX40 exhibited higher memory CTL responses against parental tumor cells. Of note, the costimulatory molecule OX-40, a member of the tumor necrosis factor receptor (TNFR) superfamily, is expressed primarily on activated CD4+ T lymphocytes. The ligand for OX40 (OX40L) is expressed on DCs, activated B-cells, endothelial cells and macrophages. Upon engagement, the OX40L delivers a potent costimulatory signal to OX40+ TLs, resulting in the production of cytokines by activated TLs, and the rescue of effector TLs from activation-induced cell death [68]. It has been postulated that, in the presence of IL-12 stimulation at the tumor site, activation of tumor-specific $CD4^+$ Th1 cells through the OX40 costimulatory pathway can enhance primary and memory CTL responses against tumors, leading to improvement in the therapeutic efficacy of IL-12 and 4-1BB costimulation in mice with a large tumor burden. Thus, combination therapy with the adenovirus encoding IL-12 (Adv. mIL-12) plus anti-4-1BB plus anti-OX40 antibodies may provide a better treatment modality for patients with advanced cancers, often associated with a state of immune suppression or tolerance.

## DCs

Murine studies suggest that the use of APCs may induce and maintain immune responses with more specificity and less toxicity than other approaches. DCs are potent APCs capable of priming T cells in an HLA-restricted fashion and initiating a T-cell response. DCs have the exceptional ability to stimulate naive or quiescent $CD4^+$ and $CD8^+$ T-cell responses both *in vitro* and *in vivo*. In particular, they are critically essential in initiating primary immune responses against self-antigens, external pathogens, allografts, and malignancies [70, 71]. In their so-called immature state, DCs reside in peripheral tissues, where they search for incoming pathogens or internal pathogens recognized as non-self. On encounter with these antigens, DCs are activated and migrate into the regional lymphoid organs to trigger a specific T-lymphocyte response [72]. Considering DCs generation in order to develop new, practical DC-based immunotherapies against cancer, immature DCs, similar to those observed in peripheral tissues, can be generated by culturing peripheral blood mononuclear cells or bone marrow cells with IL-4 and GM-CSF [73-75]. However, DCs, cultured with both IL-4 and GM-CSF, are highly endocytotic, but not fully able to stimulate antigen-specific T lymphocytes or migrating into the regional lymph nodes. In contrast, mature DCs are capable of migrating to the regional lymph nodes [76, 77] and to efficiently present antigens to specific T lymphocytes [78, 79]. A variety of stimuli induce maturation of DCs including lipopolysaccharides (LPS), CD40 ligand (CD40L), and inflammatory cytokines such as IL-1β and TNF-α [80-82]. Therefore, cumulative evidence that substantiates the essential role of CDs in mounting T-cell mediated anti-tumor immunity [8] and recent advances in cell culture techniques have prompted development of DC-based immunotherapeutic strategies for the treatment of malignancies [83-85]. In this respect, vaccination of mice with DCs, loaded with antigens in the form of peptides or proteins, results in tumor-specific CTL responses capable of rejecting implanted tumors [9]. It has been shown that DCs, generated from the peripheral blood mononuclear cell progenitors of patients with metastatic liver disease from colon cancer or melanoma, can be transfected with total tumor RNA from the autologous malignant cells and used to stimulate CTLs, capable of recognizing and lysing the patient's own tumor cells or targets expressing the patient's tumor antigens. In addition, immunization of a cancer patient with DCs, transfected with the total tumor RNA derived from his CEA-expressing tumor, resulted in tumor antigen-specific CTL responses in *vivo*. Therefore, RNA-transfected DCs, as potent APCs, can offer a broadly applicable platform to induce Ag-specific T-cell responses in patients with advanced malignancies [9]. Recently, intratumoral injection of either DCs transfected *ex vivo* with recombinant adenovirus encoding IL-12 (Ad.IL-12) or an adenovirus coding for CD40L has demonstrated an intense anti-tumor effect against experimental colorectal cancer. Moreover, combination of monocyte-derived DCs and activated T lymphocytes, which express CD40L, induce significant production of anti-tumor cytokines IL-12, INF-γ, thereby appearing to be a potentially effective approach to cancer immunotherapy [72]. Of note, stimulation of DCs is widely dependent on activation by costimulatory molecules such as B7 and CD40L [86, 87]. It has been shown that adenovirus mediated gene transfer of CD40L (AdCD40L) completely abolishes the tumorigenicity of *ex vivo* infected rat HCC cells, and that intratumoral injection of AdCD40L into established intrahepatic tumor nodules in rats results in tumor regression and prolongation of survival. Treatment of rat HCC with AdCD40L induces protective anti-tumor immunity and is devoid of significant toxicity [87], approach that may also be applied in metastatic liver disease.

## Newcastle Disease Virus (NDV)

Naturally oncolytic or non-lytic strains of NDV have been investigated for cancer therapy, and NDV infection of autologous malignant cells as immunotherapy for patients with advanced colorectal cancer was described [88, 89].

## Intralesional Gene Therapy

Direct gene delivery to the lesion to stimulate the immune system has been investigated. In a phase I study, liver metastases from colorectal carcinoma were injected, under ultrasonographic guidance, with allovectin-7, a liposomal vector containing the combination of the HLA-B7 gene with $\beta_2$-microglobulin. Among 15 evaluated patients, plasmid DNA was detected in 14 patients and there was no adverse event directly related to the study drug. There was no objective regression of injected or uninjected liver metastases. Five of 15 patients had stable disease for more than 100 days [90].

## Suicide Genes

Introduction of suicide genes, encoding enzymes that convert non-toxic substances (prodrugs) into toxic metabolites, into tumor cells is an attempt to avoid severe systemic side-effects of conventional chemotherapy. A novel strategy in targeted immunotherapy utilizes the encapsulation of cells genetically modified to express prodrug convertases, which are then implanted in an immune-protected environment in the vicinity of the tumor [13]. TNF has been shown to chemosensitize tumor cells by downregulating multidrug resistance gene expression. Direct activation of CTLs or immune modulatory support is central to several efforts in gene therapy [91].

In summary, multimodal immunotherapy appears to be a promising approach in metastatic liver disease. Having the fundamental knowledge of how immune system functions, we can design a variety of rational immunotherapeutic strategies to combat malignancy. Our challenge is to estimate the effectiveness of these immunotherapeutic approaches and to optimize their application in the clinical practice.

# References

[1] Weiss L, Grundmann E, Torhorst J, Hartveit F, Moberg I, Eder M, Fenoglio-Preiser CM, Napier J, Horne CH, Lopez MJ. Haematogenous metastatic patterns in colonic carcinoma: an analysis of 1541 necropsies. *J Pathol* 1986;150:195-203.

[2] Hughes KS, Simon R, Songhorabodi S, Adson MA, Ilstrup DM, Fortner JG, Maclean BJ, Foster JH, Daly JM, Fitzherbert D. Resection of the liver for colorectal carcinoma metastases: a multi-institutional study of patterns of recurrence. *Surgery* 1986;100:278-84.

[3] Fiorentini G, Poddie DB, Cantore M, Giovanis P, Guadagni S, De Giorgi U, Cariello A, Dazzi C, Turci D. Locoregional therapy for liver metastases from colorectal cancer: the possibilities of intraarterial chemotherapy, and new hepatic-directed modalities. *Hepatogastroenterology* 2001;48:305-12.

[4] Liu LX, Zhang WH, Jiang HC. Current treatment for liver metastases from colorectal cancer. *World J Gastroenterol* 2003;9:193-200.

[5] Staley CA. Surgical therapy of hepatic tumors. In: Zakim & Boyer (eds.) Hepatology. A textbook of liver disease. 4th Edn, Philadelphia, *Saunders* 2003, pp. 1371-81.

[6] Friedman LS. The risk of surgery in patients with liver disease. *Hepatology* 1999;29:1617-23.

[7] Lygidakis NJ, Stringaris K, Kokinis K, Lyberopoulos K, Raptis S. Locoregional chemotherapy versus locoregional combined immuno-chemotherapy for patients with advanced metastatic liver disease of colorectal origin: a prospective randomized study. *Hepatogastroenterology* 1996;43:212-20.

[8] Mayer-Kuckuk P, Banerjee D, Kemeny N, Fong Y, Bertino JR. Molecular therapies for colorectal cancer metastatic to the liver. *Mol Ther* 2002;5(5 Pt 1):492-500.

[9] Nair SK, Morse M, Boczkowski D, Cumming RI, Vasovic L, Gilboa E, Lyerly HK. Induction of tumor-specific cytotoxic T lymphocytes in cancer patients by autologous tumor RNA-transfected dendritic cells. *Ann Surgery* 2002;235:540-9.

[10] Sato T. Locoregional immuno(bio)therapy for liver metastases. *Semin Oncol* 2002;29:160-7.

[11] Saxena R, Zucker SD, Crawford JM. Anatomy and physiology of the liver. In: Zakim & Boyer (eds.) Hepatology. A textbook of liver disease. 4th Edn, Philadelphia, *Saunders* 2003, pp. 3-30.

[12] Lefkowitch JH. Histopathologic diagnosis of liver disease. In: Zakim & Boyer (eds.) Hepatology. A textbook of liver disease. 4th Edn, Philadelphia, *Saunders* 2003, pp. 721-36.

[13] Boura P, Kountouras J, Lygidakis NJ. Tumor immunity and immunotherapy. *Hepatogastroenterology* 2001;48:1040-4.

[14] Brivio F, Lissoni P, Rovelli F, Nespoli A, Uggeri F, Fumagalli L, Gardani G. Effects of IL-2 preoperative immunotherapy on surgery-induced changed in angiogenic regulation and its prevention of VEGF increase and IL-12 decline. *Hepatogastroenterology* 2002;49:385-7.

[15] Bechard DE, Gudas SA, Sholley MM, Grant AJ, Merchant RE, Fairman RP, Fowler AA, Glauser FL. Nonspecific cytotoxicity of recombinant interleukin-2 activated lymphocytes. *Am J Med Sci* 1989;298:28-33.

[16] Damle NK, Doyle LV, Bender JR, Bradley EC. Interleukin 2-activated human lymphocytes exhibit enhanced adhesion to normal vascular endothelial cells and cause their lysis. *J Immunol* 1987;138:1779-85.

[17] Damle NK, Doyle LV. IL-2-activated human killer lymphocytes but not their secreted products mediate increase in albumin flux across cultured endothelial monolayers. Implications for vascular leak syndrome. *J Immunol* 1989;142:2660-9.

[18] Rosenberg S, Lotze MT, Muul LM, Leitman S, Chang AE, Ettinghausen SE, Matory YL, Skibber JM, Shiloni E, Vetto JT, et al. Observations on the systemic administration

of autologous lymphokine-activated killer cells and recombinant interleukin-2 to patients with metastatic cancer. *N Engl J Med* 1985;313:1485-92.

[19] Lotze MT, Matory YL, Rayner AA, Ettinghausen SE, Vetto JT, Seipp CA, Rosenberg SA. Clinical effects and toxicity of interleukin-2 in patients with cancer. *Cancer* 1986;58:2764-72.

[20] Rosenstein M, Ettinghausen SE, Rosenberg SA. Extravasation of intravascular fluid mediated by the systemic administration of recombinant interleukin 2. *J Immunol* 1986;137:1735-42.

[21] Peace DJ, Cheever MA. Toxicity and therapeutic efficacy of high-dose interleukin 2. In vivo infusion of antibody to NK-1.1 attenuates toxicity without compromising efficacy against murine leukemia. *J Exp Med* 1989;169:161-73.

[22] Fisch P, Moris A, Rammensee HG, Handgretinger R. Inhibitory MHC class I receptors on gammadelta T cells in tumour immunity and autoimmunity. *Immunol Today* 2000;21:187-91.

[23] Kountouras J, Boura P, Karolides A, Zaharioudaki E, Tsapas G. Recombinant a2 interferon (a-IFN) with chemo-hormonal therapy in patients with hepatocellular carcinoma (HCC). *Hepatogastroenterology* 1995;42:31-6.

[24] Boura P, Kountouras J, Lygidakis NJ, Safioleas M, Aphinives P. Transplenic and transtumoral in vivo immunostimulation: effect on cellular immunity parameters. *Hepatogastroenterology* 1999;46:799-803.

[25] Bellone M, Iezzi G, Imro MA, Protti MP. Cancer immunotherapy: synthetic and natural peptides in the balance. *Immunol Today* 1999;20:457-62.

[26] Lode HN, Xiang R, Becker JC, Gillies SD, Reisfeld RA. Immunocytokines: a promising approach to cancer immunotherapy. *Pharmacol Ther* 1998;80:277-92.

[27] Barajas M, Mazzolini G, Genove G, Bilbao R, Narvaiza I, Schmitz V, Sangro B, Melero I, Qian C, Prieto J. Gene therapy of orthotopic hepatocellular carcinoma in rats using adenovirus coding for interleukin 12. *Hepatology* 2001;33:52-61.

[28] Narvaiza I, Mazzolini G, Barajas M, Duarte M, Zaratiegui M, Qian C, Melero I, Prieto J. Intratumoral coinjection of two adenoviruses, one encoding the chemokine IFN-gamma-inducible protein-10 and another encoding IL-12, results in marked anti-tumoral synergy. *J Immunol* 2000;164:3112-22.

[29] Mazzolini G, Qian C, Narvaiza I, Barajas M, Borras-Cuesta F, Xie X, Duarte M, Melero I, Prieto J. Adenoviral gene transfer of interleukin 12 into tumors synergizes with adoptive T cell therapy both at the induction and effector level. *Hum Gene Ther* 2000;11:113-25.

[30] Ioannides CG, Grimm EA. Tumor immunity. In: Rich RR, Fleisher TA, Schwartz BD, Shearer WT, Strober W (eds). Clinical Immunology: Principles and practice. St. Louis, Mosby, 1996; pp. 333-49.

[31] Onishi S, Saibara T, Fujikawa M, Sakaeda H, Matsuura Y, Matsunaga Y, Yamamoto Y. Adoptive immunotherapy with lymphokine-activated killer cells plus recombinant interleukin 2 in patients with unresectable hepatocellular carcinoma. *Hepatology* 1989;10:349-53.

[32] Son K, Kew M, Rabson AR. Depressed natural killer cell activity in patients with hepatocellular carcinoma. In vitro effects of interferon and levamisole. *Cancer* 1982;50:2820-5.

[33] Kuppen PJ, Gorter A, Hagenaars M, Jonges LE, Giezeman-Smits KM, Nagelkerke JF, Fleuren G, van de Velde CJ. Role of NK cells in adoptive immunotherapy of metastatic colorectal cancer in a syngeneic rat model. *Immunol Rev* 2001;184:236-43.

[34] Kountouras J, Zavos C, Chatzopoulos D. Apoptosis in hepatocellular carcinoma. *Hepatogastroenterology* 2003;50:242-9.

[35] Kountouras J, Kouklakis G, Zavos C, Chatzopoulos D, Moschos J, Molyvas E, Zavos N. Apoptosis, inflammatory bowel disease and carcinogenesis: overview of international and Greek experiences. *Can J Gastroenterol* 2003;17:249-58.

[36] Kountouras J, Zavos C, Chatzopoulos D. Apoptosis in hepatitis C. *J Viral Hepat* 2003;10:335-42.

[37] Kountouras J, Zavos C, Chatzopoulos D. Apoptosis: An overview and a proposed link between glaucoma and Helicobacter pylori infection. In: '*Progress in Glaucoma Research*', Nova Science Publishers, Inc., New York, 2004 (in press).

[38] Okuno K, Takagi H, Nakamura T, Nakamura Y, Iwasa Z, Yasutomi M. Treatment for unresectable hepatoma via selective hepatic arterial infusion of lymphokine-activated killer cells generated from autologous spleen cells. *Cancer* 1986;58:1001-6.

[39] Lygidakis NJ, Vlachos L, Raptis S, Rassidakis G, Balaskas C, Sgourakis G, Mourikis D, Kehagias D, Kittas C. New frontiers in liver surgery. Two-stage liver surgery for the management of advanced metastatic liver disease. *Hepatogastroenterology* 1999;46:2216-28.

[40] Tepetes KN, Tsamandas AC, Felekouras ES, Salakou SG, Karavias DD. Conversion of unresectable hepatoma to resectable. Report of a case and review of the literature. *Hepatogastroenterology* 2000;47:1105-9.

[41] Okuno K, Hirohata T, Nakamura K, Jinnai H, Shigeoka H, Koh K, Shindo K, Yasutomi M. Hepatic arterial infusions of interleukin-2-based immunochemotherapy in the treatment of unresectable liver metastases from colorectal cancer. *Clin Ther* 1993;15:672-83.

[42] Okuno K, Yasutomi M, Hida J, Kayama H, Nakai T, Funai S, Koh K. Longterm effects of hepatic arterial interleukin-2-based immunochemotherapy after potentially curative resection of colorectal liver metastases. *J Am Coll Surg* 1998;187:271-5.

[43] Kitayama J, Tsuno N, Yasuhara H, Nagawa H, Kimura W, Kuroda A, Shibata Y, Juji T, Muto T. Lysis of endothelial cells by autologous lymphokine-activated killer cells. Cancer *Immunol Immunother* 1994;38:317-22.

[44] Rafi AQ, Zeytun A, Bradley MJ, Sponenberg DP, Grayson RL, Nagarkatti M, Nagarkatti PS. Evidence for the involvement of Fas ligand and perforin in the induction of vascular leak syndrome. *J Immunol* 1998;161:3077-86.

[45] Kountouras J, Zavos C, Chatzopoulos D, Zavos N, Boura P, Safioleas M. Locoregional immunochemotherapy in primary and metastatic liver disease: meta-analysis and review of literature. *Hepatogastroenterology* 2003;50:1506-10.

[46] Toh U, Sudo T, Kido K, Matono S, Sasahara H, Mine T, Tanaka T, Sueyoshi S, Fujita H, Shirouzu K, Yamana H. Locoregional adoptive immunotherapy resulted in

regression in distant metastases of a recurrent esophageal cancer. *Int J Clin Oncol* 2002;7:372-5.

[47] Lygidakis NJ, Sgourakis G, Vlachos L, Raptis S, Safioleas M, Boura P, Kountouras J, Alamani M. Metastatic liver disease of colorectal origin: the value of locoregional immunochemotherapy combined with systemic chemotherapy following liver resection. Results of a prospective randomized study. *Hepatogastroenterology* 2001;48:1685-91.

[48] Ueda Y, Yamagishi H, Tanioka Y, Fujiwara H, Fuji N, Itoh T, Fujiki H, Yoshimura T, Oka T. Clinical application of adoptive immunotherapy and IL-2 for the treatment of advanced digestive tract cancer. *Hepatogastroenterology* 1999;46(Suppl 1):1274-9.

[49] Lygidakis NJ, Safioleas M, Sgourakis G, Spentzouris N, Dedemadi G, Sotiropoulou P. Metastatic melanoma: transplenic immunostimulation--a new therapeutical alternative for an ever-challenging disease. *Hepatogastroenterology* 1999;46:148-56.

[50] Okuno K, Shigeoka H, Lee YS, Son E, Kayama H, Nakai T, Koh K, Yasutomi M. Adjuvant hepatic arterial IL-2 and MMC, 5-FU after curative resection of colorectal liver metastases. *Hepatogastroenterology* 1996;43:688-91.

[51] Lygidakis NJ, Ziras N, Parissis J. Resection versus resection combined with adjuvant pre- and post-operative chemotherapy--immunotherapy for metastatic colorectal liver cancer. A new look at an old problem. *Hepatogastroenterology* 1995;42:155-61.

[52] Lygidakis NJ, Savanis G, Pothoulakis J, Kapetanakis A. Transarterial locoregional immunostimulation and chemotherapy in patients with unresectable secondary liver tumours. *Anticancer Res* 1994;14(2B):643-6.

[53] Keilholz U, Schlag P, Tilgen W, Brado B, Galm F, Gorich J, Kauffmann GW, Moller P, Schneider S, Hunstein W. Regional administration of lymphokine-activated killer cells can be superior to intravenous application. *Cancer* 1992;69:2172-5.

[54] Kountouras J, Boura P, Kouklakis G. Locoregional immunochemotherapy in hepatocellular carcinoma. *Hepatogastroenterology* 2002;49:1109-12.

[55] Saibara T, Maeda T, Miyazaki M, Onishi S, Yamamoto Y. Assessment of lymphokine-activated killer activity and γ-interferon production in patients with small hepatocellular carcinomas. *Hepatology* 1993;17:781-7.

[56] Yang YA, Dukhanina O, Tang B, Mamura M, Letterio JJ, MacGregor J, Patel SC, Khozin S, Liu ZY, Green J, Anver MR, Merlino G, Wakefield LM. Lifetime exposure to a soluble TGF-beta antagonist protects mice against metastasis without adverse side effects. *J Clin Invest* 2002;109:1607-15.

[57] Liu LX, Zhang WH, Jiang HC. Current treatment for liver metastases from colorectal cancer. *World J Gastroenterol* 2003;9:193-200.

[58] Hosch SB, Scheunemann P, Luth M, Inndorf S, Stoecklein NH, Erbersdobler A, Rehders A, Gundlach M, Knoefel WT, Izbicki JR. Expression of 17-1A antigen and complement resistance factors CD55 and CD59 on liver metastasis in colorectal cancer. *J Gastrointest Surg* 2001;5:673-9.

[59] Kim KJ, Li B, Winer J, Armanini M, Gillett N, Phillips HS, Ferrara N. Inhibition of vascular endothelial growth factor-induced angiogenesis suppresses tumour growth in vivo. *Nature* 1993;362:841-4.

[60] Warren RS, Yuan H, Matli MR, Gillett NA, Ferrara N. Regulation by vascular endothelial growth factor of human colon cancer tumorigenesis in a mouse model of experimental liver metastasis. *J Clin Invest* 1995;95:1789-97.

[61] Chattopadhyay U. Tumour immunotherapy: developments and strategies. *Immunol Today* 1999;20:480-2.

[62] Ockert D, Schmitz M, Hampl M, Rieber EP. Advances in cancer immunotherapy. *Immunol Today* 1999;20:63-5.

[63] Mach N, Dranoff G. Cytokine-secreting tumor cell vaccines. *Curr Opin Immunol* 2000;12:571-5.

[64] Grimm CF, Ortmann D, Mohr L, Michalak S, Krohne TU, Meckel S, Eisele S, Encke J, Blum HE, Geissler M. Mouse alpha-fetoprotein-specific DNA-based immunotherapy of hepatocellular carcinoma leads to tumor regression in mice. *Gastroenterology* 2000;199:1104-12.

[65] Habib NA, Hodgson HJ, Lemoine N, Pignatelli M. A phase I/II study of hepatic artery infusion with wtp53-CMV-Ad in metastatic malignant liver tumours. *Hum Gene Ther* 1999;10:2019-34.

[66] Sangro B, Qian C, Schmitz V, Prieto J. Gene therapy of hepatocellular carcinoma and gastrointestinal tumors. *Ann N Y Acad Sci* 2002;963:6-12.

[67] Havlik R, Jiao LR, Nicholls J, Jensen SL, Habib NA. Gene therapy for liver metastases. *Semin Oncol* 2002;29:202-8.

[68] Pan PY, Zang Y, Weber K, Meseck ML, Chen SH. OX40 ligation enhances primary and memory cytotoxic T lymphocyte responses in an immunotherapy for hepatic colon metastases. *Mol Ther* 2002;6:528-36.

[69] Chen SH, Pham-Nguyen KB, Martinet O, Huang Y, Yang W, Thung SN, Chen L, Mittler R, Woo SL. Rejection of disseminated metastases of colon carcinoma by synergism of IL-12 gene therapy and 4-1BB costimulation. *Mol Ther* 2000;2:39-46.

[70] Banchereau J, Steinman RM. Dendritic cells and the control of immunity. *Nature* 1998;392:245-52.

[71] Steinman RM. The dendritic cell system and its role in immunogenicity. *Annu Rev Immunol* 1991;9:271-96.

[72] Sato T, Terai M, Yasuda R, Watanabe R, Berd D, Mastrangelo MJ, Hasumi K. Combination of monocyte-derived dendritic cells and activated T cells which express CD40 ligand: a new approach to cancer immunotherapy. *Cancer Immunol Immunother* 2004;53:53-61.

[73] Romani N, Gruner S, Brang D, Kampgen E, Lenz A, Trockenbacher B, Konwalinka G, Fritsch PO, Steinman RM, Schuler G. Proliferating dendritic cell progenitors in human blood. *J Exp Med* 1994;180:83-93.

[74] Romani N, Reider D, Heuer M, Ebner S, Kampgen E, Eibl B, Niederwieser D, Schuler G. Generation of mature dendritic cells from human blood. An improved method with special regard to clinical applicability. *J Immunol Methods* 1996;196:137-51.

[75] Sallusto F, Lanzavecchia A. Efficient presentation of soluble antigen by cultured human dendritic cells is maintained by granulocyte/macrophage colony-stimulating factor plus interleukin 4 and downregulated by tumor necrosis factor alpha. *J Exp Med* 1994;179:1109-18.

[76] Dieu MC, Vanbervliet B, Vicari A, Bridon JM, Oldham E, Ait-Yahia S, Briere F, Zlotnik A, Lebecque S, Caux C. Selective recruitment of immature and mature dendritic cells by distinct chemokines expressed in different anatomic sites. *J Exp Med* 1998;188:373-86.
[77] Sozzani S, Allavena P, D'Amico G, Luini W, Bianchi G, Kataura M, Imai T, Yoshie O, Bonecchi R, Mantovani A. Differential regulation of chemokine receptors during dendritic cell maturation: a model for their trafficking properties. *J Immunol* 1998;161:1083-6.
[78] Cella M, Engering A, Pinet V, Pieters J, Lanzavecchia A. Inflammatory stimuli induce accumulation of MHC class II complexes on dendritic cells *Nature* 1997;388:782-7.
[79] Pierre P, Turley SJ, Gatti E, Hull M, Meltzer J, Mirza A, Inaba K, Steinman RM, Mellman I. Developmental regulation of MHC class II transport in mouse dendritic cells. *Nature* 1997;388:787-92.
[80] Caux C, Massacrier C, Vanbervliet B, Dubois B, Van Kooten C, Durand I, Banchereau J. Activation of human dendritic cells through CD40 cross-linking. *J Exp Med* 1994;180:1263-72.
[81] Roake JA, Rao AS, Morris PJ, Larsen CP, Hankins DF, Austyn JM. Dendritic cell loss from nonlymphoid tissues after systemic administration of lipopolysaccharide, tumor necrosis factor, and interleukin 1. *J Exp Med* 1995;181:2237-47.
[82] Sallusto F, Cella M, Danieli C, Lanzavecchia A. Dendritic cells use macropinocytosis and the mannose receptor to concentrate macromolecules in the major histocompatibility complex class II compartment: downregulation by cytokines and bacterial products. *J Exp Med* 1995;182:389-400.
[83] Caux C, Dezutter-Dambuyant C, Schmitt D, Banchereau J. GM-CSF and TNF-alpha cooperate in the generation of dendritic Langerhans cells *Nature* 1992;360:258-61.
[84] Egner W, Hart DN. The phenotype of freshly isolated and cultured human bone marrow allostimulatory cells: possible heterogeneity in bone marrow dendritic cell populations. *Immunology* 1995;85:611-20.
[85] Reid CD, Stackpoole A, Meager A, Tikerpae J. Interactions of tumor necrosis factor with granulocyte-macrophage colony-stimulating factor and other cytokines in the regulation of dendritic cell growth in vitro from early bipotent CD34+ progenitors in human bone marrow. *J Immunol* 1992;149:2681-8.
[86] Sun Y, Qian C, Peng D, Prieto J. Gene transfer to liver cancer cells of B7-1 plus interleukin 12 changes immunoeffector mechanisms and suppresses helper T cell type 1 cytokine production induced by interleukin 12 alone. *Hum Gene Ther* 2000;11:127-38.
[87] Schmitz V, Barajas M, Wang L, Peng D, Duarte M, Prieto J, Qian C. Adenovirus-mediated CD40 ligand gene therapy in a rat model of orthotopic hepatocellular carcinoma. *Hepatology* 2001;34:72-81.
[88] Schlag P, Manasterski M, Gerneth T, Hohenberger P, Dueck M, Herfarth C, Liebrich W, Schirrmacher V. Active specific immunotherapy with Newcastle-disease-virus-modified autologous tumor cells following resection of liver metastases in colorectal cancer. First evaluation of clinical response of a phase II-trial. *Cancer Immunol Immunother* 1992;35:325-30.

[89] Ockert D, Schirrmacher V, Beck N, Stoelben E, Ahlert T, Flechtenmacher J, Hagmuller E, Buchcik R, Nagel M, Saeger HD. Newcastle disease virus-infected intact autologous tumor cell vaccine for adjuvant active specific immunotherapy of resected colorectal carcinoma. *Clin Cancer Res* 1996;2:21-8.

[90] Rubin J, Galanis E, Pitot HC, Richardson RL, Burch PA, Charboneau JW, Reading CC, Lewis BD, Stahl S, Akporiaye ET, Harris DT. Phase I study of immunotherapy of hepatic metastases of colorectal carcinoma by direct gene transfer of an allogeneic histocompatibility antigen, HLA-B7. *Gene Ther* 1997;4:419-25.

[91] Farzaneh F, Trefzer U, Sterry W, Walden P. Gene therapy of cancer. *Immunol Today* 1998;19:294-6.

In: Liver Cancer: New Research
Editor: Felix Lee, pp. 185-201
ISBN 1-59454-182-5


*Chapter VIII*

# Cancer Surveillance Following Orthotopic Liver Transplantation

***James F. Trotter***[11]
Associate Professor of Medicine, Division of Gastroenterology/Hepatology, University of Colorado Health Sciences Center, Denver, CO

## Introduction

During the past 15 years, liver transplantation has emerged as an effective therapy for selected patients with end-stage liver disease. Early in the era of liver transplantation, long-term survival was uncommon and clinical efforts were focused on improving surgical techniques, immunosuppression protocols and patient selection. With greater experience, the technical aspects of liver transplantation have been refined and five-year survival rates have increased to 70 – 75 %. Consequently, the clinical care of transplant recipients is increasingly focused on the management of the long-term medical problems which occur after transplantation. Surveillance for gastrointestinal (GI) malignancy is perhaps the most important long-term management issue for the gastroenterologist attending the liver recipient. This review will present current data regarding the risk of GI cancer after liver transplantation and provide rational guidelines for cancer surveillance in this patient population.

Because of the changing demographics of liver transplantation, the incidence of GI tumors in liver transplant recipients is likely to increase in the upcoming years. The number of liver transplant recipients is increasing every year. Over the past decade, the number of

[11] Proofs and reprints to: James F. Trotter, M.D., Division of Gastroenterology/Hepatology, University of Colorado Health Sciences Center, 4200 E. 9th Avenue, B-158, Denver, CO 80262, Phone: 303-372-8866, Fax: 303-372-8868, Email: James.Trotter@uchsc.edu.

liver transplants performed in the United States increased 74 %. In 1992, 3063 patients were transplanted and this number grew to 5328 in 2002 [1]. As the cohort of liver transplant recipients grows, the number of patients at risk for developing post-transplant GI tumors will increase. In addition, older patients are being transplanted with greater frequency. The percentage of patients over the age of 50 has increased 37 % between 1992 and 2002[1]. Screening for GI malignancy in these older patients is even more important since their risk for the development of cancer is higher than younger recipients.

Five factors specific to the liver transplant population may increase the incidence of GI cancer [2]. First, some transplant recipients have a predisposing condition to the development of *de novo* carcinoma. The most common are adenomatous colonic polyps, inflammatory bowel disease (IBD) (present in 70 % of patients with primary sclerosing cholangitis (PSC)) and Barrett's esophagus which occurs in a small fraction of patients. Second, the administration of immunosuppressive agents is associated with an increased incidence of many types of cancer [3-5]. Immunosuppression impairs immune surveillance which hampers the body's ability to destroy malignant cells. Third, immunosuppression increases the prevalence of bacterial and viral infections which are associated with the development of malignancy. Most notable, Epstein-Barr virus infection is strongly linked to post-transplant lymphoproliferative disease (PTLD) [6]. Similar to lymphoma, PTLD is a systemic malignancy which may involve the GI tract. However, the only two GI malignancies which are directly linked to a viral infection are anal cancer and hepatocellular carcinoma. Human papillomavirus (HPV) is strongly associated with carcinoma of the anus, perineum, vulva and anus [7]. A proportion of transplant recipients with chronic viral hepatitis, i.e., hepatitis C and hepatitis B, develop recurrent hepatitis after transplantation [8]. Twenty-five per cent or more of liver transplant recipients with recurrent hepatitis C may evolve into cirrhosis [9]. Some patients with post-transplant cirrhosis have been reported to progress to hepatocellular carcinoma [10]. The common intestinal bacterial infection, *Helicobacter pylori* may be associated with gastric mucosa-associated lymphoid tissue-type lymphomas (see discussion below). Fourth, some liver transplant recipients have malignancy at the time of transplantation and are at risk to develop recurrent cancer after surgery. In most cases, the diagnosis of carcinoma is a contraindication for transplantation, because of the high rate of recurrence and low survival rate. However, carefully selected patients with hepatocellular carcinoma may undergo successful liver transplantation with long-term survival statistics that are not different than patients without hepatocellular carcinoma [11, 12]. (See below.) Recent changes in the organ allocation system have increased the priority for transplantation in patients with hepatocellular carcinoma. As a result, approximately 1/3 of liver transplantation recipients have hepatocellular carcinoma. In this setting, post-transplantation surveillance for recurrent hepatoma is important, since all of these patients are at risk for recurrent malignancy. Finally, there is some evidence that immunosuppressive agents including azathioprine [13] and cyclosporine A [14] may directly damage DNA and induce carcinogenesis.

There are five basic criteria for the development of any type of successful screening program [15]. These criteria provide the basis for the formulation of guidelines for cancer screening in liver transplant recipients:

1) the incidence of disease must be high enough to justify screening

2) the disease must have an asymptomatic period during which time detection of disease would have clinically important consequences
3) the disease must have serious consequences for the population
4) screening techniques must be sensitive enough to make detection likely
5) screening techniques must be specific enough to differentiate between false positive and true negatives

## Incidence of GI Carcinoma in Liver Transplant Recipients

There is a relatively little data regarding the incidence of GI malignancy in liver transplant recipients. One reason for this is that the incidence of GI cancer in the liver transplant population is relatively low. In addition, there are few liver transplant recipients with sufficient long-term follow-up to determine relative risks related to carcinogenesis. Therefore, most of the data regarding the incidence of GI tumors following solid organ transplant is derived from the renal transplant population. The cohort of renal transplant recipients far exceeds the number of liver transplant recipients. There are thousands of renal transplant recipients with decades of post-transplant follow-up. Consequently, the relative risks of developing specific GI malignancies have greater statistical certainty in the renal transplant cohort. Results from the renal transplant literature may be extrapolated to liver transplant recipients, because the immunosuppressive agents and degree of immunosuppression are similar in these patients.

Some, but not all, studies show that the incidence of GI cancers in abdominal organ transplant recipients is increased compared to the general population. This issue has been addressed in a number of studies, some of which involve renal recipients and others which involve liver recipients. Birkeland et al. reported the incidence of cancer in 5,692 renal transplant recipients transplanted between 1964 – 1982 [16]. A total of 32,392 person-years were accrued in this population. The total number of GI cancers (esophageal, stomach and colorectal) was only 27. There was no increased incidence of esophageal or gastric cancer. However, there was a significant increase in the standard incidence ratios for colon cancer (3.2) and rectal cancer (4.5). Sheil reported similar results in a cohort of 6067 renal transplant recipients followed for a mean of 7 years after transplantation in Australia and New Zealand [17]. A total of 77 cancers of the digestive organs developed in these patients. The risk ratios for all types of GI cancer were increased: esophageal (8.0), gastric (1.4), colon (2.7) and anal/rectal (2.1). The incidence of GI malignancy in 73,076 solid organ transplant recipients (62,088 kidney recipients and 10,988 heart recipients) was published by Stewart et al [18]. A total of 122 GI cancers were diagnosed in this cohort. The relative risk of developing colon cancer was increased slightly (1.2) compared to controls, but was not statistically significant. There was no difference in the risk of gastric cancer. Interestingly, rectal cancer was significantly less (relative risk = 0.36) compared to controls. Penn reported his experience in a cohort of 6233 transplant recipients of which 324 were liver recipients [3]. Colon cancer was recorded in 18 patients and gastric cancer in 3. However, no estimates of relative risk were reported for liver transplant recipients.

Four studies evaluating the risk of developing GI malignancy have been performed in liver transplant recipients. However, compared to the above studies, there are only approximately 10 % as many patients followed for the development of cancer. In addition, the length of follow-up after transplantation is relatively short compared to the natural history of malignancy. Consequently, the statistical power of these studies is low. Jain et al. reported the incidence of *de novo* non-lymphoid malignancy in 1000 consecutive liver transplant recipients followed an average of 77 months after transplant [19, 20]. Five patients developed GI malignancies (1 esophageal and 4 colorectal). The authors stated that the incidence of GI malignancies was not greater than expected. Kelly et al. reported the incidence of non-lymphoid tumors in 888 liver transplant recipients with a mean follow-up period after transplant of 52.4 months [21]. Only 3 patients developed a colon cancer which was the only GI malignancy in this patient cohort. Based on these results, there was no increase in GI cancer in the liver transplant recipients. A recent report by Jonas et al. documented the incidence of malignancy in 500 liver transplant recipients followed a median of 50 months after transplantation [22]. The only GI malignancy discovered in this cohort was one gastric cancer. No estimates of relative risk were reported. Haagsma et al. reported the incidence of gastrointestinal malignancy in 174 long-term liver transplantation survivors of whom 3 developed colon cancer [23]. Compared to the general population, these investigators estimated that the relative risk of colon cancer in liver transplantation recipients was significantly higher at 12.5.

## Pre-Transplant Evaluation

Most liver transplant recipients undergo an extensive evaluation of the GI tract during the pre-transplant evaluation. These screening procedures may reduce the subsequent risk of developing GI carcinoma in liver transplant recipients compared to the general population. The standard practice at most transplant centers for patients undergoing liver transplant evaluation is to perform screening colonoscopy for all patients over the age of 50 as well as patients with an indication for the procedure (unexplained iron-deficient anemia, lower intestinal bleeding, first-degree relative with early colon cancer or positive fecal occult test). The American College of Gastroenterology recommends that all patients with cirrhosis undergo upper endoscopy for screening for esophageal varices [24].Consequently, most patients with chronic liver disease evaluated for liver transplantation undergo colonoscopy and upper endoscopy. Pre-malignant lesions, i.e, adenomatous colonic polyps, may be removed prior to transplantation in some patients. However, in almost all cases, the discovery of an intestinal cancer is a contraindication for transplantation.

The endoscopic findings in patients undergoing evaluation for liver transplantation have been published in four separate studies. Weller et al. reported results in 118 patients with an average age of 49 years who underwent endoscopic evaluation prior to liver transplantation [25]. Colonoscopy was performed in all patients over 50 and in patients with anemia, lower intestinal bleed, positive fecal occult blood test or history of pre-disposing condition for colon cancer (e.g., polyp or inflammatory bowel disease). In addition, 74 patients had upper endoscopy which discovered 3 patients (4 %) with Barrett's esophagus, 1 (1 %) with esophageal cancer and 1 (1 %) with gastric cancer. Fifty six patients underwent colonoscopy of which 16/56 (29 %) had a screening colonoscopy and the remaining 40/56 patients (71 %) underwent colonoscopy for a specific indication: positive fecal occult blood test (19), anemia (16), lower GI bleeding (3) and chronic diarrhea (2). (Some patients had more than one indication.) Colonoscopy revealed 24/56 patients (43 %) with adenomatous polyps, one (1 %) with a dysplastic polyp and one (1 %) with colon cancer. Similar results were reported by Zaman et al, who evaluated 121 patients prior to liver transplantation whose mean age was 52 years [26]. All patients underwent upper endoscopy and 71 patients over the age of 50 had flexible sigmoidoscopy. The discovery of colitis or colon polyps during flexible sigmoidoscopy led to total colonoscopy in 24 patients. On upper endoscopy, 2 patients (2 %) had Barrett's esophagus and no patients had malignancy. Fifteen of 71 patients (21 %) had adenomatous colonic polyps on lower gastrointestinal endoscopy. Selingo et al reported colonoscopic findings in 86 patients who had colonoscopy during liver transplant evaluation [27]. The mean age of these patients was 53.8 years. At their institution, colonoscopy was performed on all patients over 45, as well as patients with a specific indication (lower GI bleeding, history of polyps, etc.). Fifty-one patients (59 %) had a specific indication for colonoscopy and 35 patients (41 %) had screening colonoscopy. Seventeen patients (19 %) had colon polyps of which 10 (12 %) were adenomatous, 1 (1 %) was dysplastic and the remaining 6 were not biopsied because of coagulopathy. Overall, 11/86 (13 %) of patients had adenomatous/dysplastic polyps and 6/86 (7 %) of the polyps were undefined. Rabinovitz et al. reported the experience at the University of Pittsburgh in 412 patients who underwent screening colonoscopy as part of their liver transplant evaluation between 1985 and 1987 [28]. This study was performed early in the era of liver transplant and does not reflect current standard screening practice for liver transplant recipients. Every patient underwent colonoscopy regardless of age or specific indication. In addition, the average age of the patients was lower than the other three studies, 45.0 years. As a result, the occurrence of polyps in this cohort was lower. Only 35/412 patients (8.5 %) had colonic polyps of which 20 (4.9 %) were adenomatous.

Based on the data from these four studies, the likelihood of finding malignant or pre-malignant disease in the upper intestinal tract in patients undergoing liver transplant evaluation is small. The incidence of gastric or esophageal cancer is $\leq$ 1 % and the risk of Barrett's esophagus is 2 – 4 %. However, the incidence of adenomatous colonic polyps in this cohort of patients is much higher. The study with the greatest proportion of adenomatous polyps (43 %) had the largest proportion of patients with an indication for colonoscopy, i.e., bleeding, positive fecal occult blood test and unexplained anemia [25]. The study with the lowest incidence of adenomatous polyps had the youngest patients and no specific indication for the procedure. In the three studies whose screening procedures most closely reflect current clinical practice, the incidence of adenomatous colon polyps was 12 – 43 %.[25-27] The proportion of adenomatous polyps in the general population is similar [29].

Some patients with chronic liver disease cannot have polypectomy because of concomitant coagulopathy related to the underlying liver disease. Following transplantation, the coagulopathy resolves and polypectomy may be performed at the appropriate interval after surgery [30]. The timing of this follow-up procedure is often predicated on the post-transplant recovery of the recipient as well as the risk of developing carcinoma in the polyp.

Patients with large polyps and rapid recovery after transplant may benefit from a colonoscopy within a few months after transplant. However, the value of repeat colonoscopy to remove a diminutive polyp in a patient with multiple, significant post-transplant complications is limited.

## ESOPHAGEAL CANCER

Esophageal cancer is relatively rare after liver transplantation. The reason for this may be that most liver transplant recipients undergo therapeutic or diagnostic upper endoscopy prior to transplantation as screening or treatment for esophageal varices. During these procedures esophageal cancer may be easily diagnosed. The finding of esophageal cancer prior to transplantation is a contraindication for liver transplantation. However, there are several case reports of esophageal cancer developing in transplant recipients. Two cases of squamous cell carcinoma of the esophagus after solid organ transplantation have been reported [31,32]. These cancers occurred in patients with no known preexisting dysplastic condition and were diagnosed 2 and 10 years after transplant, respectively. Four cases of adenocarcinoma of the esophagus after liver transplantation have been reported in which three patients had known preexisting Barrett's esophagus. Yao et al. reported a patient who developed adenocarcinoma of the esophagus 9 months after liver transplantation [33]. This patient did not have a prior diagnosis of Barrett's esophagus. However, Safadi et al. described a patient who died as a result of rapid progression from Barrett's esophagus to adenocarcinoma of the esophagus [34]. In another case, a patient with Barrett's esophagus who had no evidence of dysplasia immediately prior to transplantation progressed to adenocarcinoma within 9 months after transplant [35]. Trotter and Brazer reported a similar patient who had Barrett's esophagus with no dysplasia prior to transplantation who evolved into high-grade dysplasia and underwent esophagectomy 9 months after transplantation [36]. At our center we have recently diagnosed another patient who had evidence of pre-transplant Barrett's esophagus without dysplasia and developed high-grade dysplasia within one year after transplant.

Barrett's esophagus is recognized as a pre-malignant condition which progresses to adenocarcinoma in 10 % of patients. However, the rate of progression from Barrett's esophagus to malignancy in non-transplant recipients is slow and usually takes many years. In patients with Barrett's esophagus, adenocarcinoma develops at a rate of between 1/524 and 1/4415 malignancies/patient years [37, 38]. In transplant recipients, accelerated progression of dysplastic lesions to carcinoma has been observed in skin cancer [39]. Whether immunosuppressed liver transplant recipients progress more rapidly from Barrett's esophagus to dysplasia and subsequent adenocarcinoma is unclear. However, the collection of case reports noted above raises this concern. An earlier study in non-immunosuppressed patients, has suggested that patients with Barrett's esophagus have an intrinsic immune impairment. Oka et al. showed that patients with Barrett's esophagus had evidence of significant *in vitro* impairment of B-cell and T-cell function compared to controls [40]. In addition, monocytes from Barrett's patients had a significant 2/3 reduction interleukin-2 production compared to controls. The authors of the study speculate that depressed immunity may play a role in the progression of Barrett's to dysplasia and adenocarcinoma.

Based on these data, there is no rationale for post-transplant screening for squamous cell carcinoma of the esophagus. However, in patients who have the diagnosis of Barrett's esophagus before transplant or who develop Barrett's esophagus after transplant, surveillance endoscopy is appropriate. Current recommendations by the American College of Gastroenterology for Barrett's esophagus have recently been published [41]. Gastroenterologists screening liver transplant recipients should be aware of the reports, noted above, of rapid progression to high-grade dysplasia and cancer. However, there is currently not enough data to recommend more frequent surveillance in liver transplant recipients.

## Gastric Cancer

The risk of gastric cancer is not increased in any of the follow-up studies with the exception of one and in that cohort the increase was minimal [42]. Therefore, there is no rationale for screening post-transplant recipients for gastric cancer. However, solid organ transplantation recipients may also have a higher incidence of hyperplastic gastric polyps, although the significance of this finding is unknown [43]. In addition, there is one case series of four liver transplantation recipients who developed a mucosal-associated lymphoid tissue (MALT) lymphoma associated with *Helicobacter pylori* infection [44].

## Colon Cancer

Colon cancer is the most frequently diagnosed intestinal malignancy in liver transplant recipients. Screening recommendations for colon cancer in transplant candidates with no history of ulcerative colitis (UC) or previous adenomatous colon polyps is not different than the general population. For normal risk individuals, screening begins at age 50 and consists of colonoscopy every 10 years [45]. The recommendation for surveillance colonoscopy in patients with small adenomatous polyps is the same as the general population. Follow-up colonscopy should be performed within three years in these patients [30]. As noted above, imunosuppressive therapy increases the theoretical risk for accelerated progression of adenomatous polyps to dysplasia and malignancy. However, there currently is no data to suggest that liver transplant recipients with adenomatous polyps should have surveillance colonoscopy at more frequent intervals than the general population. The patients at the greatest risk for colorectal cancer are those with pre-existing UC. Most of these patients undergo liver transplantation for primary sclerosing cholangitis (PSC) of whom 70 % have IBD. Several studies have examined the relative risk of developing colon cancer after liver transplantation. Bleday et al. reported the incidence of colon cancer in 44 patients with PSC, of whom 33 had inflammatory bowel disease [46]. In this cohort, 27 patients had undergone colonoscopy prior to transplantation which showed no dysplasia and had at least 12 months post-transplant follow-up. Three of 27 patients (11 %) developed either colon cancer or high-grade dysplasia within 13 months of transplant. Based on historical controls, the authors showed a significant five-fold increased risk of malignant transformation in their patients. Narumi et al. published their experience in the transplantation of 33 patients with PSC [47].

Two-thirds (22/33) of the patients had inflammatory bowel disease. All patients had screening colonoscopy prior to transplantation, but no comment was made regarding the presence of dysplasia. During the follow-up interval, 2 patients developed recurrent colon cancer, one patient developed *de novo* colon cancer and one patient underwent colectomy for dysplasia. Therefore, 2/22 (9 %) developed *de novo* dysplasia or carcinoma. The authors noted that colon cancer was the most frequent cause of death in patients transplanted for PSC at their center. Higashi et al reported 2/36 (5.6 %) patients with PSC and UC who developed colon cancer after transplantation [48]. While both patients had screening colonoscopies prior to transplants, no comment was made regarding the presence of dysplasia. These patients developed colon cancer 14 and 11 months after transplantation, respectively. Knechtle et al. reported similar results in 41 patients with PSC of whom 29 had IBD [49]. No comment was made regarding pre-transplant colonoscopy. Three of 41 patients (7.3 %) developed colon cancer a mean of 20.7 months after transplantation. Loftus et al. described the Mayo Clinic experience of 57 patients with IBD and PSC followed for a median interval of 4.2 years after liver transplantation [50]. Seven patients (12 %) had dysplasia noted prior to transplantation and an additional 9 patients (16 %) developed dysplasia (8) or carcinoma (1) after transplant, respectively. The colon cancers were diagnosed 1.2, 1.5 and 6.8 years after transplant, respectively. A total of 7 patients underwent colectomy for cancer (5) or dysplasia (2). The cumulative risk of developing colon cancer was 17 % at 8 years of follow-up or 1.25 % per person-year of follow-up. However, none of the patients with dysplasia or colon cancer died as a result of their underlying malignancy. Consequently, dysplasia/cancer had no impact on long-term patient survival. While the risk of colon cancer was 4.4 times higher than non-transplant UC patients, this difference did not reach statistical significance. Interestingly, 6/15 patients diagnosed with dysplasia (7 before transplant and 8 after transplant) had no evidence of dysplasia on subsequent colonoscopy or colectomy specimen. Fabia et al. reported the incidence of colon carcinoma in 63 patients with PSC and UC following liver transplantation [51]. Fifteen patients had undergone previous colectomy and were excluded from analysis. Of the remaining 48 patients, 5 (10 %) were diagnosed with colon cancer at a mean of 48 months after transplantation. Only 1 of 1022 (0.1 %) other liver transplant recipients without PSC and IBD developed colon cancer after transplant, ($p<0.00001$ compared to IBD/PSC patients). Two patients had severe dysplasia or "low-stage colonic cancer" at the time of transplant. The remaining 4 patients who developed colon cancer had no dysplasia prior to transplantation. The UCLA group has published their experience of 127 patients with PSC with a median follow-up of 3.01 years [52]. Ninety-two (72 %) had concomitant IBD. During the follow-up interval, the patients had surveillance colonoscopy with colonic biopsies every 6 months and underwent colectomy if dysplasia was discovered. Based on these colonoscopic examinations, 27/127 patients (21 %) underwent colectomy for dysplasia or colon cancer. Fifteen patients were diagnosed with dysplasia, 6 with carcinoma in situ and 6 with colon cancer. The overall incidence of carcinoma or carcinoma in situ was 12/92 (13 %) which is similar to other reports. All patients with dysplasia were referred for colectomy. Similar to the Mayo experience, there was no difference in survival in the patients with dysplasia or cancer, compared to other patients.

The results from these studies have important implications for the screening of colon cancer in liver transplant recipients with pre-existing IBD. The mean follow-up interval after transplant in these 7 studies was 39.6 months during which time 10.5 % of patients developed dysplasia and 7.9 % were diagnosed with colon cancer. (See Table 1). The findings from the early studies suggest that colon cancer was a common cause of death in this cohort of patients [46-48]. One may speculate that high-grade dysplasia may have been present in some of these patients at the time of transplant, since this was not commented upon in these studies [47, 48]. The results from the Mayo and UCLA experience suggest that aggressive post-transplant surveillance colonoscopy may prevent the development of fatal colon cancer. Surveillance colonoscopy was performed every 6 months by the UCLA group [52] and yearly in the Mayo [50] report. If dysplasia or early colon cancer was detected, then a curative colectomy was recommended. This practice may be the reason that patients with dysplasia or colon cancer experienced no reduction in long-term survival.

**Table 1 Dysplasia or Colon Cancer in Liver Transplant Recipients with PSC and UC**

| Author | Reference | n | Mean follow-up (months) | % Dysplasia | % Colon Cancer |
|---|---|---|---|---|---|
| Bleday | 46 | 27 | 39 | 7 | 4 |
| Narumi | 47 | 22 | 38 | 5 | 5 |
| Higashi | 48 | 31 | 35 | - | 7 |
| Knechtle | 49 | 21 | - | - | 14 |
| Loftus | 50 | 57 | 50* | 14 | 2 |
| Fabia | 51 | 48 | - | - | 10 |
| Goss | 52 | 92 | 36* | 16 | 13 |
| mean | | | 39.6 | | 7.9 |

* = median follow-up

In terms of the endoscopic management of the PSC patient, the following recommendations may be made. First, all patients with PSC without a clinical history of IBD should undergo colonoscopy prior to transplantation to determine if histologic IBD is present. The diagnosis of histologic IBD increases the risk for post-transplant colon cancer and mandates that the patient undergo post-transplant surveillance colonoscopy. If histologic IBD is not present in these patients prior to transplant, then post-transplant surveillance colonoscopy is not indicated. Patients with PSC and known IBD before transplant should undergo colonoscopic examination with mandatory colonic biopsies prior to transplantation. If dysplasia is discovered, the patient should undergo colectomy before transplant, or soon after transplant, depending on the clinical situation. For patients without dysplasia before transplantation, colonoscopic examination with mandatory colonic biopsies should be performed at least once yearly. For most patients, colectomy is recommended if dysplasia is discovered [50, 52]. However, prophylactic colectomy is not recommended without the presence of dysplasia [50, 52].

For patients without PSC or IBD, screening for colon cancer after transplantation is based on current guidelines for the general population. There is preliminary evidence that liver transplantation recipients may have a higher incidence of adenomatous colon polyps after transplantation [53]. Unfortunately, many liver transplantation recipients may not receive appropriate screening for preventable malignancies after transplantation.[54]

## Anal Cancer

Compared to colorectal cancer, the incidence of anal cancer is very low. Each year approximately 129,200 new cases of colorectal cancer are diagnosed compared to only 3,400 new cases of anal cancer. However, the risk of developing anal cancer in solid organ transplant recipients is estimated to be between 40[12] – 100[5] times higher than the normal population. The Transplant Tumor Registry of the University of Cincinnati reported 65 anogenital cancers in 2299 malignancies recorded [7]. Based on these findings, anogenital cancer in transplant recipients comprises 65/2299 (2.8 %) of all malignancies which is much higher than in the general population. There are similarities between anal cancer and cervical cancer. Most anal cancers are squamous cell carcinomas and like cervical cancer arise from dysplastic intraepithelial neoplastic lesions [55]. In both cervical and anal cancer, the human papillomavirus (HPV) has been implicated as a causative agent in the development of intraepithelial neoplasia and carcinoma [56]. Women with previous cervical cancer are at higher risk for anal cancer which underscores the association of HPV with both types of cancer [57]. HPV also causes genital warts which are associated with anal cancer [58]. HPV type 16 is most often associated with the development of anal cancer and can be isolated from the majority of anal cancers [56]. Because of immunosuppression, anal HPV and early intraepithelial dysplastic lesions have been found in some transplant recipients. Ogunbiyi et al. performed screening anal biopsies in 133 renal transplant recipients who were without symptoms [59]. In the control group, 12.4 % of patient biopsies were positive for HPV (type 16) and 1 % had an intraepithelial neoplastic lesion. The incidence of HPV in transplant recipients was significantly higher. In fact, 24.1 % were positive for HPV, 14 % had intraepithelial neoplastic lesions and one patient had anal cancer.

The incidence of anal cancer is 1/100,000 in the general population. Even with 100-fold increased incidence in the solid organ transplant population, the incidence in the transplant population is 1/1000. Therefore, even though the incidence is markedly increased in the transplant cohort, anal cancer remains an uncommon problem. Because of the low incidence of anal cancer, even a transplant hepatologist who follows a large number of liver transplant recipients may rarely, if ever, see this type of malignancy. While there are no specific recommendations for screening transplant recipients for anal cancer, the following is a rational approach [55]. All patients with genital warts should be referred to a dermatologist, urologist, proctologist or gynecologist experienced in the management of venereal warts in the immunosuppressed patients. As part of this evaluation, patients with venereal warts should be screened for anal cancer with anoscopy. Any suspicious anal lesions should be excised or treated with topical agents and followed with careful surveillance. Patients with dysplastic anal lesions should be followed by a proctologist experienced in the management of anal disease in the immunosuppressed patient. In addition, because of the association of cervical cancer and anal cancer, any female with cervical dysplasia or cancer should be considered for anal cancer screening. Some authors have suggested that transplant recipients should be screened for anal cancer, because of the high risk of developing this malignancy [55].

## Hepatocellular Carcinoma

Many patients with chronic liver disease who undergo liver transplantation have concomitant hepatocellular carcinoma. Early studies of liver transplantation as a treatment for hepatocellular carcinoma reported high recurrence rates with low long-term survival rates [12]. Many of these patients had large hepatocellular carcinomas (> 5 cm) and multiple cancerous nodules in the liver. In recent years the indications for liver transplantation for patients with hepatocellular carcinoma have evolved. Current selection criteria for patients with hepatocellular carcinoma have been published by the United Network of Organ Sharing (UNOS) [1]. Patients are considered suitable for transplantation if a single lesion is $\leq$ 5.0 cm or if $\leq$ 3 lesions are present and each is < 3.0 cm. Using these careful selection criteria, favorable long-term outcomes have been reported. In fact, under the current organ allocation criteria, patients with hepatocellular carcinoma are given a higher priority for transplantation. As a result, 22 % of liver transplantation recipients currently have hepatocellular carcinoma in their explanted liver. Several centers have demonstrated that the long-term survival of patients with hepatocellular carcinoma is the same as other patients [11, 12, 60, 61].

Any patient transplanted with a hepatocellular carcinoma is at risk for recurrent disease. Consequently, patients who undergo liver transplantation with hepatocellular carcinoma should be screened for recurrent disease after transplantation. While many patients have hepatocellular carcinoma identified prior to transplantation, some hepatomas are not diagnosed before the transplant and are discovered incidentally in the explanted liver. In fact, up to 53 % of liver transplant recipients have incidental hepatocellular carcinoma [61]. There is conflicting data regarding the survival of patients with incidental hepatocellular carcinoma. One might expect that patients with incidental hepatoma have a higher long-term survival, because incidental tumors are usually smaller and less invasive. This intuitive view is supported by studies which have reported that survival is greater in patients with incidental hepatocellular carcinoma [62]. However, several studies have shown that the survival of patients with an incidental hepatocellular carcinoma is no better than when the hepatocellular carcinoma is diagnosed before transplant [12, 60, 61]. One explanation for this finding may be that patients with known hepatocellular carcinoma are less ill and those with incidental tumors with have more advanced liver disease at the time of transplant. Based on this data, patients with incidental hepatocellular carcinoma should undergo post-transplant screening for recurrent malignancy. The most likely sites of hepatocellular carcinoma recurrence are the transplanted liver and lung [12].

While there are no standardized criteria for post-transplant surveillance of hepatocellular carcinoma, the following guidelines may be used for post-transplant screening in patients for recurrent hepatoma. At our center, we study patients with known and incidental hepatocellular carcinoma by abdominal/chest CT scans and serum alpha-fetoprotein levels at 3 months, 6 months 12 months and annually thereafter. While the discovery of recurrent hepatocellular carcinoma is important for the patient and the transplant team, there is limited data on therapy for this disease in liver transplant recipients [63].

Patients who develop recurrent viral hepatitis after transplantation are at risk to develop primary hepatocellular carcinoma. While uncommon, *de novo* hepatocellular carcinoma has been reported in patients who developed recurrent viral hepatitis C after liver transplantation which subsequently evolved into cirrhosis and hepatocellular carcinoma [10]. Similar cases have been reported in renal transplant recipients infected with hepatitis B [64-66]. Therefore, patients with recurrent viral hepatitis who develop recurrent cirrhosis after transplantation should be screened for the development of primary hepatocellular carcinoma. The standard recommendations are not different than in non-transplant patients: serial alpha- fetoprotein and abdominal ultrasounds or CT scans every 6 – 12 months.

## CHOLANGIOCARCINOMA

Cholangiocarcinoma develops in 10 –15 % of patients with PSC [61]. Unfortunately, patients with cholangiocarcinoma discovered prior to transplantation have a poor outcome after transplantation. Goss et al [52]. and Knechtle et al [49]. both reported 100 % mortality within three years of transplant in patients with PSC who had known cholangiocarcinoma at the time of transplant. With few exceptions, the diagnosis of cholangiocarcinoma before transplantation is a contraindication for liver transplant. There is limited data demonstrating improved outcomes in patients undergoing liver transplantation with cholangiocarcinoma. These preliminary findings suggest measurable survival in patients who undergo extensive pre-operative staging and adjuvant chemotherapy and radiation [67, 68]. Some patients with PSC have incidental cholangiocarcinoma and may be at risk for recurrent malignancy after transplant. Unfortunately, there are no screening procedures which have uniformly been demonstrated to be effective in the detection of cholangiocarcinoma. In addition, therapies for cholangiocarcinoma are largely ineffective. As a result, there are no specific screening recommendations for the detection of cholangiocarcinoma in liver transplant recipients who have incidental cholangiocarcinoma detected at the time of transplant.

## SUMMARY

With a growing cohort of liver transplant recipients, the need for endoscopic procedures and cancer surveillance is increasing. The recommendations for cancer screening in the liver transplant recipient are summarized in Table 2. Some, but not all, studies show an increased incidence of GI malignancies in liver transplant and solid organ transplant recipients. Adenocarcinoma of the esophagus is uncommon after transplant. However, several case reports suggest that liver transplant recipients with Barrett's esophagus may progress more rapidly to adenocarcinoma than normal patients. Consequently, liver transplant recipients with Barrett's esophagus may require more vigilant post-transplant surveillance. Screening for colon cancer in liver transplant recipients without UC is not different than the general population. Liver transplant recipients with PSC and UC are at risk for developing colon cancer. These patients should have careful post-transplant surveillance colonoscopy. If dysplasia is detected, then colectomy should be recommended for most patients to prevent progression to colon cancer. Patients with hepatocellular carcinoma should have serial abdominal/chest CT scans and alpha-fetoprotein to detect recurrence. Chronic hepatitis may evolve into cirrhosis in a minority of patients after transplant. These patients should be screened for progression to hepatocellular carcinoma with abdominal CT scans and alpha-fetoprotein measurements every six to twelve months. There are no effective screening strategies for gastric cancer or cholangiocarcinoma. As a result, there are no specific recommendations regarding post-transplant screening for these malignancies.

**Table 2 Screening Recommendations for Liver Transplant Recipients**

| **Site** | **post-transplant screening recommendations** |
|---|---|
| Esophagus | Yearly screening for patients with known Barrett's esophagus |
| Stomach | No screening required |
| Colon | |
| inflammatory bowel disease | Yearly colonoscopy with mandatory colonic biopsies |
| adenomatous polyp | Colonoscopy every 3 years (more frequent if clinically indicated) |
| Anal | Anoscopy for patients with genital warts and cervical cancer |
| Hepatocellular carcinoma | |
| pre-transplant hepatocellular carcinoma | Alpha-fetoprotein/abdominal CT scan at months 3, 6, 12 and yearly thereafter |
| post-transplant cirrhosis | Alpha-fetoprotein/abdominal CT scan every 6 – 12 months |
| Cholangiocarcinoma | No screening required |

## REFERENCES

[1] UNOS. 2002 Annual Report of the U.S. Organ Procurement and Transplantation Network and the Scientific Registry of Transplant Recipients: *Transplant Data* 1992-2001 [Internet]. Rockville (MD): HHS/HRSA/OSP/DOT; 2003 [modified 2003 Feb 18; cited 2003 Aug 23]. Available from: *http://www.optn.org/data/annualReport.asp.*

[2] Tan-Shalaby J, Tempero M: Malignancies after liver transplantation: a comparative review. *Sem Liver Disease* 15:156-164, 1995.

[3] Penn I. Posttransplantation *de novo* tumors in liver allograft recipients. *Liver Transpl Surg* 2:52-9, 1996.

[4] Penn I. Cancers following cyclosporine therapy. *Transplantation* 43:32-5, 1987.

[5] Penn I. Tumors after renal and cardiac transplantation. *Heme Oncolo Clin North Am* 7:431-45, 1993.

[6] Paya CV, Fung JJ, Nalesnik MA, et al. Epstein-Barr virus-induced posttransplant lymphoproliferative disorders. *Transplantation* 68:1517-25, 1999.

[7] Penn I. Cancers of the anogenital region in renal transplant recipients. Analysis of 65 cases. *Cancer* 58:611-6, 1986.

[8] Shiffman ML: Management of posttransplantation viral hepatitis C. *Liver Transpl Surg* 4:S79-86, 1998.

[9] Gane EJ, Portmann B, Naoumov NV, et al: Long-term outcome of hepatitis C infection after liver transplantation. *New Engl J Med* 334:815-20, 1996.

[10] Saxena R, Ye MQ, Emre S, Klion F, Nalesnik MA, Thung SN: *De novo* hepatocellular carcinoma in a hepatic allograft with recurrent hepatitis C cirrhosis. *Liver Transpl Surg* 5:81-2, 1999.

[11] Mazzaferro V, Regalia E, Doci R, et al: Liver transplantation for the treatment of small hepatocellular carcinomas in patients with cirrhosis. *N Engl J Med* 334:693-9, 1996.

[12] Bismuth H, Majno PE, Adam R: Liver transplantation for hepatocellular carcinoma. *Semin Liver Dis* 19:311-22, 1999.

[13] Feczko PJ, Mexwa DG: Gastrointestinal carcinomas in renal transplant recipients. *Gastrointest Radiol* 16:351-353, 1991.

[14] Yuzawa K, Kondo I, Fukao K, Iwasaki Y, Hamaguchi H: Mutagenicity of cyclosporine. Induction of sister chromatid exchange in human cells. *Transplantation* 42:61-3, 1986.

[15] Gnauck R: World Health Organization criteria for screening. *In* Winawer SJ, Schotenfeld K, Sherlock P, (eds) Colorectal cancer: prevention, epidemiology and screening. NewYork: *Raven* 1980, 175-180.

[16] Birkeland SA, Strorm HH, Lamm LU, et al: Cancer risk after renal transplantation in the Nordic countries. *Int J Cancer* 60:183-9, 1995.

[17] Sheil AGR: Development of malignancy following renal transplantation in Australia and New Zealand. *Trans Proc* 24:1275-9, 1992.

[18] Stewart T, Henderson R, Grayson H, Opelz G: Reduced incidence of rectal cancer, compared to gastric and colonic cancer in a population of 73,076 men and women chronically immunosuppressed. *Clinical Cancer Res* 3:51-5, 1997.

[19] Jain AB, Yee LD, Nalesnik MA, et al: Comparative incidence of *de novo* nonlymphoid malignancies after liver transplantation under tacrolimus using surveillance epidemiologic end result data. *Transplantation* 66:1193-1200, 1998.

[20] Fung JJ, Jain A, Kwak EJ, Kusne S, Dvorchik I, Eghtesad B. De novo malignancies after liver transplantation: a major cause of late death. *Liver Transpl* 7:S109-18, 2001.

[21] Kelly DM, Emre S, Guy SR, Miller CM, Schwartz ME, Sheiner PA: Liver transplant recipients are not at increased risk for nonlymphoid solid organ tumors. *Cancer* 83:1237-43, 1998.

[22] Jonas S, Rayes N, Neumann U, et al: *De novo* malignancies after liver transplantation using tacrolimus-based protocols or cyclosporine-based quadruple immunosuppression with an interleukin-2 receptor antibody or antithymocyte globulin. *Cancer* 80:1141-50, 1997.

[23] Haagsma EB, Hagens VE, Schaapveld M, van den Berg AP, de Vries EG, Klompmaker IJ, Slooff MJ, Jansen PL. Increased cancer risk after liver transplantation: a population-based study. *J Hepatol* 34:84-91, 2001.

[24] Grace N: Diagnosis and treatment of gastrointestinal bleeding secondary to portal hypertension. *Am J Gastroenterol* 92:1081-91, 1997.

[25] Weller DA, DeGuide JJ, Riegler JL: Utility of endoscopic evaluations in liver transplant candidates. *Am J Gastroenterol* 93:1346-50, 1998.

[26] Zaman A, Hapke R, Flora K, Rosen H, Benner K: Prevalence of upper and lower gastrointestinal tract findings in liver transplant candidates undergoing screening endoscopic evaluation. *Am J Gastroenterol* 94:895-9, 1999.

[27] Selingo JA, Herrine SK, Weinberg DS, Rubin RA: Role of screening colonoscopy in elective liver transplantation evaluation. *Transplant Proc* 29:2506-8, 1997.

[28] Rabinovitz M, Schade RR, Dindzans VJ, Belle SH, Van Thiel DH, Gavaler JS: Colonic disease in cirrhosis. An endoscopic evaluation in 412 patients. *Gastroenterology* 99:195-9, 1990.

[29] Correa P, Strong JP, Reif A, Johnson WD. The epidemiology of colorectal polyps. *Cancer* 39:2258-64, 1977.

[30] Winawer SJ, Zauber AG, O'Brien MJ, et al: Randomized comparison of surveillance intervals after colonoscopic removal of newly diagnosed adenomatous polyps. *N Engl J Med* 328:901-6, 1993.

[31] Scobey MW, Kerr BJ, Geisinger KR, Hamilton RW, Richter JE: Squamous cell carcinoma of the esophagus in association with long-term immunosuppressive therapy. *South Med J* 80:1587-9, 1987.

[32] Feczko PJ, Mexwa DG: Gastrointestinal carcinomas in renal transplant recipients. *Gastrointest Radiol* 16:351-353, 1991.

[33] Yao F, Ahuja J, Savides T, Behling C, Li S, Hart M: Rapid progression of gastroesophageal junction adenocarcinoma after liver transplantation. *J Clin Gastroenterol* 24:54-5, 1997.

[34] Safadi R, Ilan Y, Eid A, et al: Solid tumors after liver transplantation. *Transplant Proc* 31:1894-5, 1999.

[35] Ilan Y, Shouval D, Galun E, et al: Esophageal malignancy after liver transplantation in a patient with Barrett's esophagus. *Scand J Gastro* 31:415-416, 1996.

[36] Trotter JF, Brazer SR: Rapid progression to high-grade dysplasia in Barrett's esophagus after liver transplantation. *Liver Transpl Surg* 5:332-3, 1999.

[37] Hameeteman W, Tytgat GNJ, Houthoff HJ, van der Tweel JG: Barrett's esophagus: development of dysplasia and adenocarcinoma. *Gastroenterology* 96:1249-56, 1989.

[38] Cameron AJ, Ott BJ, Payne WS: The incidence of adenocarcinoma in columnar-lined Barrett's esophagus. *N Engl J Med* 313:857-59, 1985.

[39] Marks R, Rennie G, Selwood T: The relationship of basal cell carcinomas and squamous cell carcinomas to solar keratoses. *Arch Dermatol* 124:1039-42, 1988.

[40] Oka M, Attwood SE, Kaul B, Smyrk TC, DeMeester TR: Immunosuppression in patients with Barrett's esophagus. *Surgery* 112:11-7, 1992.

[41] Sampliner RE and the Practice Parameters Committee of the American College of Gastroenterology. Practice Guidelines on the diagnosis, surveillance and therapy of Barrett's esophagus. *Am J Gastroenterol* 93:1028-32, 1998.

[42] Sheil AGR: Development of malignancy following renal transplantation in Australia and New Zealand. *Trans Proc* 24:1275-9, 1992.

[43] Amaro R, Neff GW, Karnam US, Tzakis AG, Raskin JB. Acquired hyperplastic gastric polyps in solid organ transplant patients. *Am J Gastroenterol* 97:2220-4, 2002.

[44] Shehab TM, Hsi ED, Poterucha JJ, Gunaratnam NT, Fontana RJ.Helicobacter pylori-associated gastric MALT lymphoma in liver transplant recipients. *Transplantation* 71:1172-5, 2001.

[45] Ransohoff DF, Sandler RS. Screening for colorectal cancer. *N Engl J Med* 346:40-44, 2002;.

[46] Bleday R, Lee E, Jessurun J, Heine J, Wong WD: Increased risk of early colorectal neoplasms after hepatic transplant in patients with inflammatory bowel disease. *Dis Colon Rectum* 36:908-912, 1993.

[47] Narumi S, Roberts JP, Emond JC, Lake J, Ascher NL: Liver transplantation for sclerosing cholangitis. *Hepatology* 22:451-457, 1995.

[48] Higashi H, Yanaga K, Marsh JW, Tzakis A, Kakizoe, Starzl TE: Development of colon cancer after liver transplantation for primary sclerosing cholangitis associated with ulcerative colitis. *Hepatology* 11:477-480, 1990.

[49] Knechtle SJ, D'Alessandro AM, Harms BA, Pirsch JD, Belzer FO, Kalayoglu M: Relationships between sclerosing cholangitis, inflammatory bowel disease, and cancer in patients undergoing liver transplantation. *Surgery* 118:615-20, 1995.

[50] Loftus EV, Aguilar HI, Sandborn WJ, et al: Risk of colorectal neoplasia in patients with primary sclerosing cholangitis and ulcerative colitis following orthotopic liver transplantation. *Hepatology* 27:685-90, 1998.

[51] Fabia R, Levy MF, Testa G, et al: Colon carcinoma in patients undergoing liver transplantation. *Am J Surg* 176:265-9, 1998.

[52] Goss JA, Shackleton CR, Farmer DG, et al: Orthotopic liver transplantation for primary sclerosing cholangitis. A 12-year single center experience. *Ann Surg* 225:472-83, 1997.

[53] Atassi T, Thuluvath PJ. Risk of colorectal adenoma in liver transplant recipients compared to immunocompetent control population undergoing routine screening colonoscopy. *J Clin Gastroenterol* 37:72-3, 2003.

[54] Zeldin GA, Maygers J, Klein A, Thuluvath PJ. Vaccination, screening for malignancy, and health maintenance of the liver transplant recipient. *J Clin Gastroenterol* 32:148-50, 2001.

[55] Palefsky JM, Barrasso R. HPV infection and disease in men. *Obstet Gynecol Clin North Am* 23:895-916, 1996.

[56] Palefsky JM, Holly EA, Gonzales J, Berline J, Ahn DK, Greenspan JS: Detection of human papillomavirus DNA in anal intraepithelial neoplasia and anal cancer. Cancer Res 51:1014-9, 1991.

[57] Rabkin C, Biggar R, Melbye M, Curtis R: Second primary cancers following anal and cervical carcinoma: evidence of shared etiologic factors. *Am J Epidemiol* 136:54-8, 1992.

[58] Euvrard S, Kanitakis J, Chardonnet Y, et al: External anogenital lesions in organ transplant recipients. A clinicopathologic and virologic assessment. *Arch Dermatol* 133:175-8, 1997.

[59] Ogunbiyi OA, Scholefield JH, Raftery AT, et al: Prevalence of anal human papillomavirus infection and intraepithelial neoplasia in renal allograft recipients. *Br J Surg* 81:365-7, 1994.

[60] Klintmalm GB. Liver transplantation for hepatocellular carcinoma: a registry report of the impact of tumor characteristics on outcome. *Ann Surg* 228:479-90, 1998.

[61] Min AD, Saxena R, Thung SN, et al: Outcome of hepatitis C patients with and without hepatocellular carcinoma undergoing liver transplant. *Am J Gastroenterol* 93:2148-53, 1998.

[62] Ojogho ON, Esquivel CO, Imperial J, et al: Orthotopic liver transplantation for hepatocellular carcinoma. Factors affecting long-term patient survival. *Arch Surg* 131:935-9, 1996.

[63] Schlitt HJ, Neipp M, Weimann A, et al: Recurrence patterns of hepatocellular and fibrolamellar carcinoma after liver transplantation. *J Clin Oncol* 17:324-31, 1999.

[64] Dalgeish AG, Tiller DJ, Horvath J, Tattersall MHN: Hepatocellular carcinoma associated with hepatitis B in a renal graft recipient. *Med J Aust* 2:240-1, 1983.

[65] Hiesse C, Cantarovich M, Charpentier B, Prancais P, Benoit G, Fries D: Need for hepatocellular carcinoma screening before renal transplantation in HBS+, HBE+, western african. *Clinical Nephrology* 24:209-11, 1985.

[66] Luketic VA, Shiffman ML, McCall JB, Posner MP, Mill AS, Carithers RL: Primary hepatocellular carcinoma after orthotopic liver transplantation for chronic hepatitis B infection. *Ann Intern Med* 114:212-3, 1991.

[67] De Vreede I, Steers JL, Burch PA, Rosen CB, Gunderson LL, Haddock MG, Burgart L, Gores GJ. Prolonged disease-free survival after orthotopic liver transplantation plus adjuvant chemoirradiation for cholangiocarcinoma. *Liver Transpl* 6:309-16, 2000.

[68] Sudan D, DeRoover A, Chinnakotla S, Fox I, Shaw B Jr, McCashland T, Sorrell M, Tempero M, Langnas A. Radiochemotherapy and transplantation allow long-term survival for nonresectable hilar cholangiocarcinoma. *Am J Transplant* 2:774-9, 2002.

In: Liver Cancer: New Research
Editor: Felix Lee, pp. 203-226

ISBN 1-59454-182-5


*Chapter IX*

# Angiogenesis Related Factors in Hepatocellular Carcinoma and Anti-Angiogenesis Therapy

***Baomin Shi*[*], *Xiuyan Wang*[*], *Zhen Yang*[#], *Hongjun Sun*[*], *Qingling Mu*[*], *Jian Xu* and *Taihuang Wu*[*]***

[*]Department of General Surgery, Shandong Provincial Hospital, Clinical College of Shandong University, Jinan, 250021 China[12]

[#]Department of Surgery, Tongji Hospital, Tongji Medical College, Huazhong University of Science and Technology, Wuhan, 430030, China

## Abstract

Angiogenesis is an essential process in many physiological and pathological conditions and has become the focus of researches in angiogenesis related diseases such as ischemic coronary or peripheral artery diseases and various tumors. Therapeutical angiogenesis for ischemic disease and anti-angiogenesis for tumors have partially achieved in many experimental studies and clinical trials. Hepatocellular carcinoma, as a hypervascular cancer, has been proved to be more related with angiogenesis. Vascular density and many angiogenesis related factors have been confirmed to be much involved in almost all the process of hepatocarcinogenesis, tumor growth, invasion and metastasis, recurrence and prognosis. These factors include vascular endothelial growth factor, angiopoietin-tie system, somatostatin, angiostatin and endostatin, matrix metalloproteinase, angiogenin and even nerve growth factor, macrophage migration inhibitory factor, ephrin, and rennin-angiotension system. Many strategies targeting these factors and angiogenesis process have been established and proved to be efficient in inhibiting HCC tumor growth, invasion, metastasis and recurrence and consequently promote the five-year

[12] **Tel:86-531-6655450 Fax: 86-531-7038687 Email: baomins@tom.com**

survival rate. Anti-angiogenesis may be another effective therapy for HCC besides chemotherapy and immunotherapy and also be a great benefit for both unresectable HCC patients and those after surgical operation.

## INTRODUCTION

Angiogenesis, the development of new microvascular networks, is required in many physiological and pathological conditions, including embryonic development, wound healing, tissue regeneration and tumor growth [1-3]. It plays a key role in numerous human diseases including vessel over production involved ones like malignant tumors, rheumatoid arthritis, retinal and choroidal neovascularisation and various skin diseases, and also vessel deficiency lesions such as ischemic coronary heart disease and peripheral limb ischemia.

The development of blood vessels in adult tissues is a complex process in which different growth factors and cytokines act in concert. Angiogenesis has been considered a physiological response to ischemia [4] and therapeutic angiogenesis has emerged as a promising therapy for ischemic disease [5]. Several clinical trials have succeeded in the treatment of ischemic diseases such as ischemic heart disease and peripheral limb ischemia using these angiogenic growth factors or vectors encoding for them like vascular endothelial growth factor (VEGF), angiopoietin, fibroblast growth factor (FGF), etc [6].

Anti-angiogenesis is another focus of researches on angiogenesis or vasculogeneisis especially in tumor treatment. It has been more than 30 years since the concept of anti-angiogenic therapy was first presented by Judah Folkman who suggested that cutting the blood supply of a tumor might actually destroy it [1]. During the following three decades researchers had gained essential insight into the biological mechanisms of angiogenesis. Numerous regulatory molecules have been discovered to be able to influence endothelial cell physiology in vitro and angiogenesis in vivo. They can be divided into several groups, consisting of growth factors, extracellular matrix molecules and membrane bound proteins like integrins and growth factor receptors [7].

Various strategies targeting the above three steps for anti-angiogenesis have been established in the majority of tumors including hepatocellular carcinoma (HCC). Some already known drugs like Taxol® [8], Thalidomide [9] or Interferon-a [10] are seeing a new area of therapeutic use since it was discovered that they have anti-angiogenic properties. Other drugs are already on the market to become anti-angiogenic when coupled to specific molecules which target them specifically to proliferating endothelial cells [11,12]. Anti-angiogenesis has become an important approach in treatment for various cancers and gained partially success in both experimental studies and clinical trials.

Tumor angiogenesis involves several processes, including endothelial cell activation, proliferation, migration, and tissue infiltration from preexisting blood vessels that are triggered by specific angiogenic growth factors produced by tumor cells and the surrounding stroma [3, 13–16]. Angiogenesis is thought to play a crucial role in tumor growth, invasion, and metastasis.

HCC is, in general, a hypervascular tumor, the growth of which is largely dependent on the extent of blood supply [17]. HCC vascularity varies widely according to tumor size and histological grade. In moderately or poorly differentiated HCCs with a diameter of 2 cm or larger, artery-like vessel are well developed, diffuse capillarization of blood space is present, and the HCCs are angiographically detectable. On the other hand, in small-sized and well-differentiate HCCs, vascular situations are not so prominent [18]. Other study also showed that tumor size was correlated with microvessel density [19]. Intratumoral arteriole density was found to be significantly associated with histological grade, proliferative activity, and patient survival [20]. Therefore, hypervascularity is one of the main characteristics of large and moderately or poorly differentiated HCC [21].

It has been agreed that many growth factors such as VEGF, FGF, platelet-derived endothelial cell growth factor (PDGF), angiostatin and endostatin, interleukins and tie-angiopoietin system, etc., play important roles in HCC carcinogenesis, development , invasion and recurrence and are closely related with its prognosis. Anti-angiogenesis targeting the above growth factors in HCC has been extensively investigated and gained prosperous effect in HCC treatment both experimentally and clinically.

# Vascular Endothelial Growth Factor

## VEGF and its Characteristics

VEGF, also known as vascular permeability factor (VPR), has been described and identified first by Senger et al. and Ferrara et al [22,23]. It is a major regulator of both physiological and pathological angiogenesis [24] and is an endothelial cell-specific mitogen that promotes many other events necessary for angiogenesis [25-28].

VEGF has been considered to be an important endothelial cell mitogen as well as a potent enhancer of vascular permeability present in a number of normal tissues. Its expression in mRNA level has been confirmed in various organs, such as the lung, kidney, adrenal gland, heart, liver, and gastric mucosa; and in malignant tumors, brain tumor, bladder cancer, kidney cancer, ovarian cancer, gastric cancer, esophageal cancer, colon cancer, breast cancer, and hepatocellular carcinoma [18, 29-31]. By alternating splicing of mRNA, at least five different molecular species with 121, 145, 165, 189, and 206 amino acids were determined [25], although the physiological significance of the multiple isoforms has not been fully established. The five different members of the VEGF family have been named as: VEGF [32], VEGF-B [33], VEGF-C [34], VEGF-D [35,36] and VEGF-E [37]. VEGF121 and VEGF165 are the most abundant isoforms. The first is a freely soluble protein, and the second is also secreted, although an important percentage remains bound to the cell surface and extracellular matrix. In contrast, the other isoforms are almost completely sequestered in the extracellular matrix [31].

VEGF exerts its actions by binding to tyrosine kinase receptors, VEGFR-1 (flt-1), VEGFR-2 (flk-1) and VEGF-3 (flt-4), almost exclusively expressed in endothelial cells [38-40]. Binding of VEGF to its receptors causes receptor dimerization and activation of the intrinsic kinase, followed by autophosphorylation of the receptor and subsequent signal transduction. VEGF and its receptors has become the current focus in a wide range of fields not only in angiogenesis and antineoplastic researches but also in augmentation of new collaterals in many ischemic diseases [38].

Factors that regulate VEGF expression in tumor and non-tumor cells are now being elucidated. The best-characterized mediator that induces an increase in VEGF is hypoxia [41,42]. VEGF expression in cultured cells is elevated by hypoxia due to hypoxia-responsive elements that are regulated by a putative iron-containing sensor system. VEGF expression is also regulated by numerous cytokines and growth factors such as IL-1b, IL-6, PDGF-BB, TGF-b, TGF-a, bFGF, EGF, HGF, hypoxia- inducible factor 1, insulin-like growth factor I, insulin-like growth factor II, alpha-tumor necrosis factor, nitric oxide, etc. Mutation of the ras and p53 genes has also been shown to up-regulate VEGF expression [3,4] [41-52].

Identification of VEGF both in its protein level and mRNA level and its significance have been extensively studied in various hepatic diseases, such as HCC, metastases hepatic cancer, acute and chronic hepatitis, liver cirrhosis, and other benign liver tumors [3] [53-60].

It has been testified that VEGF plays an important role in the growth of sinusoidal endothelial cells and hepatocytes , or termed liver regeneration, and in the development of primary and secondary liver carcinoma and benign liver pathological changes such as hemangioma, focal hyperplasia, and hepatitis by promoting neovascularization [1,61-64]. VEGF is expressed mainly in HCC cells, sinusoidal endothelial cells, Kupffer cells, hepatic macrophages, stellate cells, and extracellular matrix of the portal tracts [65,66].

## VEGF and Hepatocarcinogenesis

VEGF may play an important role in the early phases of hepatocarcinogenesis. The degree of VEGF expression increases gradually according to the stepwise development of hepatocarcinogenesis. It is higher in high-grade dysplastic nodules (DNs) and early HCCs than in low-grade DNs. The hepatocytes and HCC cells adjacent to peliosis and fibrous septa show stronger VEGF expression. Angiogenesis, unpaired arteries, and sinusoidal capillarization developed from low-grade DNs and gradually increased to the highest degree in HCCs. The proliferation cell nuclear antigen labeling indexes of hepatocytes and HCC cells also increase gradually as hepatocarcinogenesis progresses. Small HCCs show a higher status of neoangiogenesis and cell proliferation activity than advanced HCCs. The degree of VEGF expression is correlated with angiogenesis and cell proliferation activity [67].

Hypoxia can stimulate angiogenesis to support tumor growth by induction of angiogenic factors including VEGF. Thus hypoxia may be a major cause of hypervasculature of HCC at early stage. Recently it has been reported that several hypoxia-regulatory factors are closely involved in angiogenesis of hepatocellular carcinoma. The stability and function of these factors can be regulated by interaction with other protein factors and consequently modulate the expression of angiogenic factors depending on oxygen tension [68].

## VEGF and HCC Development and Invasion

It has been confirmed that VEGF is closely correlated to the growth of HCC cells, progression of tumor volume, invasion and metastasis. The expression levels of VEGF mRNA in tumors with PV-emboli and in poor-encapsulated tumors were higher than in those without PV-emboli and in well-encapsulated tumors. Microvascular density in HCC tissues was significantly correlated with the expression levels of VEGF mRNA . Serum VEGF concentrations could be a new marker for predicting the angiogenesis, invasion and metastasis of HCC [69].

Zhao et al revealed that the serum VEGF levels in the HCC group (465.62 +/- 336.24 pg/ml) was significantly elevated as compared with those in patients with benign liver lesions (159.54 +/- 120.58 pg/ml) and those in normal controls (123.53 +/- 51.84 pg/ml). In the 115 HCC patients, the serum VEGF levels in patients with portal vein (PV) emboli or with metastasis or with large HCC lesions (>/= 5 cm in diameter) were significantly higher than those without PV-emboli, without metastasis or with small HCC lesions. The serum VEGF levels in stage I, II, III, IVa and IVb HCC patients were become more and more from 340.6 pg/ml of stage I to 647.93 +/- 344.56 pg/ml in stage Vb HCC. So the pre-therapeutic serum VEGF levels in HCC patients reflect the disease's potential activity of vascular invasion and metastasis [70].

Yamaguchi et al [18] studied VEGF expressions by immunohistochemistry and RT-PCR analysis in the tissues of 74 cases of HCC and concluded that its expression was closely related to the histological grade. In well-differentiated HCC, its expression was the highest (100%), while in moderate one, the positive rate was 88.5%, and 67.3% in poorly differentiated HCC.

Suzuki et al reported a positive rate of 69.6% from 23 HCC patients and its expression was associated with fibrous capsule and septal formation by in situ hybridization and RT-PCR [55].

Chow et al [56] investigated VEGF expression immunohistochemistrically in tissues of 36 cases of HCC. The positive rate is only 36.1%. They showed that expression of VEGF was significantly associated with a higher proliferative index and sonographic portal vein thrombosis and but it did not correlate with a biochemical liver profile, alpha-fetoprotein levels, histological grading, gender or clinical stage of cirrhosis.

One group of immunohistochemistry study of VEGF and bFGF on 20 specimens of HCC by Mise et al [57] suggested that VEGF contributes to angiogenesis of liver tumors, whereas basic FGF may be involved in the invasion of HCC into the surrounding tissues.

Tang et al [71] summarized a decade's studies on HCC metastasis at the Liver Cancer Institute of Fudan University in China. They concluded that serum VEGF, microvessel density, and p53 scoring may be of value for the prediction of postoperative metastatic recurrence. Interferon alpha proved effective for the prevention of recurrence both experimentally and clinically. Molecular research into the invasiveness of HCC identified some factors positively related to invasiveness including epidermal growth factor receptor (EGF-R), matrix metalloproteinase-2 (MMP-2), urokinasetype plasminogen activator (uPA), its receptor (uPA-R) and inhibitor (PAI-1), intercellular adhesion molecule-1 (ICAM-1) [72].

Even in HCC patients after chemoembolization, the establishment of collateral circulation and reconstruction of blood supply of residual cancer tissue are proved to be evolved in the development of neovascularization and expression of VEGF [73].

Most of the studies have reached an agreement on VEGF effect in HCC. However, negative report also exists. In a group study of 71 cases of HCC, El-Assal et al [50]reported, that neither VEGF mRNA levels nor protein expression in HCC were statistically correlated with the tumoral microvessel density or any histopathological features of the tumor.

VEGF may also facilitate HCC tumor growth in the bone by acting as an angiogenic factor once invasion of the bone is complete. This might be another reason for the high incidence of bone metastasis in HCC [74].

## VEGF and HCC Prognosis

Tumor angiogenesis is critical to both the growth and metastasis of HCC, and has drawn much attention in recent years. Many angiogenesis-related markers, such as VEGF, bFGF, PDGF, angiogenin, pleiotrophin, and endostatin levels, as well as intratumor microvessel density (MVD) have been evaluated and found to be of valuable prognostic significance [75,76].

Serum levels of VEGF may provide useful prognostic information in patients with various types of cancers. Preoperative serum VEGF is a significant independent predictor of tumor recurrence [77]. In HCC, a serum VEGF level of more than 500 pg/mL and tumor size more than 5 cm were independent preoperative factors predictive of microscopic venous invasion. During a median follow-up of 11.6 months, 48% of patients with a serum VEGF level of more than 500 pg/mL and 27% of those with a serum VEGF level of 500 pg/mL or less developed postoperative recurrence. These results show that a high preoperative serum VEGF level is a predictor of microscopic venous invasion in HCC, suggesting that the serum VEGF level may be useful as a biologic marker of tumor invasiveness and a prognostic factor in HCC [78].

## Anti-Angiogenesis and HCC Treatment Targeting VEGF

The use of antiangiogenic agents such as suramin, BB-94 (Batimastat), TNP-470, and carboxyamido-triazole (CAI, a synthetic inhibitor of non-excitable calcium channels that reversibly inhibits angiogenesis) has become a new therapeutic strategy for treating metastasis in HCC. These agents have been used to treat metastatic model of HCC in nude mouse (LCI-D20 mouse model). Lot of studies confirmed the inhibitory effects of the drugs on tumour growth, angiogenesis, invasion and metastasis in LCI-D20 mouse models [79,80].

Different strategies have been designed to inhibit VEGF function. Using specific VEGF antibodies and antisense inhibition, coupling of a toxin to VEGF, and blocking the interaction of VEGF with its receptors are all methods for stopping the angiogenic effects of this growth factor.

Injecting a monoclonal VEGF-antibody into nude mice bearing various tumors of human origin significantly suppresses tumor growth and reduces tumor weight of treated animals up 96% [80,81]. A humanized antibody against VEGF, rhuMAb-VEGF has recently been designed [82,83] and undergoes testing in cancer patients in Phase II clinical trials.

Antisense-VEGF gene therapy could be an effective strategy to treat HCC. Endothelial cell proliferation, tubule formation and tumor growth may be diminished by down-regulation of endogenous VEGF expression in tumor cells or tissue. Suppression of VEGF led to a decrease in tumor growth at the established tumor size, whether relatively small or large [84]. Other study also indicated that expression of antisense VEGF RNA in SMMC-7721 cells could decrease the tumorigenicity [85].

The coupling of a toxin to VEGF itself could also have effective anti-angiogenesis. When active parts of diphtheria toxin (DT390) are linked to VEGF165 or VEGF121, the chimeric molecule exerts highly selective toxic effects on endothelial cells, leaving other cell types untouched. It disrupts neovascularisation in the chicken allantoic membrane assay, and it slows down the growth of the tumors in a murine Kaposi's sarcoma model [86].

PTK787/ZK 222584 (PTK/ZK) is an oral potent and selective inhibitor of VEGF-mediated Flt-1 and KDR receptor tyrosine kinases. PTK/ZK has been shown to reduce growth and microvasculature in subcutaneously implanted human tumor xenografts in nude mice. Phase I studies are under way evaluating the optimum dose and schedule of oral PTK/ZK administered continuously to patients with advanced cancers of types known to overexpress VEGF, particularly in patients with liver metastases from colorectal cancer treated with PTK/ZK [87].

Inhibition of VEGFR-2 signaling may be another way to stop angiogenesis. Such inhibitors have been identified by in vitro screening of random chemical compound libraries. One of these compounds, SU5416, is a potent and selective inhibitor of the Flk-1/KDR receptor tyrosine kinase that is presently under evaluation in Phase I clinical studies for the treatment of human cancers. It strongly inhibits growth of subcutaneous tumors in mice, converting the tumors to pale white, avascular nodes [88] suggesting the antiangiogenic property of this agent.

SU6668, a novel inhibitor of these receptors, has competitive inhibitory properties with respect to ATP. In cellular systems, SU6668 inhibited receptor tyrosine phosphorylation and mitogenesis after stimulation of cells by appropriate ligands. Oral or i.p. administration of SU6668 in athymic mice resulted in significant growth inhibition of a diverse panel of human tumor xenografts of glioma, melanoma, lung, colon, ovarian, and epidermoid origin. Furthermore, intravital multifluorescence videomicroscopy of C6 glioma xenografts in the dorsal skinfold chamber model revealed that SU6668 treatment suppressed tumor angiogenesis. Investigations of SU6668 activity in cancer patients are ongoing in Phase I clinical trials [89].

But all these trials have not been investigated in HCC.

### Hepatoblastoma

Hepatoblastoma is the most common primary hepatic malignancy of childhood, frequently presenting as advanced disease. Inhibition of VEGF effectively suppresses tumorigenesis in multiple experimental models. Specific anti-VEGF therapy inhibits neoangiogenesis and significantly suppresses tumor growth in experimental hepatoblastoma. Anti-VEGF agents may represent new therapeutic alternatives for children with advanced disease [90].

### Secondary Hepatocellular Carcinoma

The expression of VEGF and its circulating levels of secondary hepatocellular carcinoma especially from gastrointestinal and endocrine cancers have also been extensively investigated [91,92]. It has a similar increase of VEGF expression in secondary HCC and primary HCC. VEGF is associated with the progression, invasion and metastasis of colorectal cancer, and overexpression of VEGF mRNA in the primary tumor is assumed to be closely correlated with poor prognosis in colorectal cancer patients [93,94]. The results of the study of Kumar et al [94] on the preoperative serum VEGF suggested that it could be a good predictor for early colorectal cancer. In gastric cancer which has highly expression of VEGF, it has been proved to have more possibility of hepatic metastases [95]. The antibodies for VEGF has also been successfully tried to treat hepatic metastases from gastrointestinal cancer [96].

## Tie-Angiopoietin System

Beside the VEGFRs, only Tie-1 [97] and Tie-2 [98] are known so far to be endothelial cell specific surface receptors with tyrosine kinase activity and were found to hold unique functions in vascular biology as revealed by gene knockout experiments.

Tie-1 has been found in wound healing tissue and during menstruation [99,100]. Tie-2 is also present on endothelial cells in human breast cancer and glioblastoma tissues [101,102], suggesting a connection to tumor angiogenesis. The natural ligands for the Tie-2 receptor are called angiopoietins. Angiopoietin-1 binds and activates Tie-2 [103].

The signals emerging from the angiopoietin-1:Tie-2 interaction seem to be responsible for the assembly of non-endothelial cells for the vessel wall, such as pericytes and smooth muscle cells [104]. The other Tie-2 ligand, angiopoietin-2, does not activate Tie-2, suggesting an antagonist function to angiopoietin-1. These findings together underline the feasability to use the Tie:angiopoietin system to control angiogenesis and vasculogenesis.

Sugimachi K et al [105] proved that the angiopoietin-2 gene was upregulated in the hypervascular type of HCC. Angiopoietin-1, rather than angiopoietin-2, was more frequently expressed in the normal liver. Angiopoietin-1 was expressed in 68% of HCCs, whereas angiopoietin-2 was expressed in 81%, and was significantly higher in poorly differentiated HCCs characterised by high vascularity, with the similar result as Chen et al [106].

Mitsuhashi et al [107] investigated the expression of angiopoietin-1, angiopoietin-2, Tie-2, and VEGF in surgically resected specimens from 46 patients with HCC. Immunohistochemical staining showed increased angiopoietin-2 protein in HCC. Furthermore, a high angiopoietin-2/1 mRNA ratio in HCC was closely associated with tumor portal vein invasion, tumor diameter, and the microvessel density level. The survival time for patients in the high angiopoietin-2/1 mRNA ratio group was significantly poorer when compared with the low angiopoietin-2/1 mRNA ratio group.

In Peng et al [108] studies, angiopoietin-1 and angiopoietin-2 cDNA were subcloned into the pcDNA3 vector and subsequently transfected into a human SMMC7721 HCC cell line . Then HCC cells were injected subcutaneously into 30 nude mice and the tumor growth speed and amount of newborn vasculature in the HE stained tissue were observed every 2 days till 3 weeks or the death of animals. The tumor grew faster with angiopoietin-2 expression; much more blood vessels were seen in the tumor tissue than that without angiopoietin-2 expression. Angiopoietin-1 gene expression seems to have no obvious effect on the increase of vasculature and tumor growth.

Ectopic expression of angiopoietin-2 promotes the rapid development of human HCCs and produces hemorrhage within tumors in nude mice. In vitro expression of a dominant-negative construct, containing a soluble Tie2 ectodomain (sTie2), led to angiopoietin protein interaction, inhibition of endogenous Tie2 phosphorylation in vascular endothelial cells. Tumorigenicity with angiogenesis was suppressed by in vivo gene transfer and sTie2 expression in a murine HCC model, suggesting a possible role for angiopoietin/Tie2 signaling in the induction of HCC neovascularization and disease progression. It may be concluded that inhibition of the angiopoietin/Tie2 signal transduction cascade is a promising approach for HCC treatment [109]. Furthermore, angiopoietin has been proved to have a synergic effect with VEGF to increase vascularity and tumor growth in HCC [110].

## SOMATOSTATIN

Many experimental studies have shown that somatostatin or its analogues such as octreotide had antiproliferateive effects on many kinds of cancer cells mediated directly by tumoral somatostatin receptors or indirectly by down-regulation of angiogenesis growth factors or inducing apoptosis. In vitro, octreotide inhibits the proliferation, invasion, and differentiation of HCC cells elicited by VEGF. In vivo, octreotide is sufficiently potent to suppress nude mice corneal neovascularization induced by tumor tissues from HCC LCI-D20. Systemic administrations of octreotide produce a significant suppression of the growth of LCI-D20. Immunohistochemical studies of tumor tissues revealed decreased microvessel density in octreotide-treated animals. The somatostatin analogue octreotide is a potent prohibitor for tumor angiogenesis and has antiproliferative effect on tumor growth in nude mice bearing HCC xenografts by its suppressive effect on blood vessel supply [111,112].

Other studies by Guo et al [113] showed that octreotide could promote the effects of hepatic arterial occlusion therapy for transplanted cancer in rat liver. Decreasing the blood perfusion of tumor after hepatic arterial blockage might be one of its major mechanisms. The mechanism of antineoplastic action of octreotide in hepatoma also related to its inducing apoptosis in human hepatoma cells [114].

Several clinical trials proved that using somatostatin alone or combination with chemothrombosis greatly benefited HCC patients [115-117]. One study [115] showed that the median survival of the patients with inoperable HCC treated with long acting somatostatin analogues were prolonged from 8 months to 15 months. The tumor remained stable or regressed in 40% of the patients and most of patients had a supuerior quality of life. The other clinical trial showed that octreotide prolonged the meadian survival and promoted 1-year survival rate of patients with advanced HCC significantly [117].

However, there is another negative report on the effect of somatostatin. Yuan et al [118] proved by random trial that there was no difference in the cumulative survival between the sandostatin -treated group compared with the control group [median survival 1.93 months vs. 1.97 months]. There was no tumor regression and no reduction of alpha-fetoprotein (AFP) levels in patients receiving sandostatin treatment. They concluded that sandostatin monotherapy did not have survival benefit in the selected group of patients with advanced HCC. But that group of 35 cases of HCC appears too small a number to draw a convincing conclusion.

Therefore, though most of studies have proved the antiangiogenesis effect of octreotide on HCC, further studies are ought to be performed on more patients.

## ANGIOSTATIN

Angiostatin is one of the most exciting discoveries in the field of angiogenesis and cancer therapy. The mechanism of its anti-angiogenic effect is not exactly known but it probably kills endothelial cells by inducing apoptosis [119]. Systemic administration of human or recombinant human angiostatin potently inhibits the growth of human and murine primary carcinoma in mice, showing nearly a complete inhibition of tumor growth without detectable toxicity or resistance [120,121]. Angiostatin makes endothelial cells resistant to angiogenic stimuli and induces ‘dormancy’ of metastases.

Recent studies have reported that antiangiogenic gene delivery into cancer cells inhibits growth of certain tumors in vivo.

The anti-angiogenic effects of angiostatin gene transduction into HCC both in vitro and in vivo have been confirmed. Suppression of HCC tumor growth was noted in mice implanted with angiostatin gene-transfected cells, and such suppression was proportional with the percentage of transfected cells. Analysis of the vascular density in these tumors showed that the tumor growth suppression effect of angiostatin gene correlated with suppression of tumor vascularity [122].

It has been shown that gene transfer of AAV-angiostatin via the portal vein led to significant suppression of the growth of both nodular and metastatic EL-4 lymphoma tumors established in the liver and prolonged the survival time of the mice. The suppression was due to the inhibiting neovessels and inducing tumor cell apoptosis. The anti-angiogenic activity of angiostatin was independent of VEGF. AAV-mediated anti-angiogenic gene therapy is valuable for targeting unresectable liver metastases, especially after surgical removal of primary tumors [123].

# Endostatin

Endostatin is generated by proteolytic cleavage of collagen XVIII. In normal tissues, 2 variants of the endostatin precursor, namely the short and long forms, regulate tissue specificity. The long form is a hepatocyte-specific variant, and the short form is a major component of the tumor extracellular matrix in primary and metastatic liver cancers [124]. Endostatin strongly inhibits endothelial cell proliferation in vitro and angiogenesis in chicken allantoic membrane assays. It might inhibit angiogenesis by binding to the heparan sulphate proteoglycans implicated in growth factor signaling [125].

Phase I trials have now been initiated for endostatin to evaluate the usefulness of this promising new angiogenesis inhibitor in humans. It could effectively stop the growth of metastases originating from Lewis lung carcinoma as well as primary tumors (melanoma, fibrosarcoma, hemangioendothelioma, renal cell carcinoma, HCC etc.) [126,127].

Li et al [128] proved that endostatin gene could be efficiently transported into mice with TF-liposome-DNA delivery system by administration of aerosol. TF-liposome-mediated endostatin gene therapy strongly inhibited angiogenesis and the growth of mouse xenograft liver tumors.

It has also been showed by the studies of Li et al [129], that the growth of hepatoma models transplanted in the muscle of legs was suppressed by recombinant endostatin due to decreased density of vascularity and increased necrosis of tumor cells.

Partially purified endostatin secreted from Av3mEndo (a recombinant adenoviral vector encoding a secretable form of murine endostatin) transduced mammalian cells was shown to potently inhibit endothelial cell migration in vitro. A single intravenous administration of Av3mEndo in mice was shown to result in (1) prolonged and elevated levels of circulating endostatin, (2) partial inhibition of VEGF-induced angiogenesis in a VEGF implant angiogenesis model, and (3) prolonged survival and in 25% of mice the complete prevention of tumor growth in a prophylactic human colon/liver metastasis xenograft murine model. These results support the contention that adenoviral vector-mediated expression of an antiangiogenic protein (s) represents an attractive therapeutic approach to HCC and other angiogenesis-dependent diseases [130].

It has also been found the addition of angiostatin or endostatin to conventional chemotherapy could enhance antitumoral efficacy in a murine model of early colorectal liver metastasis [131].

# Other Factors

## Nerve Growth Factor (NGF)

NGF has been suggested to play a role in cancer progression. NGF is specifically elevated in mouse hepatocellular carcinomas (HCCs) by cDNA array analysis. NGF is expressed by hepatocytes during carcinogenesis, regeneration, and primary culture. TrkA expression and the abundance of nerve fibers in the walls of tumor-associated arteries suggest a possible role for NGF in angiogenesis [132]. Further studies should be done upon anti-angiogenesis effect in HCC.

## Ephrin

Ephrin ligands and their cognate receptor tyrosine kinases, Eph, mediate numerous developmental processes in both invertebrates and vertebrates. The expression level of ephrin-B1 in HCC tissues was significantly higher than that in non-tumor tissues. The overexpression of the Eph gene was shown to be oncogenic [133], indicating that the activation of the ephrin/Eph system may promote tumor growth. It has been demonstrated that ephrin-A1 and its receptor EphA2 are expressed during tumor neovascularization [134] indicating an important role of the ephrin/Eph system in tumor angiogenesis.

It has been investigated by Sawai Y et al [135] that the expression of ephrin-B1 promoted tumor growth by initiating tumor angiogenesis in HCC. The ephrin-B1 transcript was detected in HCC tissues, and that the level was significantly higher than in non-tumor tissues. The ephrin-B1 overexpressing cells showed a rapid growth in vivo and tumor vessel number was significantly increased in ephrin-B1 overexpressing tumors. These results suggest that ephrin-B1 may be involved in tumor progression by promoting neovascularization.

## Angiogenin

Angiogenin is a 14 kDa single chain protein which has been isolated from human adenocarcinoma cells. It induces angiogenesis in the rabbit cornea in the picomolar range [136,137]. Human cDNAs coding for angiogenin, were isolated from a cDNA library prepared from human liver poly (A) mRNA. The largest cDNA insert (697 base pairs) contained a short 5'-noncoding sequence followed by a sequence coding for a signal peptide of 24 (or 22) amino acids, 369 nucleotides coding for the mature protein of 123 amino acids, a stop codon, a 3'-noncoding sequence of 175 nucleotides, and a poly (A) tail [138].

Angiogenin is a potent angiogenic protein whose inhibition is known to prevent human tumor growth in athymic mice. It is secreted by both tumor and normal cells; and interacts with endothelial and smooth muscle cells to induce a wide range of cellular responses including cell migration and invasion, proliferation, and formation of tubular structures [139].

Neomycin, an aminoglycoside antibiotic, inhibits nuclear translocation of human angiogenin in human endothelial cells, an essential step for angiogenin-induced angiogenesis [140].

Immunohistochemistry and in situ hybridization showed greater increments of angiogenin protein expression and mRNA expression, respectively, in HCC tissues than in the surrounding nontumorous tissues. Microvessel density within tumorous tissues increased according to dedifferentiation of the histological grade of HCC, showing a significant correlation with angiogenin expression levels. In HCC patients, despite the cirrhotic background, serum angiogenin levels increased as the tumor vascularity increased (197.8+/- 64.9 ng/ml for hypovascular, 326.7 +/- 148.6 ng/ml for hypervascular, and 405.0 +/- 121.3 ng/ml for very hypervascular), in good accordance with histological grading, and significantly decreased after successful treatment with transcatheter arterial embolization or percutaneous ethanol injection. HCC patients with lower serum level of angiogenin have higher 5-year survival rate whearas those with higher level of angiogenin have lower 5-year survival rate [141].

However, one former study [142] of hepatocellular carcinomas showed that neither angiogenin nor bFGF production was related to angiogenesis. But that study only included four cases of HCC patients and the conclusion is not so reasonable and convincing.

## Macrophage Migration Inhibitory Factor

Macrophage migration inhibitory factor (MIF) may contribute to multiple aspects of tumor progression, including control of cell proliferation, differentiation, cell survival and angiogenesis. Recombinant MIF and the supernatants of tumor cell line culture could enhance the invasion and migration of HCC cells. This effect can be inhibited by the addition of a neutralizing anti-MIF antibody. Increased MIF serum levels correlated with higher levels of interleukin-8 (IL-8) in the sera of patients with HCC than in normal volunteers. MIF may act as an autocrine-acting factor that stimulates angiogenesis and metastasis in HCC by promoting expression of angiogenic factors and migration of tumor cells. Thus MIF suppression may be another antitumor approach by angiogenesis inhibition [143].

## IFN-Alpha

IFN-alpha inhibits metastasis and recurrence of human HCC after curative resection in nude mice mediated by antiangiogenesis through downregulating expression of vascular endothelial growth factor [144].

## Renin-Angiotensin System

The renin-angiotensin system is frequently activated in patients with chronic liver diseases. Angiotensin-II (AT-II), which is produced by angiotensin-converting enzyme (ACE), has many physiological effects, including strong pro-angiogenic activity by inducing VEGF. Studies have found that the ACE inhibitor, perindopril (PE), is a potent inhibitor of experimental HCC growth and angiogenesis, by suppression of VEGF at a clinically comparable dose [145,146].

## Matrix Metalloproteinase

Matrix metalloproteinase (MMP) family, and their natural inhibitors (TIMPs) contribute to the regulation of tumor microenvironment and play a key role in angiogenesis and tumor growth. Tissue inhibitors of metalloproteinases (TIMP) block proteolytic degradation of extracellular matrix and consequently impede tumor invasion and metastasis. In vivo studies demonstrated that genetic modulation of TIMP-1 could inhibit cellular proliferation and angiogenesis during hepatocarcinogenesis. TIMP-1 overexpression could significantly inhibit the proliferation of hepatocytes in TAg mice. TIMP-1 inhibits TAg-induced hepatocarcinogenesis by altering hepatocellular proliferation and tumor vascularization, without any effect on hepatocyte apoptosis and stromal composition [147].

Repeated injections of DNA plasmids encoding the tissue inhibitors of metalloproteinases (TIMPs) TIMP-2 or TIMP-3, were efficient in inhibiting tumor growth of human HuH7 HCC cells xenografted into nude mice with no treatment-related toxicity. An inhibition of angiogenesis and tumor necrosis accompanied the inhibitory effects of TIMP-2 or TIMP-3 on tumor expansion and invasion. Bystander effect was produced by transfected HuH7 tumor cells mixed with untransfected cells in 1:1 ratio in culture that resulted in killing 98% of cells within 96 h [148].

Su et al [149] confirmed that the vaccine based on chicken homologous MMP-2 as a model antigen could induce both protective and therapeutic antitumor immunity. There was the deposition of autoantibodies against MMP-2 within the tumor. Angiogenesis was apparently inhibited within tumor, and chick CAMs angiogenesis was also inhibited. These findings may provide a vaccine strategy for cancer therapy through the induction of an autoimmune response against MMP-2 in a cross-reaction by the immunization with the single xenogeneic homologous MMP-2 gene.

Several synthetic inhibitors of MMPs show antitumor, antimetastasis and antiangiogenesis effects in various models. A new selective MMP inhibitor, MMI-166, has significant antitumor and antimetastatic effects in tumor growth, angiogenesis and metastasis by reducing and inhibiting angiogenesis in liver with a good synergistic effect with MMC [150].

## Human Macrophage Metalloelastase

A stepwise logistic analysis revealed that human macrophage metalloelastase and VEGF mRNA expression were two independent variables significantly affecting the vascularity of HCC tumors. human macrophage metalloelastase gene expression is significantly associated with hypovascular tumors; moreover, angiogenesis in HCC is not determined by a single factor, but depends on the net balance between human macrophage metalloelastase and VEGF gene expressions [151].

## Conclusion

In tumorigenesis, a network of blood vessels must be formed to sustain the nutrient and oxygen supply that a tumor requires for continued growth [1]. There is a direct correlation between tumor microvessel density and the incidence of metastases, and long-term survival [2–4]. Anti-angiogenesis or anti-angiogenic agents have been regarded as possible therapeutic options.

Anti-angiogenesis research is being translated to the clinic. As Hegedorn reviewed, there are more than thirty angiogenesis inhibitors tested in clinical trials over the last three decades. The key targets of angio-inhibitory therapies are blocking of matrix metalloproteinases (seven trials), VEGF pathways (four trials) and avb3-integrin action (two trials). Other trials evaluate the anti-angiogenic potential of the signaling-inhibitors SU101 and SU6668 to block growth factors receptors for PDGF and:or FGF-2 [7].

In current clinical trials throughout the United States, angiogenesis inhibitors are being used against cancer in combination with conventional chemotherapy or radiotherapy. Angiogenesis inhibitors are also being used in combination with each other. This practice may increase as different angiogenesis inhibitors become more widely available [152].

Angiogenesis plays a key role in almost all the process of HCC, including early stage of hepatocarcinogenesis, development of tumor growth, tumor invasion and metastasis and it is also a valuable predictor for HCC prognosis. Therefore, HCC, a hypervascular tumor, may have a better effect under anti-angiogenesis therapy. This has already been confirmed by experimental studies and clinical trials in HCC treatment by angiogenesis inhibitors such as suramin, BB-94, TNP-740, etc [79,80]. In the future, angiogenesis inhibitors may be added to chemotherapy or to immunotherapy, or to other modalities. Combinations of angiogenesis inhibitors may also be administered together to block HCC cells growth or as an adjuvant therapy to prevent recurrences after surgical resection.

## References


[1] Folkman J. Tumor angiogenesis: therapeutic implications.*N Engl J Med,* 1971;285 (21):1182-6.

[2] Folkman J. Angiogenesis-dependent diseases. *Semin Oncol,* 2001;28 (6):536-42.

[3] Folkman J, Shing Y. Angiogenesis. *J Biol Chem*, 1992;267 (16):10931-4 1992.

[4] Folkman J. Seminars in Medicine of the Beth Israel Hospital, Boston. Clinical applications of research on angiogenesis. *N Engl J Med.* 1995;333 (26):1757-63

[5] Freedman SB, Isner JM. Therapeutic angiogenesis for ischemic cardiovascular disease. *J Mol Cell Cardiol*, 2001;33 (3):379-93.

[6] Siddiqui AJ, Blomberg P, Wardell E, et al. Combination of angiopoietin-1 and vascular endothelial growth factor gene therapy enhances arteriogenesis in the ischemic myocardium. *Biochem Biophys Res Commun,* 2003; 310 (3):1002-9.

[7] Hagedorn M, Bikfalvi A. Target molecules for anti-angiogenic therapy: from basic research to clinical trials. *Crit Rev Oncol Hematol,* 2000;34 (2):89-110. [6]

[8] Belotti D, Vergani V, Drudis T, et al. The microtubule-affecting drug paclitaxel has antiangiogenic activity. *Clin Cancer Res.* 1996 ;2 (11):1843-9,

[9] Hsu C, Chen CN, Chen LT, et al. Low-dose thalidomide treatment for advanced hepatocellular carcinoma. *Oncology,* 2003;65 (3):242-9.

[10] Wang L, Wu WZ, Sun HC, et al. Mechanism of interferon alpha on inhibition of metastasis and angiogenesis of hepatocellular carcinoma after curative resection in nude mice. *J Gastrointest Surg.* 2003;7 (5):587-94

[11] Huang X, Molema G, King S, et al. Tumor infarction in mice by antibody-directed targeting of tissue factor to tumor vasculature . *Science,* 1997;275 (5299):547–50.

[12] Arap W, Pasqualini R, Ruoslahti E. Cancer treatment by targeted drug delivery to tumor vasculature in a mouse model [see comments]. *Science* 1998;279 (5349):377–80.

[13] Plate KH, Breier G, Risau W. Molecular mechanisms of developmental and tumor angiogenesis. *Brain Pathol,* 1994;4:207–218.

[14] Hanahan D, Folkman J. Patterns and emerging mechanisms of the angiogenic switch during tumorigenesis. *Cell,* 1996;86:353–364.

[15] Nagy JA, Brown LF, Senger DR, et al. Pathogenesis of tumor stroma generation: a critical role for leaky blood vessels and fibrin deposition. *Biochim Biophys Acta1*,989;948:305–326.

[16] Sawai Y, Tamura S, Fukui K, et al. Expression of ephrin-B1 in hepatocellular carcinoma: possible involvement in neovascularization. *J Hepatol,* 2003;39 (6):991-6.

[17] Kido C, Sasaki T, Kaneko M. Angiography of primary liver cancer. *Am J Roentgenol Radium Ther Nucl Med*, 1971;113:70–81.

[18] Yamaguchi R, Yano H, Iemura A, et al. Ogasawara S, Haramaki M, Kojiro M. Expression of endothelial growth factor in human hepatocellular carcinoma. *Hepatology,* 1998;28:68-77

[19] Mise M, Arii S, Higashituji H, et al. Clinical significance of vascular endothelial growth factor and basic fibroblast growth factor liver tumor. *Hepatology,* 1996;23 (3):455-64

[20] Morinaga S, Imada T, Shimizu A, et al. Angiogenesis in hepatocellular carcinoma as evaluated by alpha smooth muscle actin immunohistochemistry. *Hepatogastroenterology,* 2001;48 (37):224-8.

[21] Sugimachi K, Tanaka S, Terashi T, et al. The mechanisms of angiogenesis in hepatocellular carcinoma: angiogenic switch during tumor progression. *Surgery,* 2002;131 (Suppl 1):S135–S141.

[22] Senger DR, Galli SJ, Dvorak AM, et al. Tumor cells secrete a vascular that promotes accumulation of ascites fluid. *Science,* 1983; 219:983-985

[23] Ferrara N, Henzel WJ. Pituitary follicular cells secrete a novel heparin-binding growth for vascular endothelial cells. *Biochem Biophys Res Commun,* 1989;161:851-858

[24] Ferrara N, Houck K, Jakeman L, Leung DW. Molecular and biological properties of the vascular endothelial growth factor family of proteins. *Endocr Rev*, 1992;13 (1):18-32.

[25] Ferrara N. Molecular and biological properties of vascular endothelial growth factor. *J Mol Med,* 1999;77 (7):527-43.

[26] Connolly DT, Heuvelman DM, Nelson R, et al. Tumor vascular permeability factor stimulates endothelial cell growth and angiogenesis. *J Clin Invest,* 1989; 84 (5):1470-8.

[27] Gospodarowicz D, Abraham JA, Schilling J. Isolation and characterization of a vascular endothelial cell mitogen producedby pituitary-derived folliculo stellate cells. *Proc Natl Acad Sci U S A,* 1989; 86 (19):7311-5.

[28] Keck PJ, Hauser SD, Krivi G, et al. Vascular permeability factor, an endothelial cell mitogen related to PDGF. *Science,* 1989; 246 (4935):1309-12.

[29] Kitadai Y, Haruma K, Tokutomi T, et al. Significance of vessel count and vascular endothelial growth factor esophageal carcinomas. *Clin. Cancer Res,* 1998;4:2195-2200

[30] Takahashi Y, Cleary KR, Mai M, et al. Significance of vessel count and vascular endothelial growth factor and its receptor (KDR) in intestinal-type gastric cancer. *Clin Cancer Res,* 1996; 2 (10):1679-84

[31] Alitalo K. VEGFR-3 and its ligand VEGF-C are associated with angiogenesis in breast. *Pathol,* 1999;154 (5):1381-90.

[32] Leung DW, Cachianes G, Kuang WJ, et al. Vascular endothelial growth factor is a secreted angiogenic mitogen. *Science,* 1989; 246 (4935):1306–9.

[33] Olofsson B, Pajusola K, Kaipainen A, et al. Vascular endothelial growth factor B, a novel growth factor for endothelial cells. *Proc Natl Acad Sci USA,* 1996; 93 (6):2576–81.

[34] Joukov V, Pajusola K, Kaipainen A, et al. A novel vascular endothelial growth factor, VEGF-C, is a ligand for the Flt4 (VEGFR-3) and KDR (VEGFR-2) receptor tyrosine kinases. *EMBO J,* 1996;15 (7):1751.

[35] Achen MG, Jeltsch M, Kukk E, et al. Vascular endothelial growth factor D (VEGF-D) is a ligand for the tyrosine kinases VEGF receptor 2 (Flk1) and VEGF receptor 3 (Flt4). *Proc Natl Acad Sci USA,* 1998;95 (2):548–53.

[36] Yamada Y, Nezu J, Shimane M, et al. Molecular cloning of a novel vascular endothelial growth factor, VEGF-D. *Genomics,* 1997;42 (3):483–8.

[37] Ogawa S, Oku A, Sawano A, et al. A novel type of vascular endothelial growth factor, VEGF-E (NZ-7 VEGF), preferentially utilizes KDR:Flk-1 receptor and carries a potent mitotic activity without heparin-binding domain. *J Biol Chem,* 1998;273 (47):31273–82

[38] Millauer B, Wizigmann-Voos S, Schnurch H, et al. High affinity VEGF binding and developmental expression suggest Flk-1 as a major regulator of vasculogenesis and angiogenesis. *Cell,* 1993; 72 (6):835-46.

[39] Quinn TP, Peters KG, De Vries C, et al. Fetal liver kinase 1 is a receptor for vascular endothelial growth factor and is selectively expressed in vascular endothelium. *Proc Natl Acad Sci U S A,* 1993;90 (16):7533-7

[40] Barleon B, Hauser S, Schollmann C, et al. Differential expression of the two VEGF receptors flt and KDR in placenta and vascular endothelial cells. *J Cell Biochem,* 1994; 54 (1):56-66.

[41] Maxwell PH, Dachs GU, Gleadle JM, et al. Hypoxia-inducible factor-1 modulates gene expression in solid tumors and influences both angiogenesis. *Proc Natl Acad Sci U S A,* 1997; 94:8104–9

[42] Frank S, Stallmeyer B, Kampfer H, et al. Differential regulation of vascular endothelial growth factor and its receptor fms-like-tyrosine kinase is mediated by nitric oxide in rat renal mesangial cells. *J. Biochem,* 1999;338 ( Pt 2):367-74.

[43] Kang SM, Maeda K, Onoda N, et al. Combined analysis of p53 and vascular endothelial growth factor expression in colorectal carcinoma for determination of tumor vascularity and liver metastasis. *Int J Cancer,* 1997; 74 (5): 502-7.

[44] Pepper MS, Ferrara N, Orci L, et al. Potent synergism between vascular endothelial growth factor and basic fibroblast growth factor in the induction of angiogenesis in vitro. *Biochem Biophys Res Commun,* 1992; 189 (2):824-31.

[45] Pertovaaara L, Kaipainen A, Mustonen T, et al. Vascular endothelial growth factor is induced in response to transforminggrowth factor-beta in fibroblastic and epithelial cells. *J Biol Chem,* 1994;269 (9):6271-4.

[46] Finkenzeller G, Marme D, Weich HA, et al. Platelet-derved growth factor-induced transcription of endothelial growth factor gene is mediated by protein kinase C. *Cancer Res,* 1992; 52: 4821-4823

[47] Paleolog EM, Young S, Stark AC, et al. Modulation of angiogenic vascular endothelial growth factor by tumor necrosis factor alpha and interleukin-1 in rheumatoid arthritis. *Arthritis Rheum,* 1998; 41 (7):1258-65

[48] Nanashima A, Ito M, Sekine I, et al. Significance of angiogenic factors in liver metastatic tumors originating from colorectal cancers. *Dig Dis Sci,* 1998;43 (12):2634-40

[49] Akiyoshi F, Sata M, Suzuki H, et al. Serum vascular endothelial growth factor levels in various liver diseases. *Dig Dis Sci,* 1998;43:41-5

[50] El-Assal ON, Yamanoi A, Soda Y, et al. Clinical significance of microvessel density and vascular endothelial growth factor expression in hepatocellular carcinoma and surrounding liver: possible involvement of vascular endothelial growth factor in the angiogenesis of cirrhotic liver. *Hepatology,* 1998;27:1554-62

[51] Jinno K, Tanimizu M, Hyodo I, et al. Circulating vascular endothelial growth factor (VEGF) is a possible tumor marker for metastasis in human hepatocellular carcinoma. *J Gastroenterol,* 1998; 33 (3):376-82

[52] Flores-Stadler EM, Chou P, Walterhouse D, et al. Hemangiopericytoma of the liver: immunohistochemical observations, expression of angiogenic factors, and review of the literature. *J Pediatr Hematol Oncol,* 1997;19 (5):449-54

[53] Li XM, Tang ZY, Zhou G, et al. Significance of vascular endothelial growth factor mRNA expression in invasion and metastasis of hepatocellular carcinoma. *J Exp Clin Cancer Res,* 1998;17 (1):13-7

[54] Mochida S, Ishikawa K, Toshima K, et al. The mechanisms of hepatic sinusoidal endothelial cell regeneration: a possible communication system associated with vascular endothelial growth factor in liver cells. *J Gastroenterol Hepatol,* 1998 ;13 Suppl:S1-5

[55] Suzuki K, Hayashi N, Miyamoto Y, et al. Expression of vascular permeability factor/vascular endothelial growth factor in human hepatocellular carcinoma. *Cancer Res* 1996 ;56 (13):3004-9

[56] Chow NH, Hsu PI, Lin XZ, et al. Expression of vascular endothelial growth factor in normal liver and hepatocellular carcinoma: an immunohistochemical study. *Hum Pathol,* 1997;28 (6):698-703

[57] Mise M, Arii S, Higashituji H, et al. Clinical significance of vascular endothelial growth factor and basic fibroblast growth factor gene expression in liver tumor. *Hepatology,* 1996;23 (3):455-64

[58] Yoshiji H, Kuriyama S, Yoshii J, et al. Vascular endothelial growth factor tightly regulates in vivo development of murine hepatocellular carcinoma cells. *Hepatology,* 1998 ;28 (6):1489-96

[59] Kanai T, Konno H, Tanaka T, et al. Anti-tumor and anti-metastatic effects of human-vascular-endothelial-growth-factor-neutralizing antibody on human colon and gastric carcinoma xenotransplanted orthotopically into nude mice. *Int J Cancer,* 1998;77 (6):933-6

[60] Konno H, Arai T, Tanaka T, et al. Antitumor effect of a neutralizing antibody to vascular endothelial growth factor on liver metastasis of endocrine neoplasm. *Jpn J Cancer Res,* 1998;89 (9):933-9

[61] Kim KJ, Li B, Winer J, et al. Inhibition of vascular endothelial growth factor-induced angiogenesis suppresses tumour growth in vivo. *Nature,* 1993;362 (6423):841-4

[62] Senger DR, Perruzzi CA, Feder J, et al. A highly conserved vascular permeability factor secreted by a variety of humanand rodent tumor cell lines. *Cancer Res,*1986 ;46 (11):5629-32

[63] Plate KH, Breier G, Weich HA, et al. Vascular endothelial growth factor and glioma angiogenesis: coordinate induction of VEGF receptors, distribution of VEGF protein and possible in vivo regulatory mechanisms. *Int J Cancer,* 1994;59 (4):520-9., 1992.

[64] Tokunaga T, Oshika Y, Abe Y, et al. Vascular endothelial growth factor (VEGF) mRNA isoform expression pattern is correlated with liver metastasis and poor prognosis in colon cancer. *Br J Cancer,* 1998; 77 (6):998-1002

[65] Ishigami SI, Arii S, Furutani M, et al. Predictive value of vascular endothelial growth factor (VEGF) in metastasis and prognosis of human colorectal cancer. *Br J Cancer,* 1998;78 (10):1379-84

[66] Kumar H, Heer K, Lee PW, et al. Preoperative serum vascular endothelial growth factor can predict stage in colorectal cancer. *Clin Cancer Res,* 1998;4 (5):1279-8

[67] Park YN, Kim YB, Yang KM, et al. Park C Increased expression of vascular endothelial growth factor and angiogenesis in the early stage of multistep. *Hepatocarcinogenesis*. 2000;124 (7):1061-5.

[68] Kim KR, Moon HE, Kim KW. Hypoxia-induced angiogenesis in human hepatocellular carcinoma. *J Mol Med,* 2002;80 (11):703-14

[69] Li XM, Tang ZY, Qin LX, et al. Serum vascular endothelial growth factor is a predictor of invasion and metastasis in hepatocellular carcinoma. *J Exp Clin Cancer Res,* 1999;18 (4):511-7.

[70] Zhao J, Hu J, Cai J, et al. Vascular endothelial growth factor expression in serum of patients with hepatocellular carcinoma. *Chin Med J (Engl),* 2003;116 (5):772-6.

[71] Tang ZY, Ye SL, Liu YK, et al. A decade's studies on metastasis of hepatocellular carcinoma. *J Cancer Res Clin Oncol,* 2003;9 (16 Pt 1):6030-7.

[72] Zhou XD. Recurrence and metastasis of hepatocellular carcinoma: progress and prospects. *Hepatobiliary Pancreat Dis Int.* 2002;1 (1):35-41.

[73] Li X, Feng GS, Zheng CS, et al. Influence of transarterial chemoembolization on angiogenesis and expression of vascular endothelial growth factor and basic fibroblast growth factor in rat with Walker-256 transplanted hepatoma: an experimental study. *World J Gastroenterol,* 2003;9 (11):2445-9.76

[74] Iguchi H, Yokota M, Fukutomi M, et al. A possible role of VEGF in osteolytic bone metastasis of hepatocellular carcinoma. *J Exp Clin Cancer Res,* 2002; 21 (3):309-13.

[75] Qin LX, Tang ZY. The prognostic molecular markers in hepatocellular carcinoma. *World J Gastroenterol,* 2002;8 (3):385-92.

[76] Ker CG, Chen HY, Juan CC, et al. Role of angiogenesis in hepatitis and hepatocellular carcinoma.VEGF and HCC carcinogenesis. *Hepatogastroenterology,* 1999;46 (26):646-50.

[77] Chao Y, Li CP, Chau GY, et al. Prognostic significance of vascular endothelial growth factor, basic fibroblast growth factor, and angiogenin in patients with resectable hepatocellular carcinoma after surgery. *Ann Surg Oncol,* 2003;10 (4):355-62.

[78] Poon RT, Ng IO, Lau C, et al. Serum vascular endothelial growth factor predicts venous invasion in hepatocellular carcinoma: a prospective study. *Ann Surg,* 2001;233 (2):227-35.

[79] Qin LX, Tang ZY, Li XM, et al. Effect of antiangiogenic agents on experimental animal models of hepatocellular carcinoma. *Ann Acad Med Singapore,* 1999;28 (1):147-51.

[80] Kin M, Torimura T, Ueno T, et al. Angiogenesis inhibitor TNP-470 suppresses the progression of experimentally-induced hepatocellular carcinoma in rats. *Int J Oncol,* 2000;16 (2):375-82.

[81] Borgstrom P, Bourdon MA, Hillan KJ, et al. Neutralizing anti-vascular endothelial growth factor antibody completely inhibits angiogenesis and growth of human prostate carcinoma micro tumors in vivo. *Prostate,* 1998;35 (1):1–10.

[82] Lin YS, Nguyen C, Mendoza JL, et al. Preclinical pharmacokinetics, interspecies scaling, and tissue distribution of a humanized monoclonal antibody against vascular endothelial growth factor. *J Pharmacol Exp Ther,* 1999;288 (1):371–8.

[83] Presta LG, Chen H, O'Connor SJ, et al. Humanization of an anti-vascular endothelial growth factor monoclonal antibody for the therapy of solid tumors and other disorders. *Cancer Res,* 1997;57 (20):4593–9.

[84] Kang MA, Kim KY, Seol JY, et al. The growth inhibition of hepatoma by gene transfer of antisense vascular endothelial growth factor. *J Gene Med,* 2000;2 (4):289-96.

[85] Tang YC, Li Y, Qian GX. Reduction of tumorigenicity of SMMC-7721 hepatoma cells by vascular endothelial growth factor antisense gene therapy. *World J Gastroenterol,* 2001;7 (1):22-7.

[86] Arora N, Masood R, Zheng T, et al. Vascular endothelial growth factor chimeric toxin is highly active against endothelial cells. *Cancer Res,* 1999;59 (1):183–8.

[87] Thomas AL, Morgan B, Drevs J, et al. Vascular endothelial growth factor receptor tyrosine kinase inhibitors:PTK787/ZK 222584. *Semin Oncol*, 2003;30 (3 Suppl 6):32-8.

[88] Fong TA, Shawver LK, Sun L, et al. SU5416 is a potent and selective inhibitor of the vascular endothelial growth factor receptor (Flk-1:KDR) that inhibits tyrosine kinase

catalysis, tumor vascularization, and growth of multiple tumor types. *Cancer Res,* 1999;59 (1):99–106.

[89] Laird AD, Vajkoczy P, Shawver LK, et al. SU6668 is a potent antiangiogenic and antitumor agent that induces regression of established tumors. *Cancer Res,* 2000;60 (15):4152-60.

[90] McCrudden KW, Hopkins B, Frischer J, et al. Anti-VEGF antibody in experimental hepatoblastoma: suppression of tumor growth and altered angiogenesis. *J Pediatr Surg,* 2003;38 (3):308-14.

[91] Konno H, Arai T, Tanaka T, et al. Antitumor effect of a neutralizing antibody to vascular endothelial growth factor on liver metastasis of endocrine neoplasm. *Jpn J Cancer Res,* 1998;89 (9):933-9.

[92] Tokunaga T, Oshika Y, Abe Y, et al. Vascular endothelial growth factor (VEGF) mRNA isoform expression pattern is correlated with liver metastasis and poor prognosis in colon cancer. *Br J Cancer*, 1998; 77 (6):998-1002.

[93] Ishigami SI, Arii S, Furutani M, Niwano M, Harada T, Mizumoto M, Mori A, Onodera H, Imamura M. Predictive value of vascular endothelial growth factor (VEGF) in metastasis and prognosis of human colorectal cancer. *Br J Cancer,* 1998;78 (10):1379-84.

[94] Kumar H, Heer K, Lee PW, et al. Preoperative serum vascular endothelial growth factor can predict stage in colorectal cancer. *Clin Cancer Res,* 1998; 4 (5):1279-8.

[95] Takahashi Y, Cleary KR, Mai M, et al. Significance of vessel count and vascular endothelial growth factor and its receptor (KDR) in intestinal-type gastric cancer. *Clin Cancer Res,* 1996; 2 (10):1679-84.

[96] Kanai T, Konno H, Tanaka T, et al. Anti-tumor and anti-metastatic effects of human-vascular-endothelial-growth-factor-neutralizing antibody on human colon and gastric carcinoma xenotransplanted orthotopically into nude mice. *Int J Cancer,* 1998;77 (6):933-6.

[97] Iwama A, Hamaguchi I, Hashiyama M, et al. Molecular cloning and characterization of mouse TIE and TEK receptor tyrosine kinase genes and their expression in hematopoietic stem cells. *Biochem Biophys Res Commun*

[98] , 1993;195 (1):301–9.

[99] Schnurch H, Risau W. Expression of tie-2, a member of a novel family of receptor tyrosine kinases, in the endothelial cell lineage. *Development,* 1993;119 (3):957–68.

[100] Korhonen J, Partanen J, Armstrong E, et al. Enhanced expression of the tie receptor tyrosine kinase in endothelial cells during neovascularization. *Blood,* 1992;80 (10):2548–55.

[101] Wong AL, Haroon ZA, Werner S, et al. Tie2 expression and phosphorylation in angiogenic and quiescent adult tissues. *Circ Res,* 1997;81 (4):567–74.

[102] Peters KG, Coogan A, Berry D, et al. Expression of Tie2:Tek in breast tumour vasculature provides a new marker for evaluation of tumour angiogenesis. *Br J Cancer,* 1998;77 (1):51–6.

[103] Stratmann A, Risau W, Plate KH. Cell type-specific expression of angiopoietin-1 and angiopoietin-2 suggests a role in glioblastoma angiogenesis. *Am J Pathol,* 1998; 153 (5):1459–66.

[104] Davis S, Aldrich TH, Jones PF, et al. Isolation of angiopoietin-1, a ligand for the TIE2 receptor, by secretion-trap expression cloning. *Cell*, 1996;87 (7):1161–9.
[105] Suri C, Jones PF, Patan S, et al. Requisite role of angiopoietin-1, a ligand for the TIE2 receptor, during embryonic angiogenesis. *Cell*, 1996; 87 (7):1171–80.
[106] Sugimachi K, Tanaka S, Taguchi K, et al. Angiopoietin switching regulates angiogenesis and progression of human hepatocellular carcinoma. *J Clin Pathol*, 2003; 56 (11):854-60.
[107] Chen L, Yang Z, Wang G, et al. Expression of angiopoietin-2 gene and its receptor Tie2 in hepatocellular carcinoma. *J Tongji Med Univ*, 2001; 21 (3):228-30, 235.
[108] Mitsuhashi N, Shimizu H, Ohtsuka M, et al. Angiopoietins and Tie-2 expression in angiogenesis and proliferation of human hepatocellular carcinoma. *Hepatology*, 2003;37 (5):1105-13.
[109] Peng L, Sun J, Wang WD, et al. Biological effect of ectopic expression of angiopoietin-1 and -2 in hepatocellular carcinoma cell line. *Hepatobiliary Pancreat Dis Int*, 2003; 2 (1):94-7.
[110] Tanaka S, Sugimachi K, Yamashita Y, et al. Angiogenic switch as a molecular target of malignant tumors.*J Gastroenterol*, 2003; 38 Suppl 15:93-7.
[111] Moon WS, Rhyu KH, Kang MJ, et al. Overexpression of VEGF and angiopoietin 2: a key to high vascularity of hepatocellular carcinoma? *Mod Pathol*, 2003;16 (6):552-7.
[112] Jia WD, Xu GL, Xu RN, et al. Octreotide acts as an antitumor angiogenesis compound and suppresses tumor growth in nude mice bearing human hepatocellular carcinoma xenografts. *J Cancer Res Clin Oncol*, 2003;129 (6):327-34.
[113] Chen X, Liu Z, Ai Z. Antineoplastic mechanism of Octreotide action in human hepatoma.*Chin Med J (Engl)*,2001;114 (11):1167-70.
[114] Guo WJ, Zhuang JY, Bai YR, et al. Octreotide augments the effects of hepatic arterial occlusion in treating a rat liver tumor model. *Hepatogastroenterology*, 2003;50 (50):349-53.
[115] Samonakis DN, Moschandreas J, Arnaoutis T, et al.Treatment of hepatocellular carcinoma with long acting somatostatin analogues. *Oncol Rep*, 2002;9 (4):903-7.
[116] Moscetti L, Saltarelli R, Giuliani R, et al.Intra-arterial liver chemotherapy and hormone therapy in malignant insulinoma:case report and review of the literature. *Tumori*, 2000;86 (6):475-9.
[117] Kouroumalis E, Skordilis P, Thermos K, et al. Treatment of hepatocellular carcinoma with octreotide: a randomised controlledstudy. *Gut*, 1998;42 (3):442-7.
[118] Yuen MF, Poon RT, Lai CL, et al.A randomized placebo-controlled study of long-acting octreotide for the treatment of advanced hepatocellular carcinoma. *Hepatology*, 2002;36 (3):687-91.
[119] Lucas R, Holmgren L, Garcia I, et al. Multiple forms of angiostatin induce apoptosis in endothelial cells. *Blood*, 1998;92 (12):4730-41.
[120] O'Reilly MS, Holmgren L, Chen C, et al. Angiostatin inducesand sustains dormancy of human primary tumors in mice. *Nat Med*, 1996;2 (6):689–92.
[121] Sim BK, O'Reilly MS, Liang H, et al. A recombinant human angiostatin protein inhibits experimental primary and metastatic cancer. *Cancer Res*, 1997;57 (7):1329–34.

[122] Ishikawa H, Nakao K, Matsumoto K, et al. Antiangiogenic gene therapy for hepatocellular carcinoma using angiostatin gene. *Hepatology,* 2003;37 (3):696-704.

[123] Xu R, Sun X, Tse LY, et al. Long-term expression of angiostatin suppresses metastatic liver cancer in mice. *Hepatology,* 2003;37 (6):1451-60.

[124] Hohenester E, Sasaki T, Olsen BR, et al. Crystal structure of the angiogenesis inhibitor endostatin at 1.5 A resolution. *EMBO J,* 1998;17 (6):1656–64.

[125] Musso O, Theret N, Heljasvaara R, et al.Tumor hepatocytes and basement membrane-Producing cells specifically express two different forms of the endostatin precursor, collagen XVIII, in human liver cancers. *Hepatology,* 2001;33 (4):868-76.

[126] O'Reilly MS, Boehm T, Shing Y, et al. Endostatin: an endogenous inhibitor of angiogenesis and tumor growth. *Cell,* 1997;88 (2):277–85.

[127] Dhanabal M, Ramchandran R, Volk R, et al. Endostatin: yeast production, mutants, and antitumor effect in renal cell carcinoma. *Cancer Res,* 1999;59 (1):189–97.

[128] Li X, Fu GF, Fan YR, et al. Potent inhibition of angiogenesis and liver tumor growth by administration of an aerosol containing a transferrin-liposome-endostatin complex. *World J Gastroenterol.* 2003;9 (2):262-6.

[129] Li P, Feng Z, Zhang G, et al.Inhibitory effect of recombinant endostatin on angiogenesis and tumor growth of hepatoma. *J Huazhong Univ Sci Technolog Med Sci,* 2003;23 (3):223-6.

[130] Chen CT, Lin J, Li Q, et al. Antiangiogenic gene therapy for cancer via systemic administration of adenoviralvectors expressing secretable endostatin. *Hum Gene Ther,* 2000;11 (14):1983-96.

[131] Ohno T, Kawano K, Sasaki A, et al. Antitumor and antivascular effects of AC-7700, a combretastatin A-4 derivative, against rat liver cancer. *Int J Clin Oncol,* 2002;7 (3):171-6.

[132] te Velde EA, Vogten JM, Gebbink MF, et al. Enhanced antitumour efficacy by combining conventional chemotherapy with angiostatin or endostatin in a liver metastasis model. *Br J Surg,* 2002;89 (10):1302-9.

[133] Kishibe K, Yamada Y, Ogawa K. Production of nerve growth factor by mouse hepatocellular carcinoma cells and expression of TrkA in tumor-associated arteries in mice. *Gastroenterology,* 2002;122 (7):1978-86.

[134] Maru Y, Hirai H, Yoshida M, Takaku F. Overexpression confers an oncogenic potential upon the eph gene. *Oncogene,* 1990;5:445–447.

[135] Ogawa K, Pasqualini R, Lindberg RA, et al. The ephrin-A1 ligand and its receptor, EphA2, are expressed during tumor neovascularization. *Oncogene,* 2000;19:6043–6052.

[136] Sawai Y, Tamura S, Fukui K, et al. Expression of ephrin-B1 in hepatocellular carcinoma: possible involvement in neovascularization. *J Hepatol,* 2003;39 (6):991-6.

[137] Vallee BL, Riordan JF. Organogenesis and angiogenin. *Cell Mol Life Sci*, 1997;53 (10):803–15.

[138] Fett JW, Strydom DJ, Lobb RR, et al. Isolation and characterization of angiogenin, an angiogenic protein from human carcinoma cells. *Biochemistry,* 1985;24 (20):5480–6.

[139] Kurachi K, Davie EW, Strydom DJ, et al. Sequence of the cDNA and gene for angiogenin, a human angiogenesis factor. *Biochemistry,* 1985;24 (20):5494-9.

[140] Xu ZP, Tsuji T, Riordan JF, et al.The nuclear function of angiogenin in endothelial cells is related to rRNA production. *Biochem Biophys Res Commun,* 2002;294 (2):287-92.

[141] Hu GF. Neomycin inhibits angiogenin-induced angiogenesis.*Proc Natl Acad Sci U S A.* 1998;95 (17):9791-5.

[142] Hisai H, Kato J, Kobune M, et al. Increased expression of angiogenin in hepatocellular carcinoma in correlation with tumor vascularity. *Clin Cancer Res,* 2003;9 (13):4852-9.

[143] Li D, Bell J, Brown A, et al. The observation of angiogenin and basic fibroblast growth factor gene expression in human colonic adenocarcinomas, gastric adenocarcinomas, and hepatocellular carcinomas. *J Pathol,* 1994;172 (2):171-5.

[144] Ren Y, Tsui HT, Poon RT, et al. Macrophage migration inhibitory factor: roles in regulating tumor cell migration and expression of angiogenic factors in hepatocellular carcinoma. *Int J Cancer,* 2003;107 (1):22-9.

[145] Wang L, Wu WZ, Sun HC, et al. Mechanism of interferon alpha on inhibition of metastasis and angiogenesis of hepatocellular carcinoma after curative resection in nude mice. *J Gastrointest Surg,* 2003;7 (5):587-94.

[146] Yoshiji H, Kuriyama S, Fukui H. Angiotensin-I-converting enzyme inhibitors may be an alternative anti-angiogenic strategy in the treatment of liver fibrosis and hepatocellular carcinoma.Possible role of vascular endothelial growth factor. *Basel Tumour Biol,* 2002;23 (6):348-56.

[147] Yoshiji H, Yoshii J, Ikenaka Y, et al.Suppression of the renin-angiotensin system attenuates vascular endothelial growth factor-mediated tumor development and angiogenesis in murine hepatocellular carcinoma cells. *Int J Oncol,* 2002;20 (6):1227-31.

[148] Martin DC, Sanchez-Sweatman OH, Ho AT, et al. Transgenic TIMP-1 inhibits simian virus 40 T antigen-induced hepatocarcinogenesis by impairment of hepatocellular proliferation and tumor angiogenesis. *Lab Invest,* 1999;79 (2):225-34.

[149] Tran PL, Vigneron JP, Pericat D, et al. Gene therapy for hepatocellular carcinoma using non-viral vectors composed of bis guanidinium-tren-cholesterol and plasmids encoding the tissue inhibitors of metalloproteinases TIMP-2 and TIMP-3. *Cancer Gene Ther,* 2003;10 (6):435-44.

[150] Su JM, Wei YQ, Tian L, et al. Active immunogene therapy of cancer with vaccine on the basis of chicken homologous matrix metalloproteinase-2. *Cancer Res,* 2003;63 (3):600-7.

[151] Ohta M, Konno H, Tanaka T, et al.Nakamura S.Effect of combination therapy with matrix metalloproteinase inhibitor MMI-166 and mitomycin C on the growth and liver metastasis of human colon cancer. *Jpn J Cancer Res,* 2001;92 (6):688-95.

[152] Gorrin-Rivas MJ, Arii S, Mori A, et al.Implications of human macrophage metalloelastase and vascular endothelial growth factor gene expression in angiogenesis of hepatocellular carcinoma. *Ann Surg,* 2000;231 (1):67-73.

[153] Folkman J, Browder T, Palmblad J. Angiogenesis research: guidelines for translation to clinical application. *Thromb Haemost*, 2001;86 (1):23-33.

In: Liver Cancer: New Research
Editor: Felix Lee, pp. 227-251
ISBN 1-59454-182-5


*Chapter X*

# Research on Angiogenesis in Liver Cancer and its Clinical Implications

***Ronnie T. Poon***
Department of Surgery and Centre for the Study of Liver Disease,
The University of Hong Kong, Pokfulam, Hong Kong, China.

## Abstract

Angiogenesis, the process by which new blood vessels are developed, is known to be fundamental to tumor growth and metastasis. Neovascularization must occur to provide oxygen and nutrients to the tumor cells, and to remove catabolites and carbon dioxide. Furthermore, the immature neovessels enhance tumor cell dissemination into the circulation.

Hepatocellular carcinoma (HCC) is a hypervascular tumor characterized by neovascularization, which plays an important role in the growth and progression of HCC. Angiogenesis provides a target for novel prognostic and therapeutic approaches to HCC. Assessment of microvessel density, which is the density of newly formed vessels, using immunohistochemical staining for specific endothelial cell markers has been shown to provide prognostic information independent of conventional pathological parameters in HCC patients. Assessment of expression of angiogenic factors like vascular endothelial growth factor (VEGF) provides an alternative way of evaluating angiogenic activity of HCC that is more objective compared with microvessel density. Tumor expression of VEGF has been shown to correlate with tumor invasiveness and intrahepatic metastasis in our previous studies. As most angiogenic factors are soluble factors, it is possible to measure the circulating angiogenic factors as an indirect measurement of tumor angiogenic factors. Our previous studies have demonstrated that serum VEGF level does correlate with tumor expression of VEGF, and serum VEGF level can be used as a novel prognostic marker in patients with HCC. Further studies have led to the discovery of new angiogenic factors such as tissue factor in HCC, which may serve as new target for antiangiogenic therapy.

Studies in animal models have also demonstrated the efficacy of antiangiogenic agents in suppressing hepatocarcinogenesis and growth of HCC. Antiangiogenic therapy has already entered clinical trials in HCC patients and holds the promise of providing an effective novel treatment for HCC, which is of great clinical significance because there is no existing effective systemic therapy for HCC. Antiangiogenic therapy also shows promise as an adjuvant or adjunctive therapy in combination with existing surgical or locoregional therapies for HCC.

## INTRODUCTION

Angiogenesis refers to the process of formation of new blood vessels from pre-existing vessels such as capillaries and postcapillary venules. The importance of angiogenesis in tumor growth and metastasis was first described by Folkman in the early 1970s [1]. Subsequent research by Folkman and others has clearly established that tumor growth is angiogenesis dependent [2-5]. The development of neovasculature in the tumor provides two essential functions for the growth and metastasis of a cancer. First, the vessels provide a route for supply of nutrient and oxygen to sustain tumor growth, and excretion of metabolic waste. Without angiogenesis, a tumor can only grow to the size of 2-3 mm [3] with total dependence of its supply of oxygen and nutrient by simple diffusion [1]. The formation of an invasive tumor requires a switch to angiogenic phenotype. Second, the neovessels provide access for tumor cells to enter the circulation. The new capillaries formed in tumors have incomplete basement membrane, facilitating penetration by tumors cells into the circulation [6]. The angiogenesis activity in the tumors has been shown to correlate with metastasis and tumor recurrence after resection in many human cancers [7-11]. The understanding of the critical role of angiogenesis in tumor growth and metastasis has led to the development of a new approach of anticancer therapy that is now under clinical trials. Figure 1 summarizes the role of angiogenesis in the various steps of tumor growth and metastasis.

Hepatocellular carcinoma (HCC) is one of the most common malignancies in the world, with a particularly high prevalence in Asia and Africa. It is one of the most lethal malignancies, and it is currently the second most common cause of cancer death in China. It is one of the most vascular human tumors, and its active neovascularization can be visualized in angiography and used as a diagnostic criterion for HCC (Figure 2). It is intuitive to speculate that tumor angiogenesis plays a critical role in the invasiveness and metastatic potential of HCC. However, research on angiogenesis in liver cancer is relatively lacking compared with other cancers [12]. In this chapter, the recent progress of research on angiogenesis in HCC is reviewed, including some research data from the author's group. The potential clinical implications of research in this area are highlighted.

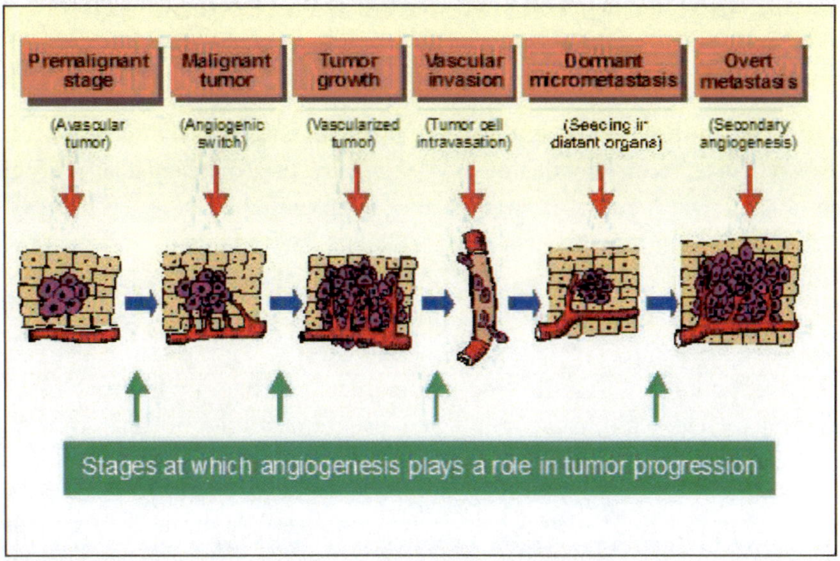


Figure 1. Role of angiogenesis in cancer development, growth and metastasis.
A switch to an angiogenic phenotype is a prerequisite for the development from a premalignant stage to an invasive tumor. The neovascularization provides not only nutrients for tumor growth but also a large surface area of leaky vessels with incomplete basement membrane that facilitate intravasation of tumor cells. Tumor cells seeding in distant organs develop initially as avascular dormant micrometastases. Angiogenic switch leads to secondary angiogenesis and tumor growth, resulting in overt metastases. (Reprinted from reference 92 with permission of American Society of Clinical Oncology)

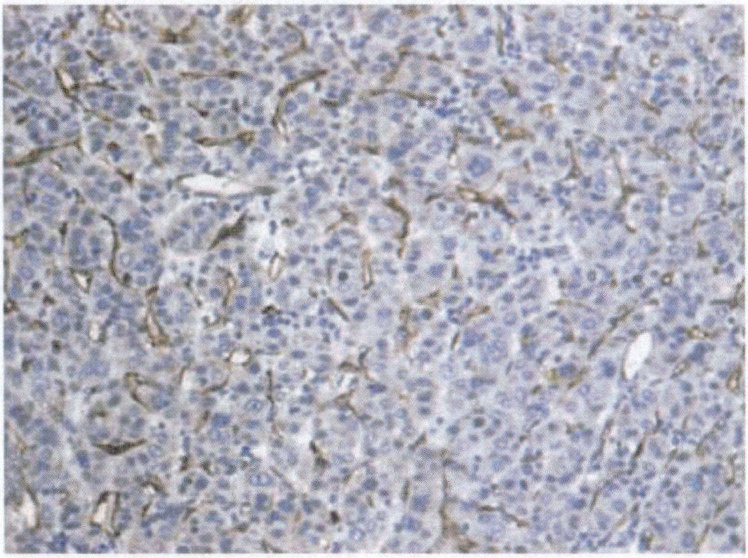

Figure 2. Numerous microvessels stained by anti-CD34 (brownish staining) in a tumor section of hepatocellular carcinoma (magnification x 100).

# General Principles of Regulation of Tumor Angiogenesis

Since the recognition of the importance of angiogenesis in tumor growth by Folkman, active research has been conducted to elucidate the mechanisms controlling tumor angiogenesis [13]. The process of angiogenesis is a complex multi-step process initiated by the release of angiogenic factors from tumor cells. The angiogenic factors bind to specific receptors of endothelial cells of pre-existing blood vessels and activate the endothelial cells, which then secrete enzymes to degrade the underlying basement membrane. Additional proteinases such as matrix metalloproteinases (MMPs) and plasminogen activators are secreted by the tumor cells to degrade the extracellular matrix in front of the sprouting vessels. The activated endothelial cells then proliferate, migrate and assemble into new capillary tubes, followed by the synthesis of a new basement membrane. For many years since the formulation of concept of angiogenesis by Folkman, the new blood vessels in tumors have been presumed to originate from endothelial cells in the pre-existing vessels in surrounding tissues. However, recent studies suggested that some of the neovessels in tumors may be derived from circulating endothelial precursor cells that originate from the bone marrow [14, 15]. There is also evidence indicating that some tumors may be vascularized without significant angiogenesis, probably by using existing vessels through a process described as vascular co-option, or even by forming vascular channels on their own through a non-endothelial cell process called "vascular mimicry" [16]. However, it is still widely accepted that angiogenesis by the sprouting of new blood vessels from pre-existing vessels in surrounding tissues plays the most important role in tumor growth and metastasis in most cancers.

The development of a tumor from an initially dormant phase to a vascularized, rapidly growing phase requires the coordinated activation of genes that results in a switch to an angiogenic phenotype [13]. Tumor cells can secrete a group of proangiogenic polypetides, known as angiogenic factors, which trigger the formation of neovasculature from host vessels. However, tumor cell-derived angiogenic factors are not the only regulators of angiogenesis. The extent of angiogenesis in a tumor is the result of complex interactions of factors released from tumor cells, capillary endothelial cells and infiltrating host cells such as macrophages and fibroblasts. There are also negative regulators of angiogenesis known as antiangiogenic factors. Tumor angiogenesis is the net balanced result of actions of multiple angiogenic and antiangiogenic factors from both tumor cells and host cells in the tumor.

To date, there are more than 30 known endogenous inducers of angiogenesis, and this list is continuously growing. Similarly, there is an expanding list of endogenous inhibitors of angiogenesis. Table 1 lists some of the relatively well-characterized angiogenic and antiangiogenic factors. Vascular endothelial growth factor (VEGF) is one of the first isolated angiogenic peptides, and is also the most potent directly acting angiogenic protein known so far [17]. It has a specific mitogenic effect on endothelial cells, and it also increases vascular permeability (hence also known as vascular permeability factor) and promotes extravasation of proteins from tumor vessels, leading to the formation of a fibrin matrix that supports the growth of endothelial cells and allows invasion of stromal cells into the developing tumor [18]. Tumor-derived VEGF appears to play a central role in the regulation of angiogenesis in tumors. VEGF is the central mediator of tumor angiogenesis stimulated by hypoxia. The secretion of VEGF by tumor cells is stimulated by hypoxia [19]. As solid tumors expand, the cells within the expanding mass frequently become hypoxic because of the increasing distance from the nearest blood vessels, and the VEGF-mediated angiogenesis in response to hypoxia appears to be a general mechanism involved in tumor growth of many types of tumors. The expression of VEGF by tumor cells is also stimulated by activation of oncogenes like *ras* or inactivation of tumor suppressor genes like *p53* [20, 21]. The high endothelial cell specificity of VEGF is related to the expression of its receptors, Flt-1 and KDR, by endothelial cells [22]. However, recent evidence suggested that some tumor cells may also express VEGF receptors, and VEGF may act as an autocrine growth factor in stimulating the proliferation of such cancer cells [23]. Suppression of VEGF-mediated angiogenesis by an anti-VEGF monoclonal antibody has been shown to result in inhibition of tumor growth [24].

**Table 1. Endogenous Angiogenic and Antiangiogenic Factors That Regulate Angiogenesis**

| Angiogenic factors | Antiangiogenic factors |
|---|---|
| Vascular endothelial growth factor | Thrombospondin-1, 2 |
| Acidic and basic fibroblast growth factors | Endostatin |
| Transforming growth factor-α/β | Angiostatin |
| Platelet-derived endothelial cell growth factor | Interferon-α/β |
| Hepatocyte growth factor | Interleukin-12 |
| Tumor necrosis factor-α | Platelet factor 4 fragment |
| Epidermal growth factor | Tissue inhibitor of metalloproteinase -1/2 |
| Placental growth factor | Human macrophage metalloelastase |
| Tissue factor | Anti-thrombin III fragment |
| Interleukin-6/8 | Vascular endothelial growth inhibitor |
| Angiogenin | Vasostatin |
| Angiopoietin-1 | |
| Cyclooxygenase-2 | |
| Macrophage migration inhibitory factor | |
| Nitric oxide | |

Another potent angiogenic factor involved in tumor angiogenesis is fibroblast growth factor (FGF), in particular basic fibroblast growth factor (bFGF). A variety of tumors have been found to express bFGF, and blockade of bFGF receptors also results in suppression of solid tumor growth [25]. Apart from tumor cell-derived bFGF that acts as a paracrine endothelial mitogen, endothelial cells themselves produce and release bFGF, which acts in an autocrine fashion independently [26]. bFGF appears to act synergistically with VEGF in the induction of angiogenesis [27].

In addition to VEGF and bFGF, the process of neovascularization is stimulated by some proangiogenic cytokines known to be secreted by host cells, such as platelet-derived endothelial cell growth factor (PD-ECGF) found in platelets [28], and transforming growth factor β 1 (TGF β 1) produced by macrophages and activated platelets [29]. PD-ECGF stimulates endothelial cell migration rather than proliferation, and its angiogenic effect is mediated by the release of 2-deoxy-D-ribose as a result of breakdown of thymidine by its thymidine phosphorylase activity. TGF β 1 appears to act in a dose-dependent manner, with low concentrations exhibiting a stimulatory and high concentrations exhibiting an inhibitory effect on angiogenesis [30]. Epidermal growth factor (EGF) is a mitogenic growth factor important in the proliferation of both normal and tumor cells, and it has also been found to have a proangiogenic activity [31]. Angiopoietin 1 and 2 belong to a new family of angiogenic factors recently identified [32, 33]. It has been shown to function as ligands for the Tie-2 vascular endothelial-specific receptor, which regulates endothelial interactions with periendothelial support cells and is required for vascular maturation to occur [34]. Recently, it has been discovered that cyclooxygenase-2 (Cox-2), an enzyme known to regulate cellular processes such as apoptosis, also has an angiogenic effect via thromboxane-A2 pathway [35]. Several proteins generated by the hemostatic system are now recognized to play a regulatory role in angiogenesis [36]. For example, tissue factor is a primary physiological initiator of blood coagulation that has been shown to enhance tumor angiogenesis. Although tissue factor normally safeguards vascular integrity by inducing hemostasis in wounds, abnormal expression of tissue factor in different tumors and related vascular endothelial cells contributes to unnecessary clot formation in cancer patients and plays a key role in the thrombotic tendency observed in many cancer patients [37]. Clotting-dependent induction of tumor angiogenesis is primarily mediated by tissue factor induced generation of thrombin and subsequent deposition of a cross-linked fibrin network, which provides a proangiogenic matrix that facilitates blood vessel infiltration.

Among the antiangiogenic factors, thrombospondin is one that has been relatively well characterized. It is a glycoprotein that is secreted by many cells, such as endothelial cells, fibroblasts, monocytes and macrophages [38]. It is a potent inhibitor of endothelial cell growth, and has been shown to be downregulated during tumorogenesis [39]. However, recent evidence suggested that thrombospondin has a dose-dependent bi-phasic effect on angiogenesis; it stimulates endothelial cell migration at low concentrations and is inhibitory at high concentrations [40]. Another two important antiangiogenic factors isolated from tumors are angiostatin and endostatin [41, 42]. Angiostatin is a 38-kDa internal fragment of plasminogen, [41] and endostatin is a protein fragment of collagen XVIII [42]. Administration of either agent has been shown to inhibit the growth of metastasis [41, 42].

# REGULATION OF ANGIOGENESIS IN HCC

## Epidermal Growth Factor

A Japanese group first reported overexpression of two angiogenic factors, EGF and FGF in human HCC in 1991 [43]. In the nontumorous tissue, EGF was not expressed, whereas FGF was weakly positive. Another Japanese group confirmed overexpression of EGF protein by Northern hybridization in tumor cells of 17 specimens of human HCC, whereas none of another 10 specimens of metastatic adenocarcinoma in the liver expressed EGF [44]. This suggested that EGF might play a role in the development or progression of HCC. A recent experimental study showed that inhibition of EGF activity by an EGR receptor tyrosine kinase inhibited the growth of implanted HCC and intrahepatic metastasis in a murine HCC model [45]. However, the role of EGF in angiogenesis of HCC remains unclear because EGF can also promote tumor growth by directly stimulating tumor cell proliferation.

## Basic Fibroblast Growth Factor

Motoo et al [46]. showed that expression of von Willebrand factor, an endothelial cell marker, was significantly higher in FGF-positive tumors compared with FGF-negative tumors. The expression of von Willebrand factor is not usually seen in sinusoids in normal liver but is frequently found in HCC, which is referred to as 'capillarization' of sinusoids, and its expression increases stepwise in the process of hepatocarcinogenesis [47]. Motoo's finding suggested that FGF may be involved in the angiogenesis during hepatocarcinogenesis. Mise et al. demonstrated overexpression of bFGF but not acidic FGF in 9 of 20 HCC specimens, and their study also showed a positive correlation between bFGF mRNA levels and capsular infiltration by tumor cells, but there was no significant correlation between bFGF mRNA levels and the intensity of tumor staining in angiograms [48]. El-Assal et al. found that expression of bFGF protein in human HCC specimens correlated with tumor angiogenesis, suggesting that bFGF is a potent angiogenic factor in HCC [49]. Recently bFGF has also been shown to act as a mitogen for HCC cell proliferation via an autocrine mechanism in addition to its angiogenic effect [50]. bFGF plays a significant role in the development and progression of HCC, and it appears that bFGF has both an autocrine effect on HCC cell proliferation and a paracrine effect on endothelial proliferation. A study in murine HCC showed that bFGF synergistically augments VEGF-mediated HCC development and angiogenesis at least partly by induction of VEGF through KDR/Flk-1 [51].

## Vascular Endothelial Growth Factor

The most widely studied angiogenic factor in HCC is VEGF, which is one of the most important angiogenic factors in tumor angiogenesis. Mise et al [48]. first reported overexpression of VEGF by Northern blot analysis and immunohistochemical staining in 12 of 20 human HCC specimens compared with nontumorous liver tissue, and the level of

VEGF mRNA was found to be significantly correlated with the intensity of angiographic tumor staining. A subsequent study also demonstrated a strong association between VEGF immunostaining and angiographic vascularity, which suggested an important role of VEGF in the development of neovascularization in HCC [52]. Another study using the technique of in-situ hybridization confirmed the expression of VEGF mRNA by HCC tumor cells, especially in areas adjacent to tumor necrosis, where the VEGF expression may be stimulated by local hypoxia [53]. The expression of VEGF in hypoxic area of HCC may be upregulated through the hypoxia inducible factor 1-alpha pathway [54]. Chow et al. examined the correlation between VEGF expression and clinicopathologic features in 36 cases of HCC using a logistic regression model and found a significant association between high VEGF expression and a high proliferative index and portal vein thrombosis [55]. Their findings suggested that VEGF might be an important mediator in the progression and vascular invasion of HCC. A study by another Chinese group also demonstrated that high tumor VEGF expression was associated with venous tumor emboli or poor encapsulation of tumors in HCC [56]. More recently, it has been demonstrated that overexpression of VEGF in tumor cells correlated strongly with tumor angiogenesis in HCC [57]. Another recent study showed that tumor angiogenesis in HCC was significantly higher than that in metastatic liver tumors, and VEGF mRNA expression correlated significantly with angiogenesis only in HCC [54]. The critical role of VEGF in angiogenesis was also demonstrated in an experimental model in which the VEGF gene expression was manipulated in murine HCC cells transfected with a retroviral vector system carrying the gene [58]. In this experiment, the growth and neovascularization of the HCC tumor was shown to correspond directly to the level of VEGF gene expression.

While the above studies have provided strong evidence for the role of VEGF in the development and progression of HCC, conflicting results have been reported by some studies. Torimura et al. reported a significant association between high VEGF immunostaining and poorly differentiated HCCs [52], whereas Yamaguchi et al. found that VEGF expression was the highest among well-differentiated HCCs [59]. In a study of 71 patients with resection of HCC, El-Assal et al. found that neither VEGF mRNA nor VEGF protein expression in tumors correlated with any histopathologic features such as histological grade, tumor encapsulation and venous invasion [60]. Another study found no significant difference in VEGF expression between HCC tumor and adjacent nontumorous liver in patients with chronic hepatitis C [61]. The discrepancies in results among various studies remain unresolved. The use of tumor specimens of different size and etiology in these studies could be one factor.

The effect of VEGF on angiogenesis depends not only on tumor cell expression of VEGF, but also on the VEGF receptors in the endothelial cells. There are two VEGF receptors expressed in endothelial cells, flk-1 or flt-1 [17]. A recent study from our group demonstrated differential upregulation of Flt-1 receptor in 50 specimens of HCC [62]. The level of Flt-1 mRNA but not Flk-1 mRNA significantly correlated with the VEGF mRNA level and intrahepatic metastasis in HCC. Our findings suggested that Flt-1 may play a more important role in VEGF-receptor interaction in the angiogenesis of HCC. The requisite role of VEGF receptors in angiogenesis of HCC was supported by a study of another group [63].

## Angiopoietin-2

Angiopoietin-2 appears to be another important regulator of angiogenesis in HCC. Tanaka et al. showed that angiopoietin-2 was highly expressed in HCC tumors but not in nontumorous liver tissues, and high expression of angiopoietin-2 was associated with clinically hypervascular tumors [64]. The same group reported expression of the receptor for angiopoietin-2, Tie-2 receptor, in 80% of neovascular endothelium in HCC. Furthermore, the authors demonstrated that inhibition of Tie-2 receptor in a murine HCC model resulted in suppression of tumorigenicity and neovascularization [65]. Subsequently, another group confirmed upregulation of angiopoietin-2, but not angiopoietin-1, in HCC, and it was demonstrated that increased expression of angiopoietin-2 correlated with tumor angiogenesis and portal vein invasion [66]. The positive correlation between angiopoietin-2 expression and tumor angiogenesis in HCC was reproduced in another study, which also reported a strong positive correlation between VEGF and angiopoietin-2 expression in HCC [57]. Zhao et al. reported that both angiopoietin-2 and VEGF were upregulated in HCC and the margin of the tumor, and so were their respective receptors Tie2 and KDR [67]. However, the mechanism responsible for regulation of angiopoietin-2 expression appears to be different from that of VEGF in HCC. In one study that also reported a positive correlation between expression of angiopoietin-2 and tumor vascularity in HCC, hypoxia was found to stimulate the expression of VEGF but not that of angiopoietin-2 in HCC [68].

## Other Angiogenic Factors

Two studies have reported a positive correlation between PD-ECGF expression and portal vein tumor thrombosis in HCC [69, 70]. A further study showed that PD-ECGF expression positively correlated with tumor angiogenesis in HCC [71]. Our group has recently demonstrated the role of tissue factor in tumor angiogenesis of HCC [72]. We studied 58 resected HCC specimens and showed that expression of tissue factor in the tumors correlated significantly with tumor angiogenesis. A significant positive correlation was found between tissue factor and VEGF levels in the tumor cytosol, and high tumor cytosolic tissue factor level was associated with venous invasion, microsatellite nodules, unencapsulated tumor and advanced tumor stage. The role of tissue factor in progression of HCC was corroborated in a study of HCC in a transgenic mouse model, in which tumor angiogenesis was observed to be associated with expression of tissue factor in endothelial cells and invading macrophage in the tumor [73]. Our group has also demonstrated a possible role of macrophage migration inhibitory factor in inducing angiogenesis in HCC via upregulation of VEGF and interleukin-8 [74]. Other authors have demonstrated a role of angiogenin [75] and Cox-2 [76] in angiogenesis of HCC.

### Antiangiogenic Factors

Angiogenesis in HCC is regulated by a number of different angiogenic and antiangiogenic factors. A recent study has shown that angiogenesis in HCC depends on a net balance between expression of VEGF and human matrix metalloelastase, a matrix metalloproteinase responsible for the generation of angiostatin [77]. The role of thrombospondin-1 in HCC is unclear. One study reported that thrombospondin-1 expression in cholangiocarcinoma was higher than that in hypervascular HCC and suggested that enhanced expression of thrombospondin-1 may contribute to the hypovascularity of cholangiocarcinoma [78]. However, in that study, tumor expression of VEGF but not thrombospondin-1 was related to tumor vascularity in HCC. However, in a study by our group, increased expression of thrombospondin-1 was associated with features of tumor invasiveness and advanced tumor stage in HCC [79]. Furthermore, the expression of thrombospondin-1 positively correlated with that of VEGF in the tumors, suggesting that thrombospondin-1 may play a proangiogenic rather than an antiangiogenic role in HCC. Further studies are needed to clarify the role of antiangiogenic factors in HCC.

## Clinical Significance of Angiogenic Activity in HCC

### Prognostic Significance of Tumor Microvessel Density

Since angiogenic activity is closely related to the biological aggressiveness in a cancer, assessment of tumor angiogenesis may predict the risk of metastasis, recurrence and survival after resection of the tumor. Microvessel density (MVD) is a commonly used index of tumor angiogenic activity, in which the density of neovessels is counted in histological sections of the tumor after immunohistochemical staining of certain endothelial markers to visualize the tumor endothelial cells [80]. MVD has been shown to be a prognostic factor independent of conventional tumor pathological features in cancers such as colonic carcinoma [81], gastric carcinoma [82], and breast carcinoma [83].

In HCC, tumor microvessels can be visualized after staining for endothelial cell markers like CD34 (Figure 2) and von Willebrand factor that are specific for tumor endothelial cells, and hence differentiate sinusoid-like tumor vessels from normal sinusoids. In a study of 43 resected HCC specimens, Tanigawa et al. showed that intense staining of sinusoid-like vessels was obtained in all of the tumors using CD34 staining, whereas anti-von Willebrand factor only reacted with large vessels in 18 tumors and stained only a few of sinusoid-like vessels [84]. The same study demonstrated that MVD by CD34 staining was an independent prognostic factor of patient survival after resection of HCC. However, another study of MVD by CD34 staining in 40 patients with resection of HCC did not reveal any significant correlation between tumor MVD and pathological features dictating the aggressiveness of the tumor, such as portal vein invasion and tumor stage [85]. A recent study of 71 patients with HCC by El-Assal et al., however, has demonstrated that the MVD as assessed by staining using factor VIII-related antigen was a significant predictor of intrahepatic recurrence after curative resection, and was an independent prognostic factor for disease-free survival [60].

The same group reported in another study that MVD assessed by factor VIII-related antigen staining but not by CD34 staining was a significant prognostic factor of disease-free survival after resection of HCC [86]. Ker et al. also studied MVD in HCC using staining for factor VIII-related antigen, and they showed a trend toward early recurrence after resection of HCC in patients with a high tumor MVD [87]. Whether MVD evaluated by CD34 or MVD evaluated by von Willebrand factor staining provides better prognostic information in HCC remains debatable. Two studies using CD34 as the endothelial marker, one from the author's group and the other from a Shanghai group, both reported that a high MVD was a significant predictor of poor disease-free survival after resection of small HCC ≤ 5 cm in diameter (Figure 3) [88, 89]. The use of an angiogenic index to predict recurrence is not only important for prognostic information, but it may also help select patients at high-risk of early recurrence for adjuvant therapy. A recent study showed that enhancement imaging features of HCC on spiral contrast computed tomography scan correlated with tumor MVD observed with immunohistochemical staining, suggesting that in vivo imaging assessment of tumor neovascularity may provide an alternative to study of MVD in evaluating tumor angiogenesis [90].

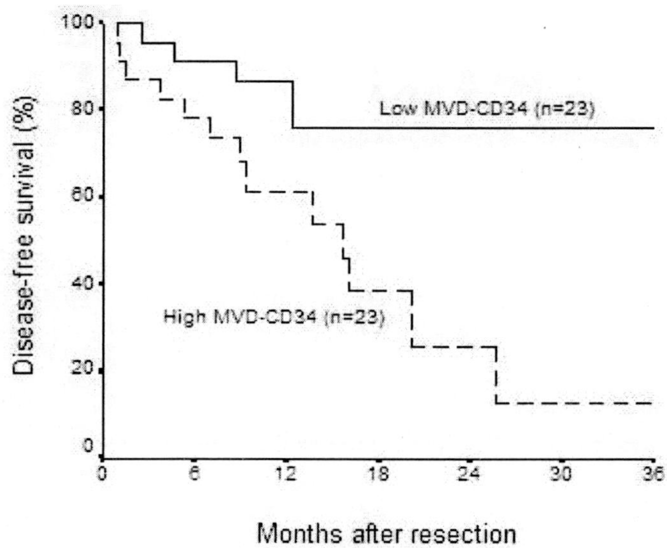


Figure 3. Disease-free survival after hepatic resection in patients with hepatocellular carcinoma ≤ 5 cm in diameter stratified into low and high microvessel density by CD34 immunostaining (MVD-CD34), respectively ($P = 0.002$). (Reprinted from reference 89 with permission of American Society of Clinical Oncology)

## Prognostic Significance of Tumor Expression of Angiogenic and Antiangiogenic Factors

Apart from direct histological evaluation of tumor MVD, evaluation of tumor expression of angiogenic factor may also provide useful prognostic information. This method may potentially reduce the subjective bias associated with the counting of microvessels for MVD evaluation, A high VEGF expression in HCC was reported to be associated with portal vein tumor thrombosis [56, 69]. A recent study has demonstrated that tumor expression of VEGF mRNA correlated significantly with risk of tumor recurrence after resection of HCC by multivariate analysis [91].

Measurement of serum or plasma concentration of angiogenic factors has been used as an indirect measure of tumor angiogenic activity. The majority of angiogenic factors are soluble and diffusible peptides. Hence, the circulating level of angiogenic factors could theoretically reflect the angiogenic activity of the tumor. Compared with the evaluation of tumor MVD or tumor expression of angiogenic factors, the measurement of circulating angiogenic factors has the advantage of being a convenient and non-invasive approach that does not require tumor specimens. Furthermore, repeated measurements before and after therapy is possible. Several studies have revealed a predictive value of serum VEGF level for disease progression and prognosis in human cancers of different origins [92]. A study by Jinno et al. has shown that the plasma VEGF level was significantly elevated in patients with HCC compared with normal control or patients with benign chronic liver disease, and patients with distant metastasis had significantly elevated plasma VEGF level compared with those who had earlier stage disease [93]. The same group also demonstrated that plasma PD-ECGF was significantly elevated in patients with HCC, and the level was higher in advanced stage disease compared with earlier stage disease [94]. Hsu et al. found that serum bFGF level was significantly higher in patients with HCC compared with normal control or chronic liver disease, and they also showed a higher bFGF level in association with advanced HCC stage [95]. Several studies have recently reported the prognostic value of the circulating levels of VEGF in patients undergoing hepatectomy for HCC. Our group has demonstrated in a prospective study of 100 patients with HCC undergoing hepatic resection that a high preoperative serum VEGF level is predictive of microscopic venous invasion [96]. Our findings corroborated with those of a retrospective study previously reported by another Chinese group, who found that high serum VEGF levels were significantly associated with portal vein tumor emboli [97]. In a more recent study, we confirmed that the serum VEGF level could be used as a surrogate marker to reflect tumor expression of VEGF in HCC (Figure 4) [98]. Another group has shown that a high preoperative serum VEGF level was a predictor of disease-free and overall survival after resection of HCC independent of conventional clinicopathological features [99]. While most studies measured the level of VEGF protein in the circulation by enzyme-linked immunosorbent assay, a recent study reported that the circulating VEGF mRNA level measured by a reverse- transcription polymerase chain reaction based assay could also predict tumor recurrence [100].

There are few data on the prognostic significance of other angiogenic or antiangiogenic factors in HCC. Our group showed that a high preoperative serum bFGF level predicted invasive tumor and early postoperative recurrence independent of tumor size [101]. One study reported that high serum endostatin level was inversely correlated with tumor angiogenic score and was positively correlated with tumor endostatin expression, suggesting that serum endostatin level may reflect the antiangiogenic activity of endostatin in HCC tumors [102]. However, another study reported that serum endostatin level was not significantly elevated in HCC patients compared with healthy control subjects, and serum endostatin levels did not correlate with tumor stage [103]. In accordance with the finding of the later study, our group found that serum endostatin level in HCC patients was not significantly higher than that of healthy controls and did not provide any prognostic value in HCC patients, whereas serum VEGF level was a significant prognostic factor in HCC patients after tumor resection [104].

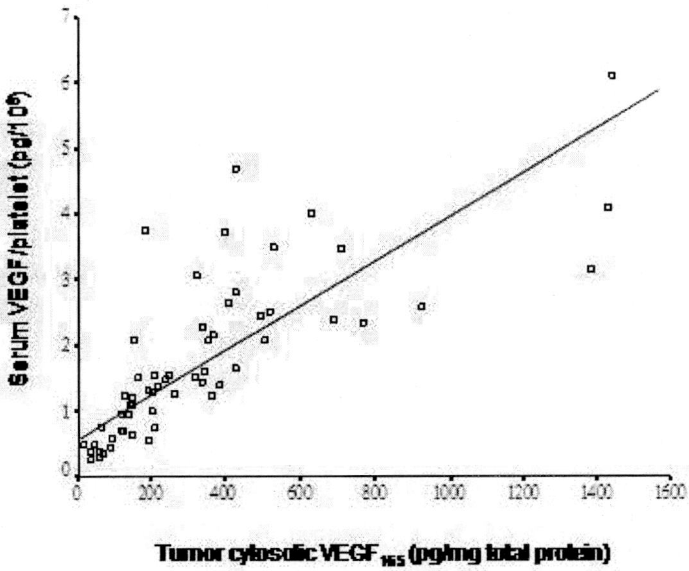


Figure 4. Positive correlation between serum VEGF/platelet and tumor cytosolic VEGF protein content in 60 patients with hepatocellular carcinoma (r = 0.447, $P = 0.006$). Serum VEGF/platelet is used instead of serum VEGF because platelet appears to serve as storage of circulating VEGF, and serum VEGF level correlates positively with platelet count. (Reprinted from reference 98 with permission of American Association for Cancer Research)

As tumor growth depends on angiogenesis, the rate of tumor cell proliferation is related to angiogenic activity. Hence, there may be a relationship between the angiogenic activity of a tumor and its responsiveness to cytotoxic drugs or radiotherapy. One potential clinical application of assessing tumor angiogenic activity is to predict tumor response to conventional chemotherapy or radiotherapy. A recent study showed that high pre-treatment serum VEGF levels were predictive of poor response and survival in patients undergoing chemoirradiation for esophageal squamous cell carcinoma [105]. We recently evaluated the pretreatment serum VEGF levels of 80 patients with HCC undergoing transarterial chemoembolization and observed that a high pretreatment serum VEGF level was predictive of poor response to chemoembolization [106]. Serum VEGF level may be a useful biological marker for selection of patients for the various treatment available for HCC.

The current staging systems, such as the widely used tumor-node-metastasis system based on conventional pathological features for HCC, are suboptimal as the survival of patients can vary widely within the same stage [107]. The assessment of tumor angiogenesis can provide supplementary prognostic information. It may have a particular value in identifying a subset of patients with early HCC, such as those with small HCC < 5 cm in diameter, who may in fact run a more malignant clinical course [89]. The ability to assess tumor angiogenic activity before surgery by measuring circulating angiogenic factors may help select patients for preoperative neoadjuvant therapies, which may include antiangiogenic therapy. It may also aid in selection of patients for the most suitable treatment among various options such as liver transplantation, resection and locoregional therapies.

## Antiangiogenic Therapy and its Potential Role in HCC

Tumor cells were the target of conventional cytotoxic chemotherapy. The proliferating endothelial cells provide a second target for a novel anticancer therapy that may have the following theoretical advantages over cytotoxic chemotherapy: 1. The microvascular endothelial cells are genetically stable cells with an extremely low mutation rate, and hence drugs targeted at the endothelial cells are less likely than cytotoxic drugs to induce drug resistance; 2. Since antiangiogenic therapy targets specific immature characteristics of tumor vasculature, which differs from normal quiescent vasculature, little or no toxicity has been demonstrated in pre-clinical studies; 3. Endothelial cells are directly exposed to blood borne agents, circumventing the problem of drug delivery to tumor cells, which is a major obstacle to conventional anticancer therapy. Antiangiogenic treatment is potentially applicable to all solid tumors irrespective of the origin of the tumor cells.

The discovery of two potent endogenous inhibitors of angiogenesis produced by the tumor itself, angiostatin and endostatin, has generated great interest in the clinical use of antiangiogenic therapy in recent years [41, 42]. In an animal study, endostatin has been demonstrated to suppress tumor growth in mice without inducing acquired drug resistance [108]. This study also showed that antiangiogenic therapy may lead to tumor regression, although antiangiogenic therapy is predominantly a cytostatic rather than cytotoxic treatment.

There are different approaches that can be employed in antiangiogenic therapy. The first approach is to block the effect of angiogenic factors, of which VEGF has been most commonly targeted. A group of investigators have successfully inhibited growth of HCC xenotransplant in nude mice model using VEGF-targeted gene therapy by gene transfer of antisense VEGF [109]. Some clinically available drugs previously known for other effects are now recognized to have an antiangiogenic effect as well. For example, interferon-alpha is an immunomodulatory agent that has been used in the treatment of unresectable hepatocellular carcinoma, and it has been recently reported that interferon-alpha inhibits the growth of human hepatocellular carcinoma implanted in nude mice by an antiangiogenic effect probably mediated by inhibition of bFGF and VEGF production [110]. Our group has studied the effect of PTK 787, an tyrosine kinase inhibitor of VEGF receptors currently under clinical trial in colorectal cancer [111], on HCC xenografts in nude mice. We found that PTK 787 significantly inhibited growth of tumor xenografts derived from inoculation PLC and Hep3B HCC cells, and PTK 787 resulted in a significant decrease in tumor MVD compared with untreated control group (unpublished data).

A second approach of antiangiogenic therapy is to use drugs that directly inhibit the proliferation of endothelial cells. TNP-470, a fumagillin analogue that can inhibit endothelial cell proliferation, has been shown to suppress the growth and metastasis of human HCC xenotransplant in animal model [112].

A third approach is to use drugs that prevent the degradation of extracellular matrix and basal membrane, a step essential for angiogenesis. For example, Batimastat is a MMP inhibitor that has been shown to be effective in inhibiting growth, invasion and metastasis of human HCC in nude mice model [113].

A fourth approach is to inhibit vascular cellular adhesion molecules such as integrin $\alpha_v\beta_3$ [114]. Finally, naturally occurring antiangiogenic factors such as angiostatin and endostatin may also be used in antiangiogenic therapy. A recent study has shown that tumor growth of implanted HCC in athymic mice was suppressed in mice implanted with angiostatin gene-transfected cells, and such suppression was proportional with the percentage of transfected cells [115]. Analysis of the vascular density in the tumors showed that the tumor growth suppression effect of angiostatin gene correlated with suppression of tumor vascularity.

The main aim of antiangiogenic therapy is to reduce tumors to relatively small dormant clusters of cells which have low metastatic potential, and which may be more susceptible to other anticancer therapies like chemotherapy and radiotherapy.

In the context of surgical resection of a primary tumor, antiangiogenic therapy may be useful in maintaining dormancy of micrometastasis and preventing the development of overt recurrence or metastatic lesions. Antiangiogenic therapy may also have a potential role of preventing the development of premalignant or dysplastic lesions into malignant tumors, as angiogenic switch is an essential step during multistage tumorigenesis. Kin et al [116] demonstrated suppression of the development and progression of HCC in cirrhotic liver by TNP-470 in an animal model without any influence on the underlying cirrhosis or liver function. Another study also showed that TNP-470 was effective in suppressing the development of carcinogen-induced hepatic nodules into HCC [117]. These studies suggest that antiangiogenic therapy could be useful as chemoprevention of HCC in patients with underlying cirrhosis apart from its potential role in treating established HCC. Of interest is the recent finding that VEGF may play an important role in the progression of cirrhosis. In a study on an animal model of cirrhosis induced by carbon tetrachloride, neutralizing antibodies of VEGF significantly reduced the development of fibrosis associated with suppression of neovascularization in the liver [118].

The use of antiangiogenic therapy for cancer has been translated from animal studies to clinical trials in recent years. Many antiangiogenic agents have already entered phase I, II or III clinical trials in patients with various kinds of cancer [119]. There is preliminary evidence that clinical use of antiangiogenic agents such as thalidomide may inhibit the progression of HCC [120]. Preliminary data from a phase II study of thalidomide for unresectable hepatocellular carcinoma showed that, among 20 patients who received the treatment, one (5%) complete response, one (5%) partial response and seven (35%) stable diseases for more than two months were observed [121]. Currently there is no effective systemic chemotherapy for HCC [122]. The development of a novel effective systemic therapy for HCC is of paramount clinical importance. However, the search for an effective antiangiogenic treatment for advanced HCC in humans is going to be much more difficult that what could be expected from animal studies. Antiangiogenic drugs that work on animal tumor models may not work in human cancer patients because the drugs are usually given in the early stage of tumor development in animal models, whereas the large tumor load and end-stage tumors in patients with inoperable HCC may defy an antiangiogenic drug that works in animal HCC models.

For example, octreotide has been shown to inhibit HCC growth in nude mice via an antiangiogenic effect [123]. However, a human trial conducted by our group showed that it was not effective in prolonging survival of patients with inoperable advanced HCC. [124] Since antiangiogenic therapy is mainly a cytostatic therapy, it is reasonable to speculate that it may work better when combined with a cytotoxic therapy. Transarterial chemoembolization is a proven effective therapy for HCC localized to the liver [122]. However, response to TACE is still suboptimal and this may be related to upregulated expression of VEGF by the surviving tumor cells in response to hypoxia, which causes continuous tumor growth in some cases [125]. Addition of antiangiogenic therapy may enhance the therapeutic efficacy of chemoembolization. According to the National Cancer Institute Database of clinical trials, a trial on the use of thalidomide as an adjunctive therapy to transarterial chemoembolization for unresectable HCC is underway in the United States. Such trials will provide important data on the role of antiangiogenic therapy in HCC. Currently, the recurrence rate is high after resection of HCC due to a high incidence of vascular invasion and intrahepatic metastasis, and chemotherapy has not been shown to be effective in preventing tumor recurrence [126]. An area of potential application of antiangiogenic therapy for HCC is as an adjuvant therapy to prevent recurrence after hepatic resection.

## Conclusions

Overall, the current evidence suggests that angiogenesis plays an important role in the aggressive biological behavior of HCC. However, the exact regulatory mechanism remains to be clarified. Further studies elucidating the mechanism involved in angiogenesis of HCC are not only crucial to our understanding of the tumor biology of HCC, but also helps provide guidance to the use of appropriate antiangiogenic agents for HCC. Study of angiogenesis in HCC may also afford a novel approach for prognostication. Antiangiogenic therapy is one of the most promising novel strategies for treating cancers, and the results of the on-going clinical trials in patients with HCC will help clarify the role of antiangiogenic therapy in this highly vascular and invasive malignancy.

## References

[1] Folkman J. Tumor angiogenesis: therapeutic implications. *N Engl J Med* 1971; 285: 1182-1186.
[2] Folkman J. What is the evidence that tumors are angiogenesis dependent? *J Natl Cancer Inst* 1990; 82: 4-6.
[3] Hori A, Sasada R, Matsutani E. Suppression of solid tumor growth by immunoneutralizing monoclonal antibody against human basic fibroblast growth factor on tumor growth in vivo. *J Natl Cancer Inst* 1993; 85: 121-131.

[4] Kim KJ, Li B, Winer J, Armanini M, Gillett N, Phillips HS, Ferrara N. Inhibition of vascular endothelial growth factor-induced angiogenesis suppresses tumour growth in vivo. *Nature* 1993; 362: 841-844.

[5] Millauer B, Shawver LK, Plate KH, Risau W, Ullrich A. Glioblastoma growth inhibited in vivo by a dominant-negative Flk-1 mutant. *Nature* 1994; 367: 576-579.

[6] Liotta LA, Stracke ML. Tumor invasion and metastases: biochemical mechanisms. *Cancer Treat Res* 1988; 40: 223-238.

[7] Weidner N, Semple JP, Welch WR, Folkman J. Tumor angiogenesis and metastasis-correlation in invasive breast carcinoma. *N Engl J Med* 1991; 324: 1-8.

[8] Macchiarini P, Fontanini G, Hardin MJ, Squartini F, Angeletti CA. Relation of neovascularization to metastasis of non-small-cell lung cancer. *Lancet* 1992; 340: 145-146.

[9] Weidner N, Carroll PR, Flax J, Blumenfeld W, Folkman J. Tumor angiogenesis correlates with metastasis in invasive prostate carcinoma. *Am J Pathol* 1993; 143: 401-409.

[10] Olivarez D, Ulbright T, DeRiese W, Foster R, Reister T, Einhorn L, Sledge G. Neovascularization in clinical stage A testicular germ cell tumor: prediction of metastatic disease. *Cancer Res* 1994; 54: 2800-2802.

[11] Tanigawa N, Amaya H, Matsumura M, Shimomatsuya T, Horiuchi T, Muraoka R, Iki M. Extent of tumor vascularization correlates with prognosis and hematogenous metastasis in gastric carcinomas. *Cancer Res* 1996; 56: 2671-2676.

[12] Poon RT, Fan ST, Wong J. Clinical significance of angiogenesis in gastrointestinal cancers: a target for novel prognostic and therapeutic approaches. *Ann Surg* 2003; 238: 9-28.

[13] Hanahan D, Folkman J. Patterns and emerging mechanisms of the angiogenic switch during tumorigenesis. *Cell* 1996; 86: 353-364.

[14] Shi Q, Rafii S, Wu MH, Wijelath ES, Yu C, Ishida A, Fujita Y, Kothari S, Mohle R, Sauvage LR, Moore MA, Storb RF, Hammond WP. Evidence for circulating bone marrow-derived endothelial cells. *Blood* 1998; 92: 362-367.

[15] Asahara T, Masuda H, Takahashi T, Kalka C, Pastore C, Silver M, Kearne M, Magner M, Isner JM. Bone marrow origin of endothelial cell progenitor cells responsible for postnatal vasculogenesis in physiological and pathological neovascularization. *Circ Res* 1999; 85: 221-228.

[16] Ribatti D, Vacca A, Dammacco F. New non-angiogenesis dependent pathways for tumour growth. *Eur J Cancer* 2003; 39: 1835-1841.

[17] Neufeld G, Cohen T, Gengrinovitch S, Poltorak Z. Vascular endothelial growth factor (VEGF) and its receptors. *FASEB J* 1999; 13: 9-22.

[18] Dvorak HF, Nagy JA, Berse B, Brown LF, Yeo KT, Yeo TK, Dvorak AM, van de Water L, Sioussat TM, Senger DR. Vascular permeability factor, fibrin, and the pathogenesis of the tumor stroma formation. *Ann N Y Acad Sci* 1992; 667: 101-111.

Shweiki D, Neeman M, Itin A, Keshet E. Induction of vascular endothelial growth factor expression by hypoxia and by glucose deficiency in multicell spheroids: implications for tumor angiogenesis. *Proc Natl Acad Sci USA* 1995; 92: 768-772.

[19] Rak J, Mitsuhashi Y, Bayko L, Filmus J, Shirasawa S, Sasazuki T, Kerbel RS. Mutant ras oncogenes upregulate VEGF/VPF expression: implications for induction and inhibition of tumor angiogenesis. *Cancer Res* 1995; 55: 4575-4580.

[20] Kieser A, Weich HA, Brandner G, Marme D, Kolch W. Mutant p53 potentiates protein kinase C induction of vascular endothelial growth factor expression. *Oncogene* 1994; 9: 963-969.

[21] Veikkola T, Karkkainen M, Cleasson-Welsh L, Alitalo K. Regulation of angiogenesis via vascular endothelial growth factor receptors. *Cancer Res* 2000; 60: 203-212.

[22] Masood R, Cai J, Zheng T, Smith DL, Hinton DR, Gill PS. Vascular endothelial growth factor (VEGF) is an autocrine growth factor for VEGF receptor-positive human tumors. *Blood* 2001;98:1904-1913.

[23] Kim KJ, Li B, Winer J, Armanini M, Gillett N, Phillips HS, Ferrara N. Inhibition of vascular endothelial growth factor-induced angiogenesis suppresses tumour growth in vivo. *Nature* 1993; 362: 841-844.

[24] Hori A, Sasada R, Matsutani E, Naito K, Sakura Y, Fujita T, Kozai Y. Suppression of solid tumor growth by immunoneutralizing monoclonal antibody against human basic fibroblast growth factor. *Cancer Res* 1991; 51: 6180-6184.

[25] Schweigerer L, Neufeld G, Friedman J, Abraham JA, Fiddes JC, Gospodarowicz D. Capillary endothelial cells express basic fibroblast growth factor, a mitogen that promotes their own growth. *Nature* 1987; 325: 257-259.

[26] Asahara T, Bauters C, Zheng LP, Takeshita S, Bunting S, Ferrara N, Symes JF, Isner JM. Synergistic effect of vascular endothelial growth factor and basic growth factor on angiogenesis in vivo. *Circulation* 1995; 92(9 Suppl): 365-371.

[27] Griffiths L, Stratford IJ. Platelet-derived endothelial cell growth factor thymidine phosphorylase in tumour growth and response to therapy. *Br J Cancer* 1997; 76: 689-693.

[28] Sporn MB, Roberts AB, Wakefield LM, de Crombrugghe B. Some recent advances in the chemistry and biology of transforming growth factor-β. *J Cell Biol* 1987; 105: 1039-1045.

[29] Pepper MS, Vassali JD, Orci L, Montesano R. Biphasic effect of transforming growth factor-β 1 on in vitro angiogenesis. *Exp Cell Res* 1993; 204: 356-363.

[30] Goldman CK, Kim J, Wong WL, King V, Brock T, Gillespie GY. Epidermal growth factor stimulates vascular endothelial growth factor production by human malignant glioma cells: a model of glioblastoma multiforme pathophysiology. *Mol Biol Cell* 1993; 4: 121-133.

[31] Davis S, Aldrich TH, Jones PF, Acheson A, Compton DL, Jain V, Ryan TE, Bruno J, Radziejewski C, Maisonpierre PC, Yancopoulos GD. Isolation of angiopoietin-1, a ligand for TIE2 receptor, by secretion-trap expression cloning. *Cell* 1996; 87: 1161-1169.

[32] Maisonpierre PC, Suri C, Jones PF, Bartunkova S, Wiegand SJ, Radziejewski C, Compton D, McClain J, Aldrich TH, Papadopoulos N, Daly TJ, Davis S, Sato TN, Yancopoulos GD. Angiopoietin-2, a natural antagonist for Tie2 that disrupts in vivo angiogenesis. *Science* 1997; 277: 55-60.

[33] Vikkula M, Boon LM, Carraway KL 3rd, Calvert JT, Diamonti AJ, Goumnerov B, Pasyk KA, Marchuk DA, Warman ML, Cantley LC, Mulliken JB, Olsen BR. Vascular dysmorphogenesis caused by activating mutation in the receptor tyrosine kinase TIE2. *Cell* 1996; 87: 1181-1190.

[34] Daniel TO, Liu H, Morrow JD, Crews BC, Marnett LJ. Thromboxane A2 is a mediator of cyclooxygenase-2-dependent endothelial migration and angiogenesis. *Cancer Res* 1999; 59: 4574-4577.

[35] Nakagawa K, Zhang Y, Tsuji H, Yoshizumi M, Kasahara T, Nishimura H, Nawroth PP, Nakagawa M. The angiogenic effect of tissue factor on tumors and wounds. *Semin Thromb Hemost* 1998; 24: 207-210.

[36] Fernandez PM, Patierno SR, Rickles FR. Tissue factor and fibrin in tumor angiogenesis. *Semin Thromb Hemost* 2004; 30: 31-44.

[37] Raugi GJ, Mumby SM, Abott-Brown D, Bornstein P. Thrombospondin: synthesis and secretion by cells in culture. *J Cell Biol* 1982; 95: 351-354.

[38] Rastinejad F, Polverini PJ, Bouck NP. Regulation of the activity of a new inhibitor of angiogenesis by a cancer suppressor gene. *Cell* 1989; 56: 345-355.

[39] Motegi K, Harada K, Pazouki S, Baillie R, Schor AM. Evidence of a bi-phasic effect of thrombospondin-1 on angiogenesis. *Histochem J* 2002; 34: 411-421.

[40] O'Reilly MS, Holmgren L, Shing Y, Chen C, Rosenthal RA, Moses M, Lane WS, Cao Y, Sage EH, Folkman J. Angiostatin: a novel angiogenesis inhibitor that mediates the suppression of metastases by a Lewis lung carcinoma. *Cell* 1994; 79: 315-328.

[41] O'Reilly MS, Boehm T, Shing Y, Fukai N, Vasios G, Lane WS, Flynn E, Birkhead JR, Olsen BR, Folkman J. Endostatin: an endogenous inhibitor of angiogenesis and tumor growth. *Cell* 1997; 88: 277-285.

[42] Motoo Y, Sawabu N, Nakanuma Y. Expression of epidermal growth factor and fibroblast growth factor in human hepatocellular carcinoma: an immunohistochemical study. *Liver* 1991; 11: 272-277.

[43] Inui Y, Higashiyama S, Kawata S, Tamura S, Miyagawa J, Taniguchi N, Matsuzawa Y. Expression of heparin-binding epidermal growth factor in human hepatocellular carcinoma. *Gastroenterology* 1994; 107: 1799-1804.

[44] Matsuo M, Sakurai H, Saiki I. ZD1839, a selective epidermal growth factor receptor tyrosine kinase inhibitor, shows antimetastatic activity using a hepatocellular carcinoma model. *Mol Cancer Ther* 2003; 2: 557-561.

[45] Motoo Y, Sawabu N, Yamaguchi Y, Terada T, Nakanuma Y. Sinusoidal capillarization of human hepatocellular carcinoma: possible promotion by fibroblast growth factor. *Oncology* 1993; 50: 270-274.

[46] Terada T, Nakanuma Y. Expression of ABH blood group antigens, receptors of Ulex europaeus agglutinin I, and factor VIII-related antigen on sinusoidal endothelial cells in adenomatous hyperplasia in human cirrhotic livers. *Hum Pathol* 1991; 22: 486-493.

[47] Mise M, Arii S, Higashituji H, Furutani M, Niwano M, Harada T, Ishigami S, Toda Y, Nakayama H, Fukumoto M, Fujita J, Imamura M. Clinical significance of vascular endothelial growth factor and basic fibroblast growth factor gene expression in liver tumor. *Hepatology* 1996; 23: 455-464.

[48] El-Assal ON, Yamanoi A, Ono T, Kohno H, Nagasue N. The clinicopathological significance of heparanase and basic fibroblast growth factor expressions in hepatocellular carcinoma. *Clin Cancer Res*. 2001; 7: 1299-1305.

[49] Kin M, Sata M, Ueno T, Torimura T, Inuzuka S, Tsuji R, Sujaku K, Sakamoto M, Sugawara H, Tamaki S, Tanikawa K. Basic fibroblast growth factor regulates proliferation and motility of human hepatoma cells by an autocrine mechanism. *J Hepatol* 1997; 27: 677-687.

[50] Yoshiji H, Kuriyama S, Yoshii J, Ikenaka Y, Noguchi R, Hicklin DJ, Huber J, Nakatani T, Tsujinoue H, Yanase K, Imazu H, Fukui H. Synergistic effect of basic fibroblast growth factor and vascular endothelial growth factor in murine hepatocellular carcinoma. *Hepatology* 2002; 35: 834-842.

[51] Torimura T, Sata M, Ueno T, Kin M, Tsuji R, Suzaku K, Hashimoto O, Sugawara H, Tanikawa K. Increased expression of vascular endothelial growth factor is associated with tumor progression in hepatocellular carcinoma. *Hum Pathol* 1998; 29: 986-991.

[52] Suzuki K, Hayashi N, Miyamoto Y, Yamamoto M, Ohkawa K, Ito Y, Sasaki Y, Yamaguchi Y, Nakase H, Noda K, Enomoto N, Arai K, Yamada Y, Yoshihara H, Tujimura T, Kawano K, Yoshikawa K, Kamada T. Expression of vascular permeability factor/vascular endothelial growth factor in human hepatocellular carcinoma. *Cancer Res* 1996; 56: 3004-3009.

[53] Yasuda S, Arii S, Mori A, Isobe N, Yang W, Oe H, Fujimoto A, Yonenaga Y, Sakashita H, Imamura M. Hexokinase II and VEGF expression in liver tumors: correlation with hypoxia-inducible factor 1 alpha and its significance. *J Hepatol* 2004; 40: 117-123.

[54] Chow NH, Hsu PI, Lin XZ, Yang HB, Chan SH, Cheng KS, Huang SM, Su IJ. Expression of vascular endothelial growth factor in normal liver and hepatocellular carcinoma: an immunohistochemical study. *Hum Pathol* 1997; 28: 698-703.

[55] Li XM, Tang ZY, Zhou G, Lui YK, Ye SL. Significance of vascular endothelial growth factor mRNA expression in invasion and metastasis of hepatocellular carcinoma. *J Exp Clin Cancer Res* 1998; 17: 13-17.

[56] Moon WS, Rhyu KH, Kang MJ, Lee DG, Yu HC, Yeum JH, Koh GY, Tarnawski AS. Overexpression of VEGF and angiopoietin 2: a key to high vascularity of hepatocellular carcinoma? *Mod Pathol* 2003; 16: 552-557.

[57] Yoshiji H, Kuriyama S, Yoshi J, Yamazaki M, Kikukawa M, Tsujinoue H, Nakatani T, Fukui H. Vascular endothelial growth factor tightly regulates in vitro development of murine hepatocellular carcinoma cells. *Hepatology* 1998; 28: 1489-1496.

[58] Yamaguchi R, Yano H, Iemura A, Ogasawara S, Haramaki M, Kojiro M. Expression of vascular endothelial growth factor in human hepatocellular carcinoma. *Hepatology* 1998; 28: 68-77.

[59] El-Assal ON, Yamanoi A, Soda Y, Yamaguchi M, Igarashi M, Yamamoto A, Nabika T, Nagasue N. Clinical significance of microvessel density and vascular endothelial growth factor expression in hepatocellular carcinoma and surrounding liver: possible involvement of vascular endothelial growth factor in the angiogenesis of cirrhotic liver. *Hepatology* 1998; 27: 1554-1562.

[60] Shimoda K, Mori M, Shibuta K, Banner BF, Barnard GF. Vascular endothelial growth factor/vascular permeability factor mRNA expression in patients with chronic hepatitis C and hepatocellular carcinoma. *Int J Oncol* 1999; 14: 353-359.

[61] Ng IO, Poon RT, Lee JM, Fan ST, Ng M, Tso WK. Microvessel density, vascular endothelial growth factor and its receptors Flt-1 and Flk-1/KDR in hepatocellular carcinoma. *Am J Clin Pathol* 2001; 116: 838-845.

[62] Dhar DK, Naora H, Yamanoi A, Ono T, Kohno H, Otani H, Nagasue N. Requisite role of VEGF receptors in angiogenesis of hepatocellular carcinoma: a comparison with angiopoietin/Tie pathway. *Anticancer Res* 2002; 22: 379-386.

[63] Tanaka S, Mori M, Sakamoto Y, Makuuchi M, Sugimachi K, Wands JR. Biologic significance of angiopoietin-2 expression in human hepatocellular carcinoma. *J Clin Invest* 1999; 103: 341-345.

[64] Tanaka S, Sugimachi K, Yamashita Yi Y, Ohga T, Shirabe K, Shimada M, Wands JR, Sugimachi K. Tie2 vascular endothelial receptor expression and function in hepatocellular carcinoma. *Hepatology* 2002; 35: 861-867.

[65] Mitsuhashi N, Shimizu H, Ohtsuka M, Wakabayashi Y, Ito H, Kimura F, Yoshidome H, Kato A, Nukui Y, Miyazaki M. Angiopoietins and Tie-2 expression in angiogenesis and proliferation of human hepatocellular carcinoma. *Hepatology* 2003; 37: 1105-1113.

[66] Zhao ZC, Zheng SS, Wan YL, Jia CK, Xie HY. The molecular mechanism underlying angiogenesis in hepatocellular carcinoma: the imbalance activation of signaling pathways. *Hepatobiliary Pancreat Dis Int* 2003; 2: 529-536.

[67] Sugimachi K, Tanaka S, Taguchi K, Aishima S, Shimada M, Tsuneyoshi M. Angiopoietin switching regulates angiogenesis and progression of human hepatocellular carcinoma. *J Clin Pathol* 2003; 56: 854-860.

[68] Zhou J, Tang ZY, Fan J, Wu ZQ, Li XM, Liu YK, Liu F, Sun HC, Ye SL. Expression of platelet-derived endothelial cell growth factor and vascular endothelial growth factor in hepatocellular carcinoma and portal vein tumor thrombus. *J Cancer Res Clin Oncol* 2000; 126: 57-61.

[69] Guo L, Kuroda N, Toi M, Miyazaki E, Hayashi Y, Enzan H, Jin Y. Increased expression of platelet-derived endothelial cell growth factor in human hepatocellular carcinomas correlated with high Edmondson grades and portal vein tumor thrombosis. *Oncol Rep* 2001; 8: 871-876.

[70] Morinaga S, Yamamoto Y, Noguchi Y, Imada T, Rino Y, Akaike M, Sugimasa Y, Takemiya S, Takanashi Y. Platelet-derived endothelial cell growth factor (PD-ECGF) is up-regulated in human hepatocellular carcinoma (HCC) and the corresponding hepatitis liver. *Hepatogastroenterology* 2003; 50: 1521-1526.

[71] Poon RT, Lau CP, Ho J, Yu WC, Fan ST, Wong J. Tissue factor expression correlates with tumor angiogenesis and invasiveness in human hepatocellular carcinoma. *Clin Cancer Res* 2003; 9: 5339-5345.

[72] Dupuy E, Hainaud P, Villemain A, Bodevin-Phedre E, Brouland JP, Briand P, Tobelem G. Tumoral angiogenesis and tissue factor expression during hepatocellular carcinoma progression in a transgenic mouse model. *J Hepatol* 2003; 38: 793-802.

[73] Ren Y, Tsui HT, Poon RT, Ng IO, Li Z, Chen Y, Jiang G, Lau C, Yu WC, Bacher M, Fan ST. Macrophage migration inhibitory factor: roles in regulating tumor cell

migration and expression of angiogenic factors in hepatocellular carcinoma. *Int J Cancer* 2003; 107: 22-29.

[74] Hisai H, Kato J, Kobune M, Murakami T, Miyanishi K, Takahashi M, Yoshizaki N, Takimoto R, Terui T, Niitsu Y, Increased expression of angiogenin in hepatocellular carcinoma in correlation with tumor vascularity. *Clin Cancer Res* 2003; 9: 4852-4859.

[75] Cheng AS, Chan HL, To KF, Leung WK, Chan KK, Liew CT, Sung JJ. Cyclooxygenase-2 pathway correlates with vascular endothelial growth factor expression and tumor angiogenesis in hepatitis B virus-associated hepatocellular carcinoma. *Int J Oncol* 2004; 24: 853-860.

[76] Gorrin-Rivas MJ, Arii S, Mori A, Takeda Y, Mizumoto M, Furutani M, Imamura M. Implications of human macrophage metalloelastase and vascular endothelial growth factor gene expression in angiogenesis of hepatocellular carcinoma. *Ann Surg* 2000; 231: 67-73.

[77] Kawahara N, Ono M, Taguchi K, Okamoto M, Shimada M, Takenaka K, Hayashi K, Mosher DF, Sugimachi K, Tsuneyoshi M, Kuwano M. Enhanced expression of thrombospondin-1 and hypovascularity in human cholangiocarcinoma. *Hepatology* 1998; 28: 1512-1517.

[78] Poon RT, Chung KK, Cheung ST, Lau C, Tong SW, Leung KL, Yu WC, Tuszynski GP, Fan ST. Clinical significance of thrombospondin 1 expression in hepatocellular carcinoma. *Clin Cancer Res* 2004; 10:4150-4157.

[79] Weidner N. Intratumor microvessel density as a prognostic factor in cancer. *Am J Pathol* 1995; 147: 9-19.

[80] Frank RE, Saclarides TJ, Leurgans S, Speziale NJ, Drab EA, Rubin DB. Tumor angiogenesis as a predictor of recurrence and survival in patients with node-negative colon cancer. *Ann Surg* 1995; 222: 695-699.

[81] Maeda K, Chung YS, Takatsuka S, Ogawa Y, Onoda N, Sawada T, Kato Y, Nitta A, Arimoto Y, Kondo Y, Sowa M. Tumour angiogenesis and tumour cell proliferation as prognostic indicators in gastric carcinoma. *Br J Cancer* 1995; 72: 319-323.

[82] Gasparini G, Weidner N, Bevilacqua P, Maluta S, Dalla Palma P, Caffo O, Barbareschi M, Boracchi P, Marubini E, Pozza F. Tumor microvessel density, p53 expression, tumor size, and peritumoral lymphatic vessel invasion are relevant prognostic markers in node-negative breast carcinoma. *J Clin Oncol* 1994; 12: 454-466.

[83] Tanigawa N, Lu C, Mitsui T, Miura S. Quantitation of sinusoid-like vessels in hepatocellular carcinoma: its clinical and prognostic significance. *Hepatology* 1997; 26: 1216-1223.

[84] Kimura H, Nakajima T, Kagawa K, Deguchi T, Kakusui M, Katagishi T, Okanoue T, Kashima K, Ashihara T. Angiogenesis in hepatocellular carcinoma as evaluated by CD34 immunohistochemistry. *Liver* 1998; 18: 14-19.

[85] Yamamoto A, Dhar DK, El-Assal ON, Igarashi M, Tabara H, Nagasue N. Thymidine phosphorylase (platelet-derived endothelial cell growth factor), microvessel density and clinical outcome in hepatocellular carcinoma. *J Hepatol* 1998; 29: 290-299.

[86] Ker CG, Chen HY, Juan CC, Lo HW, Shen YY, Chen JS, Lee KT, Sheen PC. Role of angiogenesis in hepatitis and hepatocellular carcinoma. *Hepatogastroenterology* 1999; 46: 646-650.

[87] Sun HC, Tang ZY, Li XM, Zhou YN, Sun BR, Ma ZC. Microvessel density of hepatocellular carcinoma: its relationship with prognosis. *Cancer Res Clin Oncol* 1999; 125: 419-426.

[88] Poon RT, Ng IO, Lau C, Yu WC, Yang ZF, Fan ST, Wong J. Tumor microvessel density as a predictor of recurrence after resection of hepatocellular carcinoma: a prospective study. *J Clin Oncol* 2002; 20: 1775-1785.

[89] Chen WX, Min PQ, Song B, Xiao BL, Liu Y, Ge YH. Single-level dynamic spiral CT of hepatocellular carcinoma: correlation between imaging features and density of tumor microvessels. *World J Gastroenterol* 2004; 10: 67-72.

[90] Jeng KS, Sheen IS, Wang YC, Gu SL, Chu CM, Shih SC, Wang PC, Chang WH, Wang HY. Is the vascular endothelial growth factor messenger RNA expression in resectable hepatocellular carcinoma of prognostic value after resection? *World J Gastroenterol* 2004; 10: 676-681.

[91] Poon RT, Fan ST, Wong J. Clinical implications of circulating angiogenic factors in cancer patients. *J Clin Oncol* 2001; 19: 1207-1225.

[92] Jin-no K, Tanimizu M, Hyodo I, Nishikawa Y, Hosokawa Y, Doi T, Endo H, Yamahita T, Okada Y. Circulating vascular endothelial growth factor (VEGF) is a possible tumor marker for metastasis in human hepatocellular carcinoma. *J Gastroenterol* 1998; 33: 376-382.

[93] Jin-no K, Tanimizu M, Hyodo I, Nishikawa Y, Hosokawa Y, Endo H, Doi T, Mandai K, Ishitsuka H. Circulating platelet-derived endothelial growth factor increases in hepatocellular carcinoma patients. *Cancer* 1998; 82: 1260-1267.

[94] Hsu PI, Chow NH, Lai KH, Yang HB, Chan SH, Lin XZ, Cheng JS, Huang JS, Ger LP, Huang SM, Yen MY, Yang YF. Implications of serum basic fibroblast growth factor levels in chronic liver diseases and hepatocellular carcinoma. *Anticancer Res* 1997; 17: 2803-2809.

[95] Poon RT, Ng IO, Lau C, Zhu LX, Yu WC, Lo CM, Fan ST, Wong J. Serum vascular endothelial growth factor predicts venous invasion in hepatocellular carcinoma: a prospective study. *Ann Surg* 2001; 233: 227-235.

[96] Li XM, Tang ZY, Qin LX, Zhou J, Sun HC. Serum vascular endothelial growth factor is a predictor of invasion and metastasis in hepatocellular carcinoma. *J Exp Clin Cancer Res* 1999; 18: 511-517.

[97] Poon RT, Lau CP, Cheung ST, Yu WC, Fan ST. Quantitative correlation of serum levels and tumor expression of vascular endothelial growth factor in patients with hepatocellular carcinoma. *Cancer Res* 2003; 63: 3121-3126.

[98] Chao Y, Li CP, Chau GY, Chen CP, King KL, Lui WY, Yen SH, Chang FY, Chan WK, Lee SD. Prognostic significance of vascular endothelial growth factor, basic fibroblast growth factor, and angiogenin in patients with resectable hepatocellular carcinoma after surgery. *Ann Surg Oncol* 2003; 10: 355-362.

[99] Jeng KS, Sheen IS, Wang YC, Gu SL, Chu CM, Shih SC, Wang PC, Chang WH, Wang HY. Prognostic significance of preoperative circulating vascular endothelial growth factor messenger RNA expression in resectable hepatocellular carcinoma: a prospective study. *World J Gastroenterol* 2004; 10: 643-648.

[100] Poon RT, Ng IO, Lau C, Yu WC, Fan ST, Wong J. Correlation of serum basic fibroblast growth factor levels with clinicopathologic features and postoperative recurrence in hepatocellular carcinoma. *Am J Surg* 2001; 182: 298-304.

[101] Dhar DK, Ono T, Yamanoi A, Soda Y, Yamaguchi E, Rahman MA, Kohno H, Nagasue N. Serum endostatin predicts tumor vascularity in hepatocellular carcinoma. *Cancer* 2002; 95: 2188-2195.

[102] Yamagata M, Shiratori Y, Dan Y, Shiina S, Takayama T, Makuuchi M, Omata M. Serum endostatin levels in patients with hepatocellular carcinoma. *Ann Oncol* 2000; 11: 761-762.

[103] Poon RT, Ho JW, Tong CS, Lau CP, Fan ST, Wong J. Prognostic significance of serum vascular endothelial growth factor and endostatin in patients with hepatocellular carcinoma. *Br J Surg* (In press)

[104] Shimada H, Takeda A, Nabeya Y, Okazumi SI, Matsubara H, Funami Y, Hayashi H, Gunji Y, Kobayashi S, Suzuki T, Ochiai T. Clinical significance of serum vascular endothelial growth factor in esophageal squamous cell carcinoma. *Cancer Br J Surg* 2004; 91: 1354-1360.

[105] Poon RT, Lau CP, Yu WC, Fan ST, Wong J. High serum levels of vascular endothelial growth factor predict poor response to transarterial chemoembolization in hepatocellular carcinoma: A prospective study. *Oncol Rep* 2004;11:1077-1084.

[106] Poon RT, Fan ST. Evaluation of the new AJCC/UICC staging system for hepatocellular carcinoma after hepatic resection in Chinese patients. *Surg Oncol Clin N Am* 2003; 12: 35-50.

[107] Boehm T, Folkman J, Browder T, O'Reilly MS. Antiangiogenic therapy of experimental cancer does not induce acquired drug resistance. *Nature* 1997; 390: 404-407.

[108] Kang MA, Kim KY, Seol JY, Kim KC, Nam MJ. The growth inhibition of hepatoma by gene transfer of antisense vascular endothelial growth factor. *J Gene Med* 2000; 2: 289-296.

[109] Wang L, Tang ZY, Qin LX, Wu XF, Sun HC, Xue Q, Ye SL. High-dose and long-term therapy with interferon-alfa inhibits tumor growth and recurrence in nude mice bearing human hepatocellular carcinoma xenografts with high metastatic potential. *Hepatology* 2000; 32: 43-48.

[110] Morgan B, Thomas AL, Drevs J, Hennig J, Buchert M, Jivan A, Horsfield MA, Mross K, Ball HA, Lee L, Mietlowski W, Fuxuis S, Unger C, O'Byrne K, Henry A, Cherryman GR, Laurent D, Dugan M, Marme D, Steward WP. Dynamic contrast-enhanced magnetic resonance imaging as a biomarker for the pharmacological response of PTK787/ZK 222584, an inhibitor of the vascular endothelial growth factor receptor tyrosine kinases, in patients with advanced colorectal cancer and liver metastases: results from two phase I studies. *J Clin Oncol* 2003; 21: 3955-3964.

[111] Xia JL, Yang BH, Tang ZY, Sun FX, Xue Q, Gao DM, Inhibitory effect of the angiogenesis inhibitor TNP-470 on tumor growth and metastasis in nude mice bearing human hepatocellular carcinoma. *J Cancer Res Clin Oncol* 1997; 123: 383-387.

[112] Qin LX, Tang ZY, Li XM, Bu W, Xia JL. Effect of antiangiogenic agents on experimental animal models of hepatocellular carcinoma. *Ann Acad Med Singapore* 1999; 28: 147-151.

[113] Lode HN, Moehler T, Xiang R, Jonczyk A, Gillies SD, Cheresh DA, Reisfeld RA. Synergy between an antiangiogenic integrin alphav antagonist and an antibody-cytokine fusion protein eradicates spontaneous tumor metastases. *Proc Natl Acad Sci U S A* 1999; 96: 1591-1596.

[114] Ishikawa H, Nakao K, Matsumoto K, Ichikawa T, Hamasaki K, Nakata K, Eguchi K. Antiangiogenic gene therapy for hepatocellular carcinoma using angiostatin gene. *Hepatology* 2003; 37: 696-704.

[115] Kin M, Torimura T, Ueno T, Nakamura T, Ogata R, Sakamoto M, Tamaki S, Sata M. Angiogenesis inhibitor TNP-470 suppresses the progression of experimentally-induced hepatocellular carcinoma in rats. *Int J Oncol* 2000; 16: 375-382.

[116] Ikebe T, Yamamoto T, Kubo S, Hirohashi K, Kinoshita H, Kaneda K, Sakurai M. Suppressive effect of the angiogenesis inhibitor TNP-470 on the development of carcinogen-induced hepatic nodules in rats. *Jpn J Cancer Res* 1998; 89: 143-149.

[117] Yoshiji H, Kuriyama S, Yoshii J, Ikenaka Y, Noguchi R, Hicklin DJ, Wu Y, Yanase K, Namisaki T, Yamazaki M, Tsujinoue H, Imazu H, Masaki T, Fukui H. Vascular endothelial growth factor and receptor interaction is a prerequisite for murine hepatic fibrogenesis. *Gut* 2003; 52: 1347-1354.

[118] Kerbel RS. Clinical trials of antiangiogenic drugs: opportunities, problems and assessment of initial results. *J Clin Oncol* 2001; 19: 45S-51S.

[119] Patt YZ, Hassan MM, Lozano RD, Ellis LM, Peterson JA, Waugh KA. Durable clinical response of refractory hepatocellular carcinoma to orally administered thalidomide. *Am J Clin Oncol* 2000; 23: 319-321.

[120] Schwartz JD, Sung MW, Lehrer A. Thalidomide for unresectable hepatocellular carcinoma (HCC) with optional interferon-α upon disease progression. *Proc Am Soc Clin Oncol* 2002; 21:1847.

[121] Poon RT, Fan ST, Tsang FH, Wong J. Locoregional therapies for hepatocellular carcinoma: a critical review from the surgeon's perspective. *Ann Surg* 2002; 235: 466-486.

[122] Jia WD, Xu GL, Xu RN, Sun HC, Wang L, Yu JH, Wang J, Li JS, Zhai ZM, Xue Q. Octreotide acts as an antitumor angiogenesis compound and suppresses tumor growth in nude mice bearing human hepatocellular carcinoma xenografts. *J Cancer Res Clin Oncol* 2003; 129: 327-334.

[123] Yuen MF, Poon RT, Lai CL, Fan ST, Lo CM, Wong KW, Wong WM, Wong BC. A randomized placebo-controlled study of long-acting octreotide for the treatment advanced hepatocellular carcinoma. *Hepatology* 2002; 36: 687-691.

[124] Suzuki H, Mori M, Kawaguchi C, Adachi M, Miura S, Ishii H. Serum vascular endothelial growth factor in the course of transcatheter arterial embolization of hepatocellular carcinoma. *Int J Oncol* 1999; 14: 1087-1090.

[125] Poon RT, Fan ST, Wong J. Risk factors, prevention, and management of postoperative recurrence after resection of hepatocellular carcinoma. *Ann Surg* 2000; 232: 10-24.

# Index

## 5



## A

## B



## C

## D

## E



## F

## G



## H

## I

## J



## K



## L

## M

## N



## O



## P

## T

## U



## V

## W



## X



## Y



## Z